ASSESSING PSYCHOSIS

This second edition of *Assessing Psychosis: A Clinician's Guide* offers both a practical guide and a rich clinical resource for a broad audience of mental health practitioners seeking to sharpen their understanding of diagnostic issues, clinical concepts, and assessment methods that aid in detecting the presence of psychotic phenomena. Case vignettes deepen clinical understanding, and all chapters include a summary of practical clinical guidelines. This new edition includes two new chapters and updated diagnostic criteria considering the new DSM-5-TR. Practicing psychiatrists, psychologists, social workers, psychiatric nurses, and students will find this a valuable resource for clinical practice, training, and teaching purposes.

Ali Khadivi, Ph.D., ABAP, received his Bachelor of Science in Psychology from Tufts University and his Ph.D. in Clinical Psychology from The New School for Social Research. He completed his training at New York Hospital-Cornell Medical Center, Westchester Division, with distinction. He has been practicing clinical and forensic psychology since 1991. Dr. Khadivi is board-certified in assessment psychology and holds the rank of professor of psychiatry and behavioral sciences at Albert Einstein College of Medicine in Bronx, New York. He teaches clinical and forensic psychological assessment at several hospitals and universities and provides training workshops nationally and internationally in the evaluation of major mental illnesses. Dr. Khadivi has been a clinical and forensic consultant for numerous institutions and offers expert testimony in criminal and civil forensic cases.

James H. Kleiger is a native of Colorado and a graduate of Harvard University. He received his doctorate at the University of Denver. Dr. Kleiger completed postdoctoral training at The Menninger Clinic in Topeka, Kansas, and eventually became Training Director of the Postdoctoral Fellowship Program. While at Menninger, he completed his psychoanalytic training at the Topeka Institute for Psychoanalysis and, after moving to Maryland, served as President of the Washington-Baltimore Society for Psychoanalysis. He has authored and edited many books, such as *Assessing Psychosis. A Clinician's Guide*, 1st and 2nd Editions, 2015 and 2024 (Routledge, co-authored with Ali Khadivi), and *Rorschach Assessment of Psychotic Phenomena*, 2017 (Routledge).

ASSESSING PSYCHOSIS

A Clinician's Guide

2nd edition

Ali Khadivi and
James H. Kleiger

Routledge
Taylor & Francis Group
NEW YORK AND LONDON

Designed cover image: © Getty

First published 2024
by Routledge
605 Third Avenue, New York, NY 10158

and by Routledge
4 Park Square, Milton Park, Abingdon, Oxon OX14 4RN

Routledge is an imprint of the Taylor & Francis Group, an informa business

British Library Cataloguing-in-Publication Data

A catalogue record for this book is available from the British Library

Library of Congress Cataloging-in-Publication Data
Names: Kleiger, James H., 1952– author. | Khadivi, Ali, author.
Title: Assessing psychosis : a clinicians guide / Ali Khadivi and James H. Kleiger.
Description: Second edition. | Abingdon, Oxon ; New York, NY : Routledge, 2024. | James H. Kleiger appeared as the first named author on the earlier edition. | Includes bibliographical references and index.
Identifiers: LCCN 2024006759 (print) | LCCN 2024006760 (ebook) | ISBN 9781032541129 (hardback) | ISBN 9781032540856 (paperback) | ISBN 9781003415206 (ebook)
Subjects: LCSH: Psychoses—Diagnosis.
Classification: LCC RC469 .K528 2024 (print) | LCC RC469 (ebook) | DDC 616.89/075—dc23/eng/20240408
LC record available at https://lccn.loc.gov/2024006759
LC ebook record available at https://lccn.loc.gov/2024006760

ISBN: 978-1-032-54112-9 (hbk)
ISBN: 978-1-032-54085-6 (pbk)
ISBN: 978-1-003-41520-6 (ebk)

DOI: 10.4324/9781003415206

Typeset in Sabon
by Apex CoVantage, LLC

For my daughters, Ana and Leila (AK)
For my parents, Nannette, Nike, Katie, and Margy (JHK)

CONTENTS

ACKNOWLEDGMENTS

Like any successful relationship, co-authorship requires openness, honesty, and trust. What began as a shared passion fortuitously evolved into a lasting friendship, which has deepened since our book was first published in 2015. Each of us remains grateful to the other for sharing a difficult but gratifying journey.

Nothing is possible without those who parent and teach. We have been fortunate to have the best of both. We thank our parents and a legion of teachers, supervisors, and mentors.

Dr. Kleiger expresses his gratitude to Nelson Jones, Irwin Rosen, Len Horwitz, Rosemary Segalla, Marty, and Lui Leichtman. Each has served as a guide, mentor, or friend. I also have heartfelt appreciation for the many colleagues and supervisors at the Menninger Clinic in Topeka, Kansas, during the 1980s and 1990s, all providing incredible intellectual nourishment, support, and friendship. Of course, thanks would be incomplete without mentioning the brotherhood of the Topeka Men's Group – most notably Steve Lerner, Thomas Averill, Tom Murphy, Frank Barthell, and Mahasen DeSilva.

Dr. Khadivi wishes to acknowledge and express his gratitude to his mentor, Dr. David Shapiro, whose perspective on psychopathology and understanding of the "dynamic of the working of the mind" influenced his development as an assessment psychologist in addition, special thanks to Dr. Jeffrey Levine, the former Chair of the Department of Psychiatry at Bronx-Lebanon Hospital Center, whose critical clinical thinking has been inspiring, and for his continued support over the years. Dr. Khadivi also wants to thank his students and colleagues in New York, including Drs. Shana Grover and Andreas Evdokas, for their continued encouragement.

Finally, Dr. Khadivi would like to express deep appreciation and gratitude to his wife, Dr. Yasmine Saad, whose continued support was instrumental in finishing the second edition of the book.

We are grateful to the army of like-minded friends and colleagues in the Society of Personality Assessment, whom we have known, laughed with, and learned from over the years. Special acknowledgment is owed to Jed Yalof, Don Viglione, Joni Mihura, Tony Bram, Irv Weiner, Odile Hussein, Marvin Acklin, Leslie Morey, Dave Nichols, Phil Keddy, Barton Evans, Greg Meyer, Bob Bornstein, and Virginia Brabender. And, of course, we remember the contributions of our friends Phil Erdberg and Bruce Smith, whose untimely passing still fills us with sadness.

None of this would have been possible without our families' loving presence, quiet support, patience, and encouragement.

CHAPTER CONTRIBUTORS

Dr. Gary Brucato is a clinical and forensic psychologist, researcher, and author in the areas of psychotic illness and other severe mental illnesses, as well as violence, including serial, spree, mass murder, and sexual offenses. He previously served as the Assistant Director of the Center of Prevention and Evaluation and an Associate Research Scientist at Columbia University Irving Medical Center and The New York State Psychiatric Institute in New York City, where he helped to elucidate the features and phenomenology of attenuated psychotic illness and was the co-creator of the Columbia Mass Murder Database, the largest and most definitive study of mass murder ever conducted. Dr. Brucato is a Visiting Scholar at Boston College, where he collaborates with Dr. Ann W. Burgess on research into diverse forensic topics and is on the expert panel for the Cold Case Foundation, which assists law enforcement throughout the world with challenging unsolved cases and provides educational resources. He is also in private clinical practice and conducts forensic evaluations. He has co-authored two books and nearly 100 book chapters and peer-reviewed articles on psychotic illness and violence, given over 350 professional presentations on these subjects, and been highly active as a consultant on cases and in the media.

Mark D. Cunningham, Ph.D., ABPP, is a board-certified clinical and forensic psychologist, researcher, and prolific scholar. His practice is national in scope. Dr. Cunningham has authored more than 70 publications and provided innumerable scholarly symposiums at regional and national conferences. He has published, presented, and testified regarding the differential between delusional disorders and extreme political beliefs. His research and practice have garnered regional, national, and international recognition and awards. Dr. Cunningham earned his doctorate in clinical psychology at Oklahoma State University, with a clinical psychology internship at the National Naval Medical Center. He completed a two-year NIMH-sponsored postdoctoral program at Yale University School of Medicine.

ABBREVIATIONS

AHRS	Auditory Hallucination Rating Scale
APSS	Attenuated Positive Symptom State
ASRM	Altman Self-Rating Mania
BABS	Brown Assessment of Beliefs Scale
BAVQ	Belief About Voices Questionnaire-Revised
BCIS	Beck Cognitive Insight Scale
BNSS	Brief Negative Symptom Scale
BPRS	Brief Psychiatric Rating Scale
BSABS	Bonn Scale for the Assessment of Basic Symptoms
CAARMS	Comprehensive Assessment of At-Risk Mental States
CAHQ	Characteristics of Auditory Hallucinations Questionnaire
CAINS	Clinical Assessment Interview for Negative Symptoms
CASH	Comprehensive Assessment of Symptoms and History
CAT	Children's Apperception Test
CDRS	Characteristics of Delusions Rating Scale
CDSS	Calgary Depression Scale for Schizophrenia
CFI	Cultural Formulation Interview
DDE	Dimensions of Delusional Experience
DICA	Diagnostic Interview Schedule for Children and Adolescents
DSSI	Delusions Symptoms State Inventory
EPOS	European Prediction of Psychosis Study
FTD	Formal thought disorder
ICD	International Classification of Diseases
MDS	Major Depression Rating Scale
MMSE	Mini-Mental Status Exam
MOCA	Montreal Cognitive Assessment
PANSS	Positive and Negative Syndrome Scale
PDI	Peters Delusional Inventory
PQ	Prodromal Questionnaire
PSE	Present State Examination
PTSD	Post-traumatic stress disorder
RDC	Research Diagnostic Criteria

SANS	Scale for the Assessment of Negative Symptoms
SAPS	Scale for the Assessment of Positive Symptoms
SCID	Structured Clinical Interview for DSM-IV
SCoRS	Schizophrenia Cognition Rating Scale
SDSS	Simple Delusional Syndrome Scale
SG	Story Game
SIPS	Structured Interview of Prodromal Symptoms
SIS	Structured Interview for Schizotypy
SMVQ	Southampton Mindfulness of Voices Questionnaire
SOPS	Scale of Prodromal Symptoms
SPQ	Schizotypal Personality Questionnaire
SSPI	Signs and Symptoms of Psychotic Illness
SSRS	Schizophrenia Suicide Risk Scale
SUMD	Scale to Assess Unawareness of Mental Disorder
TCO	Threat/control override
TDI	Thought Disorder Index
TDQ	Thought Disorder Questionnaire
TLC	Thought, Language Communication
TLI	Thought and Language Index
ToM	Theory of Mind
TP	Thought Problem
VAAS	Voices Acceptance and Action Scale
VAY	Voice and You
VPD	Voice Power Differential
WMAPLE	Wisconsin Manual for Assessing Psychotic-Like Experiences
YMRS	Young Mania Rating Scale

INTRODUCTION

As we noted in our previous edition of *Assessing Psychosis: A Clinician's Guide,* psychosis is one of the most studied areas in psychopathology. Scientific investigations continue to discover new information about the nature, clinical manifestations, and underlying causes of psychoses so that better treatments can be developed to address the suffering of patients and their families. Because of these discoveries and the changes in how psychosis is understood and diagnosed, we thought it would be timely to write a second edition.

Having listened to those to whom we have presented and our colleagues' comments, we have kept the structure of the Second Edition much the same. Part I includes three chapters on conceptual issues and the nature of key symptoms of psychosis. We have added additional references to reflect advances in how psychosis and its symptom manifestations are understood.

In Part II, we delve into diagnostic issues with three chapters focusing on current diagnostic classification, distinctions between diagnostic categories, dimensions, and spectra, and differential diagnosis of psychotic conditions. In terms of differential diagnosis, we have expanded our discussion of substance and medication-induced psychosis and the relationship between psychosis and PTSD.

Consistent with the First Edition, Part III includes three chapters on multi-method assessment of psychotic phenomena. We have updated our chapters on clinical interviewing, psychological assessment methods, and rating scales in assessing psychotic symptom dimensions. We are keenly interested in clinical interviewing as a method of assessment, which many clinicians overlook. At the same time, we value the role psychological assessment and, where appropriate, empirically validated structured interviews and rating scales. We stress a multimethod approach, as opposed to relying on a single form of information gathering.

DOI: 10.4324/9781003415206-1

We are most excited about our expanded Part IV. Like before, we include chapters on assessing suicide and violence risk, cultural context, and assessing psychosis in children and adolescents. Where appropriate, we have included new references. We have also added a chapter on assessing malingered psychosis in forensic settings and two new chapters written by distinguished colleagues, Drs. Gary Brucato and Mark D. Cunningham. In Chapter 11, Dr. Brucato greatly expanded the original chapter on attenuated psychosis and included much of his original research. In Chapter 13, Dr. Cunningham writes about differentiating delusions from the radicalization of extreme beliefs and conspiracy theories. Dr. Cunningham reviews his model and instrument *MADDD-or-RAD-17* for differentiating delusional disorder from extreme beliefs.

Although we take a broad look at the phenomenology and symptomatology of psychosis, as in the First Edition, we have not included a neurobiological perspective in our multi-method approach to assessing psychosis. As previously stated, we are not neuroscientists or medical researchers. Instead, we are clinicians interested in developing a more practical understanding of psychosis and detailing assessment methods available to the clinical practitioner in a routine office or hospital setting. Consistent with our efforts in the original edition, we strive to communicate directly and in a straightforward manner with practicing mental health professionals from various disciplines to clarify areas of diagnostic murkiness and provide a current review of the more salient issues involved in understanding and assessing psychosis.

Furthermore, this is not a book about psychological assessment. While we are both experienced psychological assessors, we wanted to write an inclusive text that would be helpful to a broad range of mental health professionals at different levels of training and experience. Psychological assessment and traditional use of psychological tests are important, and we have devoted a chapter to this subject; however, our goal was to approach testing in a way that would make it more accessible for the non-psychologist, who has less experience with traditional assessment instruments.

Moreover, we have not written a book for an audience of psychosis researchers. Although we cite hundreds of references drawn from current and past scientific investigations, this book is intended as a clinical guide, not a research treatise. We reference countless studies but provide no original research of our own.

The core mission of the Second Edition of *Assessing Psychosis* remains the same: To clarify diagnostic issues and focus on effective methods of assessing psychosis that will be useful to the clinical and forensic practitioner.

The case examples we cite are based on our joint clinical experience. Most are actual patients, while others are composite sketches used for teaching purposes. In all cases, the material has been heavily disguised.

As before, we have elected to use gender pronouns in a random fashion throughout this text to avoid the cumbersome "he/she, him/her" verbiage.

Ali Khadivi, Ph.D., ABAP
James H. Kleiger, Ph.D., ABAP, ABPP

Part I

CLINICAL FEATURES OF PSYCHOSIS

1

UNDERSTANDING PSYCHOSIS

Consider the following clinical encounters and answer, "Is this patient psychotic?"

Tricia is a 24-year-old grad student who describes hearing voices and seeing visions. Her experiences are vivid, but she states that the voices and visions are not real. Instead, she tells us they are products of her mind. Tricia does not tell others about these daily experiences for fear that they will think she is mentally ill. She used to believe she had magical powers; her voices and visions made her feel special and provided constancy in her life. However, over time, she realized, with both sadness and relief, that these experiences were not real.

Nonetheless, she continues to hear voices and see visions. She is hallucinating, so her therapist concludes that she must be psychotic. Do you agree?

Didia was born in an African village and moved to a large American city to study. She recently told a psychiatric resident that she had been haunted by the spirit of a tribal elder from back home after she had had sex with her boyfriend. She heard a spirit voice at night, telling her she was bad. The resident worried that she was becoming psychotic and phoned her supervisor to see if she should arrange hospitalization.

Brian, a 30-something single man, anxiously reports that an unnamed organization has hacked his computer and is sending him coded messages to get him to target government buildings, yet describes all of this without odd language or a disturbance in the focus, filtering, or pacing of his speech. He denies hearing voices or having other unsubstantiated perceptual experiences. On psychological testing, he shows no classic signs of a thought disorder. Is he delusional? Does he have a thought disorder?

The police were called when a neighbor spotted 14-year-old Kelvin covered in green paint, crouching down to examine insects in the middle of a busy street. When questioned about his odd behavior and appearance, he smiles but does not speak. His behavior is bizarre enough to suspect psychosis, right?

DOI: 10.4324/9781003415206-3

Laurel, a 32-year-old former teacher, joined the anti-vax movement and was convinced that recent elections were stolen. She believes that COVID-related deaths are exaggerated. Laurel severed contact with her family and recently quit her job. Friends have repeatedly tried to present evidence to refute her claims and recently staged an intervention to help her accept consensual reality. However, when they speak with her, she cites new evidence to support her beliefs. She accuses them of being politically motivated to silence her and those with similar ideas. Do you agree that Laurel is demonstrating fixed delusions and should be referred for an evaluation?

The parents brought their 18-year-old son, Martin, to the emergency room. Over the past three months, his grades have declined. He stopped going out with his friends and refused to leave his room. He complains that he cannot sleep and typically stays up past 1:00 a.m. playing Dungeons and Dragons online. He stopped showering and wore the same clothes. Parents found a vaping pen and suspect regular use of cannabis. When questioned about his loss of motivation and changes in behavior and appearance, Martin's answers are brief, and his affect is flat. Are we correct in viewing him as at risk for a psychotic episode?

Eleven-year-old Timmy speaks in a distracted and unfocused manner. We see similar looseness and fluidity in his Rorschach responses, which contain some odd, invented words. Timmy's mother reports that he has ADHD and was previously evaluated by a speech pathologist. Since he demonstrates disorganized speech, his therapist suspects he might be psychotic. Do you agree?

A 33-year-old male, Willum, was evaluated by a forensic psychologist after reporting to his defense counsel that he heard voices telling him to assault his girlfriend's teenage son. At the time of the assault, he was using cocaine and cannabis daily for several months. He had been free of all substances for the last ten months when he met with the psychologist. During the interview, he seemed eager to discuss the voices he was still reportedly hearing. As the psychologist asked more questions, Willum explained that the voices came from "Shadowman," who hid in the corners of his cell and directed him to commit violence. Willum said that Shadowman visited him at night and terrified him. Collateral sources, including family members and prison personnel, did not report observing odd, disorganized, anxious, or aggressive behavior. Is there enough evidence to infer that Willum has a drug-induced psychosis or that he may be feigning his symptoms? Should he be referred for further evaluation? What would we look for in psychological assessment?

Finally, 16-year-old Marie becomes violent when she sees two classmates, who do not know each other, sitting in the same row at an assembly. She immediately concludes that because they are sitting close to each other, they must be gossiping about her. How do we understand the conclusion she made? She is given the Rorschach, which shows significant signs of disordered thinking and impaired perception. Might she be delusional?

How familiar are these brief vignettes? How often have we experienced similar clinical encounters when the chief diagnostic decision is whether a patient might be psychotic? In each example cited, the patient presented with unusual behavioral signs (including speech) or shared atypical beliefs and perceptions, raising the question of whether they might be psychotic. Critical features seemed to be present in some cases, whereas, in others, they were absent. For example, Tricia and Didia complained of hearing voices and seeing visions, while Brian spoke so clearly about what sounded like a delusional belief. Laurel also described her beliefs coherently and rejected the evidence to refute her fixed beliefs. There was no mistaking that Martin's behavior had deteriorated, but should we conclude that he was at risk for becoming psychotic, or might there be an alternative explanation? What about Kelvin, whose behavior appears grossly impaired? Is this sufficient to conclude that he is psychotic? Then, there is young Timmy, who uses idiosyncratic language and has trouble conveying his ideas in a coherent and organized manner. Regarding Willum, the forensic psychologist needs to understand which behavioral features might help distinguish clinical from feigned psychosis.

Finally, what do we make of Marie, who immediately assumed that the physical proximity of two people *must* mean that they have a relationship that has negative implications for how they both feel about her? Also, are positive findings on psychological tests sufficient to identify Marie as psychotic?

Answering these questions about our hypothetical patients requires more information, but our answers also depend on how we understand the concepts, symptoms, and disorders associated with psychosis. Often, we begin with simple ideas about psychosis and assume that the diagnostic task will be a binary and straightforward one – that the individual either is or is not psychotic. However, the reality can be more complex and confusing. This confusion is due to a lack of conceptual clarity about the terms "psychosis" and "psychotic," as well as the difference between different symptom dimensions, such as delusions, hallucinations, and thought disorders. Symptoms are often conflated with syndromes, and terms are used interchangeably, leading to a lack of conceptual clarity and diagnostic confusion. Even among more experienced diagnosticians, it is easy for concepts to become confused and for terms to be used in a fuzzy manner.

Clinicians ask about the threshold or boundaries between what we consider psychotic and what we do not. Further, they seek to understand the differences between active psychotic states, psychotic dimensions, psychotic disorders, and psychotic-like experiences and how to assess them. For clarity purposes, we use the term "psychotic phenomena" to refer to a broad range of experiences, symptoms, and disorders related to psychosis. To sharpen our conceptual and diagnostic understanding, we approach psychotic phenomena from multiple perspectives, including (1) The Sense of Reality and Reality Testing, (2) Symptom Dimensions, (3) Psychotic Disorders, and (4) Risk and Vulnerability Factors.

Sense of Reality and Reality Testing

The term "psychosis" is derived from the Greek words *psyche* (mind or soul) and *osis* (abnormal or deranged). Thus, psychosis is an abnormal state of mind that refers to sensory-perceptual experiences, beliefs, and behaviors occurring outside the bounds of consensual reality. Phenomenologically, psychotic experiences may involve alterations in the experience of external reality and the self (Parnas & Henriksen, 2014), a loss of reality testing, and the absence of insight.

Although it has been eclipsed by newer definitions, DSM-III (American Psychiatric Association, 1980) defined the term "psychotic" as a gross impairment in reality testing in which an individual incorrectly judges the accuracy of their perceptions and thoughts and reaches erroneous conclusions about reality despite the presence of contradictory evidence. This explanation changed in DSM-IV and beyond to a descriptive definition based on the presence of "abnormalities in one or more of the following symptom domains: delusions, hallucinations, disorganized thinking, grossly disorganized or abnormal motor behavior (including catatonia), and negative symptoms" (American Psychiatric Association, 2022, p. 101).

However, discussing psychotic experience only in terms of symptom dimensions or diagnostic categories, without considering the ego psychology concepts of sense of reality and reality testing, leaves us with a sterile and incomplete understanding. *Sense of reality* is based on one's immediate emotional, perceptual, and intuitive experiences of the world and the self. Anomalous experiences of reality include altered perceptions, senses of self, and feelings about reality. The sense of reality is based on raw sensory-perceptual and intuitive-emotional experiences, which are "complete events in themselves, absolute and unequivocal" (Weisman, 1958, p. 246). Hallucinations are a prime example of an anomalous subjective experience of reality. Taken by themselves, hallucinations are considered a psychotic phenomenon.

In contrast to how one experiences reality, *reality testing* provides a cognitive, evaluative component whereby one judges and interprets one's experience of reality. Thus, reality testing speaks to how individuals judge or understand their anomalous experience of reality and their capacity to differentiate what they experience as real, on the one hand, from what they know to be real, on the other.

The experience and testing of reality are related but distinct mental functions. How one experiences reality and then interprets or tests the validity of this experience forms a two-part process. The essential question regarding reality testing is whether individuals can distinguish the products of their mind and imagination (i.e., what is inside) from what is objectively perceived and consensually verifiable in the external world. While avoiding a philosophical discussion about who gets to decide what is reality, mental health professionals (and most people) generally agree that there is a meaningful distinction between fantasy and reality.

The interpretation of anomalous experiences of reality (i.e., reality testing) becomes a key factor in determining whether the individual might be actively psychotic. While the presence of an anomalous perceptual experience like auditory hallucination is considered a psychotic phenomenon, it does not, by itself, indicate that the individual is in an actively psychotic mental state. Another way of thinking about this is that hallucination represents a psychotic (distorted, inaccurate, unrealistic) experience of reality, whereas delusion reflects a psychotic judgment or interpretation of this experience. Our patient Tricia was having vivid hallucinations (a psychotic experience), but she knew they were not real (intact reality testing). Thus, we may conclude that while Tricia demonstrates clear psychotic phenomena, she would not be considered actively psychotic because her reality testing remains intact.

Reality testing relates to the concept of insight. Jaspers (1963) described psychosis as incompatible with insight. Thus, as described in the next chapter, impairment in reality testing and insight are central to understanding psychosis. By defining psychosis in terms of its symptoms dimensions, DSM-5-TR and ICD-11 focus primarily on anomalous experiences of reality and not on reality testing, per se. However, reality testing and insight are critical features that help sharpen the definition of psychosis. Impaired insight implies that an individual cannot determine the nature, source, or locus of her psychotic experiences and, by extension, know whether she has a mental illness and if the symptoms are "real" or abnormal. Impairment in insight is also associated with willingness to undergo treatment, which, in turn, may influence the prognosis for recovery.

As with other phenomena associated with psychosis, loss of insight is not a binary capacity. However, like most of the phenomena we discuss, insight exists along a continuum ranging from fully intact to psychotically impaired. Additionally, while most patients experiencing psychosis lack insight into the nature of their symptoms and beliefs, not all individuals lacking in insight are considered psychotic.

Psychotic Symptom Dimensions

The question of whether psychotic phenomena are best conceptualized from categorical, dimensional, and continuum perspectives is addressed in Chapter 5. However, there are several preliminary questions to ask. Is psychosis best understood as separate forms of illnesses or groups of symptoms? Additionally, are psychotic symptoms categorically distinct from those experiences that occur in nonclinical or normal subjects, or are psychotic phenomena distributed across a broad population? It is also important to note that categorical, dimensional, and continuum perspectives are not mutually exclusive. Thus, how we understand psychotic phenomena depends on which point of view we take.

Positive, Negative, and Disorganization Symptoms

It is generally agreed that psychotic symptoms can be grouped into different categories. Andreasen described the symptoms of schizophrenia as multidimensional, falling into diverse psychological domains, including perception (hallucinations), inferential thinking (delusions), language and attention (disorganized speech), social interaction, emotion expression, and volition (Andreasen et al., 1995). An early attempt to categorize diverse symptoms was based on Crow's original distinction of positive and negative symptoms (1980). Factor analytic studies subsequently identified three broad groupings of symptoms: positive, negative, and cognitive disorganization (Liddle, 1987).

Positive symptoms have traditionally included hallucinations, delusions, and disordered thinking. Positive symptoms can be thought of as *adding* something to the repertoire of normal range behavior and experience. In contrast, negative symptoms include loss of will and motivation (avolition), anhedonia (absence of pleasure), asociality (absence of normal socializing), alogia (restricted speech or speech content), anergia (lack of energy), and apathy. Negative symptoms *subtract* something from the range of normal experiences.

Cognitive disorganization was added as a third major factor (Liddle, 1987). Liddle described a three-cluster model comprised of reality distortion, psychomotor poverty (negative symptoms), and disorganization. Reality distortion pertains to sensory-perceptual and ideational experiences that depart from consensual reality. Reality distortions include hallucinations and delusions (Kotov et al., 2016; Liddle, 1987) and are considered vital but not core features. Disorganization includes behavior, thinking, and speech and, consistent with earlier models, is considered a core feature of schizophrenia (Bleuler, 1911/1950).

As noted above, contemporary DSM and ICD diagnostic criteria shifted from conceptual to operational definitions of psychosis. Although forms of psychosis continued to be described separately, the defining characteristics involve six overlapping phenomena. Some are observable signs, and others are symptoms reported by the individual. We infer or judge other features to be present from how a patient talks about his experiences. The following five phenomena are hallmark features of psychosis: (1) hallucinations, (2) delusions, (3) disorganized thinking and speech or formal thought disorder, (4) negative symptoms, and (5) grossly disorganized or abnormal motor behavior (including catatonia). To this list of defining features, ICD-11 added a criterion involving experiences of passivity and control (World Health Organization, 2019). Experiences of passivity and external control are viewed as delusional thinking in DSM-5-TR.

The first three signs and symptoms (hallucination, delusions, and disorganized speech) are considered the core positive features of psychosis. However, the DSM-5-TR specifies that any of these symptoms are sufficient to define a psychotic disorder (DSM-5, APA, 2013).

Hallucinations

Hearing voices, seeing visions, feeling bodily sensations, and tasting or smelling things without corresponding sensory stimuli are the defining characteristics of hallucinatory experiences. Beyond clinical definitions, the perceptual experience for the individual is completely real. In Humpston's words, her voices "were my reality. Who is to deny my reality when all I need to do is to perceive. The thoughts and voices were as self-evident as 'reality' would be to any otherwise 'normal' person" (2014, p. 242).

The nature and content of the voices may vary considerably. For one individual, they may be abusive, threatening, and controlling, while for others, they may provide encouragement and comfort. Still, others may experience both positive and negative voices or a shift in the quality of the voices over time. In a moving first-person account of her experience with psychosis, Lampshire (2012) spoke poetically about her experience as a person hearing voices, which provided both a sense of comfort and a source of torment:

> Madness can be an enticing siren, calling from many ragged shores with a promise of tranquility hidden amongst the rocks; unfortunately, we are just as likely to find ourselves shattered and impaled on the rocks as we are to find a safe and serene harbour.
>
> (p. 139)

Just as with Tricia, Lampshire's voices offered comfort and safety but could also turn on her intrusive and tauntingly.

Delusions

Whereas hallucinations represent false sensory-perceptual experiences, delusions are ideational phenomena that reflect an individual's false beliefs. The defining feature of a delusional conviction is that it is held as an irrefutable truth that cannot be disconfirmed. Delusions are essentially efforts to explain something confusing, threatening, or anxiety-provoking. Whereas hallucinations may reflect an altered experience of reality, delusions reflect a loss of reality testing.

More than 100 years ago, Freud concluded that Schreber's delusion about being turned into a woman was not only an effort to explain confusing internal experiences but that by alleviating anxiety, it became a restorative process (Freud, 1958). Delusional explanations may decrease anxiety by explaining the source or nature of the voices that an individual has begun to hear. In any case, anxiety reduction is achieved at the expense of a regressive shift in reality testing. Symptomatically, it is most often the simultaneous presence of hallucinations and delusions that characterize an active psychotic state. Delusions may develop as a way of explaining anomalous perceptual experiences. Unfortunately, while this explanation may reduce anxiety associated with hallucinatory experiences, it does so at the cost of reality. Delusions involve impaired insight and loss of reality testing.

Humpston called her delusions "an instinctive search for meaning in the face of the confusion," describing psychosis as "an unfortunate endpoint of one's desperate search for explanations and understanding. The psychotic person is perpetually trapped in a cul-de-sac" (2014, p. 241). Later, Humpston shared that her delusional beliefs occurred after she began hearing voices as a desperate means of explaining her sense of perplexity.

Also writing from a first-person perspective, Chadwick (2014) described his "shift to psychosis" in terms of his delusional thinking: "As psychosis approached in the summer of 1979, the verificationist tendency (confirmation bias) also started to gallop and in madness was unstoppable. I could always confirm my delusions but not refute them" (p. 485).

Then, there was Nick Lotz, whose story of psychosis was told in the *New Yorker* (Marantz, 2013). As a college student, Nick grew increasingly anxious and self-conscious. He went out and drank nightly to the point of having blackouts. Friends seemed to stop returning his calls. He stayed up all night, snorting Adderall and Focalin, worrying that people might post embarrassing videos of him online. Like Brian, he began to suspect that people were tracking him online. He anxiously searched internet sites for coded messages about him, though he could not find any. Then, one night at a concert, he heard the Dave Matthews Band sing the lyrics, "One year of crying and the words creep up inside." At that instant, it all became clear; Nick had solved the puzzle of his life. He concluded that he had been the star of a reality TV show since starting college. In this clarifying moment, everything made sense to him.

Whereas a patient who hears voices has a psychotic symptom, the delusional patient has become actively psychotic. While not all who exhibit psychotic symptoms (or psychotic phenomena, more generally) may demonstrate explicit delusional beliefs, once they become delusional, such individuals may reasonably be considered to have passed the threshold of an actual psychotic state.

Thought Disorder

Disorganized thinking, traditionally called "formal thought disorder," is another dimension associated with psychosis. We may regard thought disorder in two ways: objectively, as a formal characteristic of how individuals express their ideas through their speech or writing (disorganized speech and linguistic peculiarities) and inferentially, as the silent way in which they reason, form concepts, and make connections between their observations and ideas (leading to errors in thinking and reasoning). In this regard, Chadwick (2014) reflected on his confusing cognitive processes during his pre-psychotic and psychotic states. He focused on his tendency to collapse boundaries between different categories. "This – perhaps through over-connectivity of thought – leads to categories merging and coalescing into a totality rather than being separated and distinct. The result is enhanced similarity perception and hence the often mentioned overinclusive thinking of thought-disordered patients" (2014, p. 484). Chadwick also described how the blurring of boundaries resulted in his being unable to write up research from Ph.D. studies because "every topic I had worked on seemed to *merge* and blend with every other topic" (2014, p. 484).

Along with hallucinations and bizarre behavior, psychotic individuals may or may not demonstrate these disturbances in formulating or expressing their ideas. For example, a person may talk about delusional beliefs clearly and coherently. Conversely, an individual may speak in a disorganized, distracted, and loose manner without expressing any delusions or hallucinations.

Negative Symptoms

If hallucinations, delusions, disordered speech and thinking, and bizarre behavior are considered the "positive" or florid signs and symptoms of psychosis, "negative" features reflect an absence of various psychological functions. In some psychotic disorders, absences or deficits are apparent in cognitive functioning, speech, emotional expressiveness, and social relatedness.

Subjective accounts of negative symptoms question the deficit hypothesis and raise questions about the defensive function of negative symptoms. For example, Longden (2012) described her withdrawal from the world as a coping strategy:

> My own experience of this reflected a fundamental need to disconnect from a world with which I had ceased to identify or desire to know. Or, at other times, it protected me from the shocking, unsettling impact of voices or flashbacks.
>
> (p. 185)

Disorganized and Bizarre Behavior

Oddities of behavior may be a sign of psychosis. The patient's manner of dress and grooming, facial expressions, posture, and social and psychomotor behavior may deviate considerably from conventional norms. Patients may behave in socially inappropriate ways, crossing normative boundaries that threaten those around them. They may dress or adorn their body peculiarly. Such was the case with Martin, who was found on his hands and knees covered with green paint in the middle of a busy street.

Some individuals may speak at an inappropriate volume or not speak at all. However, like hallucinations and disturbances in reality testing, bizarre behavior is not necessarily associated with psychosis. Someone may behave bizarrely and not be psychotic. Conversely, some suffering from a psychotic disorder may not behave in floridly bizarre ways.

Experiences of Passivity and Control

Passivity symptoms involve the experience of external or "alien" control, in which the individual reports an inability to control their actions (behavior, thinking, and speech). Instead, they believe an external force has replaced their will and intentions. Passivity symptoms were one of the nine symptom dimensions described as "first-rank symptoms" (FRS) by Kurt Schneider (1959), which were initially regarded as pathognomonic of schizophrenia. This continued to be the case through ICD-10 (WHO, 1994) and DSM-IV (American Psychiatric Association, 2000). Contrary to established practice, the diagnostic specificity of FRS did not receive sufficient research support and was downgraded as a diagnostic sign in DSM-5 (American Psychiatric Association, 2013). FRS was subsequently viewed as a transdiagnostic feature of psychotic states. However, this conclusion has recently been challenged by researchers who argue that FRS can still be a useful clinical indicator of schizophrenia (Picardi, 2019; Soares-Weiser et al., 2015). Waters (2015) presented studies showing higher prevalence rates in schizophrenia compared to psychotic states in other conditions. She also suggested that the heterogeneity among the nine types of FRS contributes to the lower specificity and sensitivity in identifying schizophrenia.

As noted earlier, DSM-5 and -TR downgraded passivity symptoms and all FRS in terms of diagnostic specificity and their existence as a separate symptom dimension, where they are subsumed under delusions. However, ICD-10 and -11 include them as a distinct dimension within the domain of positive symptoms, separate from delusions.

Cognitive Impairment

Although cognitive impairment has been studied in other conditions, it is viewed as a key feature of schizophrenia (Wilk et al., 2005; Heinrichs et al., 2013). Slow processing speed, deficits in verbal learning, and executive functioning are most severe in schizophrenia (Abramovitch et al., 2021; East-Richard et al., 2020). Patients with schizophrenia are even more likely to have widespread cognitive impairment than other psychoses (Zanelli et al., 2019). For example, a comparison of patients with schizophrenia and psychotic bipolar disorders showed that over 80% of those with schizophrenia demonstrated impairment on neuropsychological measures compared to 40–58% of individuals with remitted and psychotic bipolar disorders (Reichenberg et al., 2009). However, in terms of severity and progressive deterioration in cognitive functioning, bipolar patients may not show long-term impairment (Samamé et al., 2022).

Severity of Psychology: Psychotic Disorders

Psychosis is also understood as a severe form of psychopathology. As a diagnostic category, Schizophrenia Spectrum and Related Psychotic Disorders is a superordinate class of mental disturbances characterized by clinical signs and symptoms, some or all of which may be present in a given patient. Onset and course are key components in diagnostic decision-making. Psychosis is a primary feature of disorders in the schizophrenia spectrum, or it may be an associated feature secondary to other conditions, such as bipolar and depressive disorders.

The most common examples of psychotic disorders include schizophrenia, schizoaffective, bipolar, and delusional disorders. Other psychiatric syndromes may be associated with psychotic features (bipolar and depressive disorders, OCD, body dysmorphic disorder) or the emergence of transient symptoms, typically arising under increased stress (e.g., schizotypal, paranoid, borderline personality disorders, severe post-traumatic stress disorder, and dissociative identity disorder). Finally, psychotic states may stem from toxic or metabolic factors or result from neurological damage.

In addition to classifying psychosis as either a primary or secondary feature of an illness, psychotic disorders vary in course and progression over time. For example, psychotic episodes may be acute and time-limited. Alternatively, they may be intermittent or chronic and deteriorate in progression. Chapter 3 reviews the course and phases of psychotic episodes.

Losing contact with reality can be either a state or trait-like phenomenon. Psychotic conditions can be brought about by extreme stress or trauma or be the product of psychobiological vulnerabilities. Breaks with reality can be brief and episodic, develop over time, or occur continuously. In some cases, a psychotic state might develop rapidly, emerging as a discrete symptomatic expression for a patient in a catastrophic state of stress. For others, it may creep up quietly and sinisterly, laying its experiential groundwork beyond one's conscious awareness. Such was the case with Humpston (2014), who said that the onset of her psychosis was

> an insidious one, perhaps because the increase in perplexity was so gradual that even I did not notice it at first. The salience of my surroundings and thoughts slowly heightened each gesture from strangers in the street had become a signal and a message to me. (p. 241)

Finally, for some individuals, psychosis becomes a daily reality, eroding the person's sense of self and adaptation to the world.

Psychotic-like Experiences, Risk, and Vulnerability

Diagnostic decision-making when there are questions concerning the presence or absence of psychosis is often not binary. Sometimes, diagnosticians cannot affirmatively determine whether an individual is experiencing a psychotic state, demonstrating psychotic symptoms, or meets the criteria for a primary or secondary psychotic disorder. Subclinical psychotic-like experiences (PLE) are attenuated positive symptoms without levels of impairment and disruption in adaptive functioning. Some individuals demonstrate PLEs without transitioning to clinical psychosis. For others, PLEs may indicate a high risk for a psychotic episode.

Understanding risk and vulnerability factors is critical in assessing psychosis. When might an individual demonstrate a vulnerability for a future psychotic episode? What risk factors might alert the evaluator that the individual might be a high risk? Thus, in addition to the presence or absence of psychotic phenomena, clinicians need to learn about the continuum of psychotic-like symptoms and the cognitive and psychosocial characteristics that might indicate an individual is at risk for converting to an active psychotic state. Dr. Brocato will amplify issues related to assessing individuals at risk for psychotic episodes.

With these conceptual and diagnostic issues in mind, let us return to the patients at the beginning of this chapter and see if we can sharpen our diagnostic focus. We have already noted that while Tricia demonstrates psychotic symptoms, she does not appear to be actively psychotic.

Didia's spirit voices deserve more consideration before concluding she is psychotic. The supervisor should encourage the resident therapist to think more about the cultural context of his patient's symptoms before concluding that she is psychotic and needs hospitalization.

Even though Brian seems lucid when discussing most aspects of his day-to-day life and does not show clear evidence of disordered thinking or reasoning on testing, he has a simple delusion. All efforts by family members to reassure him that his beliefs are false have been met with denial and suspicion. Brian has crossed the threshold and suffers from a psychotic disorder.

It did not take a trained mental health professional to determine that Kelvin's behavior was dangerous and highly bizarre. In the absence of other explanations, his behavior is likely a manifestation of a psychotic state. Further observation, history-taking, toxic screens, and psychological testing will help substantiate our conclusions and establish a more precise diagnosis.

Laurel's beliefs might seem delusional. After all, she doggedly defends her beliefs despite being presented with contradictory evidence. However, does this meet the criteria for diagnosing a psychotic disorder? Later in this book, Dr. Cunningham discusses distinguishing between extreme beliefs, conspiracy theories, and delusions.

Martin did not present with marked reality distortion or positive symptoms, but aspects of his behavior raised questions about his risk profile. The evaluating clinician should explore how much Martin has been using drugs like cannabis. Additionally, it would be essential to find out more about the family's history of mental illness, specifically whether relatives might have had disorders within the schizophrenia spectrum.

With Timmy, it may be an error to take the presence of disorganized and distractible speech and inventive language as an indication of a psychotic condition. Loss of focus and lack of filtering in speaking can be features of ADHD. A history of speech and language difficulties also merits further investigation. Although Timmy demonstrates disordered thought processes, is this synonymous with the psychiatric term "thought disorder"? We are unlikely to have enough information to conclude that he is psychotic.

The forensic psychologist was correct to suspect possible feigning in the case of Willum. We review factors related to the differential diagnosis of actual versus feigned psychosis in Chapter 11 on forensic assessment of psychotic phenomena.

Finally, from this brief vignette, we have enough information to determine where Marie might fall along the continuum of psychotic phenomena. There appears to be something diagnostically important about Marie's reasoning that might lead us to wonder about her potential for developing a psychotic condition. Also, how should we weigh evidence from psychological assessment measures? We return to this question in Chapter 8 when we discuss the role that psychological testing plays in the diagnostic process and how to think about positive testing signs and clinical signs and symptoms.

Although we have a clearer definition of the parts and the whole, the concept of what constitutes psychosis is still not as clear-cut as we would like it to be. In the following chapter, we explore in-depth features of each core symptom that make up the psychotic experience. However, achieving a better understanding of each symptom realm also requires an appreciation of the continuous nature of psychotic phenomena. Thus, in subsequent chapters, we discuss the continuum of psychotic symptomatology in clinical and nonclinical populations, making our job as assessors and diagnosticians even more difficult.

Clinical Assessment Points

1. Psychosis can present with varying signs and symptoms, requiring different assessment methods.
2. Diversity in the clinical presentation of psychosis necessitates adopting a multi-method assessment approach.
3. In clinical assessment, understanding the meaning and function of the person's signs, symptoms, and behavior is essential.
4. Individuals with psychotic disorder have varying degrees of insight into their condition's symptoms, signs, or causation.

2

UNDERSTANDING CORE PSYCHOTIC SYMPTOMS

Each core symptom briefly introduced in Chapter 1 has a large body of supporting research. Beyond cataloging them as diagnostic criteria, each can be unpacked by reviewing seminal research and contemporary theories to understand the conceptual underpinnings and diagnostic implications of these core symptoms of psychosis.

Hallucinations

Hallucinations are simply defined as false sensory experiences in the absence of any external stimuli (Sims, 1995). They are conceptualized as a disturbance or abnormality in perception. Researchers and scholars have made numerous attempts to define hallucinations more precisely (see Aleman & Larøi, 2008). The most comprehensive definition is from a cognitive neuropsychiatric perspective, in which hallucinations are defined as

> a sensory experience that occurs in the absence of corresponding external stimulation of the relevant organ. It has a sufficient sense of reality to resemble a veridical perception, over which the subject does not feel s/he has direct and voluntary control and occurs in the awake state.
>
> (David, 2004, p. 110)

A similar conceptualization of hallucinations has been adapted from the previous and the current diagnostic classification manuals (American Psychiatric Association, 2013, 2022).

An important clinical aspect of the experience of hallucinations is the cognitive interpretation of the sensory distortion. When individuals experience false sensory experiences, they try to make sense of that experience cognitively. For instance, in the case of a person who hears the voice of a dead relative, he might believe that the relative is no longer deceased and is actually talking to him (a false and delusional interpretation of the

DOI: 10.4324/9781003415206-4

experience), or he may recognize that the voice. However, what appears real is not, in fact, real (an accurate and reality-based interpretation of the experience). The extent to which a person considers hallucinatory experiences to be true or false is clinically seen to reflect a capacity for reality testing or, more broadly, as having insight into the hallucinatory experience. Clinicians may wonder what happened to the concept of reality testing. Is this not a key component of psychosis? It is not only a key concept but a lynchpin in the understanding of psychotic phenomena. Unlike the individual symptoms or dimensions already described, reality testing is a superordinate concept that defines the essence of the psychotic experience. When reality testing is impaired, one loses the distinction between what is real and not real. Reality testing is an active process of determining the origin or location of a particular stimulus. It is a necessary condition for the broader concept of insight. Therefore, clinicians must assess the two aspects of hallucinations: first, the presence of a false sensory experience, and second, the interpretation of that experience by the person. As such, individuals who experience hallucinations may have varying degrees of reality testing or insight into their experiences (Berrios & Brook, 1984).

Early Conceptualization of Hallucinations

Both Kraepelin (1896) and Bleuler (1950) considered hallucinations as symptoms of psychosis, though not specific to schizophrenia. They believed hallucinations occurred in other psychotic disorders. From their perspective, hallucinatory experiences did not carry diagnostic weight in differentiating schizophrenia from other psychotic conditions.

In contrast, Kurt Schneider (1959) argued that some specific types of hallucinations had diagnostic significance. He identified two types of auditory hallucinations, including hearing two or more voices in a running commentary on the person or hearing two or more voices talking with each other. He believed that these types of hallucinations were "first-rank" symptoms and pathognomonic of schizophrenia. Before the DSM-5, the presence of one of these types of hallucinations was sufficiently clinically significant to satisfy Criteria A of schizophrenia. In the DSM-5, the diagnostic weight of Schneiderian hallucinations has been removed (Black & Grant, 2014). In addition, research studies have demonstrated that these types of hallucinations do not occur exclusively in schizophrenia (see Chapter 4 on classification).

Different Types of Hallucinations

Hallucinations can occur in all sensory modalities; however, auditory hallucinations are the most common and most frequent in psychotic disorders (Bleuler, 1950; Shergill et al., 1998). Other types of hallucinations include visual, olfactory, tactile, somatic, and gustatory. There is considerable evidence that many types of hallucinations – including visual, olfactory, and tactile – can occur under the influence of drugs, in medical and neurological conditions, or be caused by a brain disease (see Ali et al., 2011). The focus of this chapter, however, is on the types of hallucinations that occur in psychotic disorders, including affective disorders and schizophrenia-spectrum disorders.

Hallucinations in the Mentally Healthy

To understand psychotic forms of hallucinations, it is essential to understand the hallucinatory experiences that occur under normal conditions. A comprehensive review of hallucinations in mentally healthy individuals indicated that a large number of individuals without any history of psychiatric or neurological conditions experience hallucinations (see Aleman & Larøi, 2008). The prevalence rate from these studies ranges from a low of 1.7% to a high of 38.7%, depending on the study sample and methodology used (questionnaire- or interview-based measures). A more recent study indicated that 15% of individuals reported auditory hallucinations under stress or in response to sleep deprivation (Beavan et al., 2011). Although the subjects in the study did not meet the full criteria for a thinking disorder, some of the samples showed evidence of subclinical levels of a thought disorder or delusions.

Hypnagogic and hypnopompic are also normative types of hallucinations that occur when a person is falling asleep and waking up. In this sleep-related phase, a person can experience auditory, visual, and tactile hallucinations and other psychotic-like experiences (Cheyne et al., 1999). Although these sleep-related hallucinations are more common in individuals with a sleep disorder, they can also be experienced by normal individuals with no history of medical, psychiatric, or sleep problems (Ohayon, 2000; Ohayon et al., 1996).

Visual, auditory, and tactile hallucinations can also occur during the process of normal grief in individuals of varying ages (Reese, 1971). For example, hearing or seeing a dead spouse has been commonly found to occur in elderly nonpsychiatric samples who had experienced the death of a spouse (Grimby, 1993, 1998; Olson et al., 1985).

Cultural beliefs may also play a role in the experience of hallucinations. In Chapter 10, we discuss assessing hallucinations within a multicultural context.

Hallucinations in Psychotic Conditions

Individuals with psychotic disorders may experience hallucinations in any of their senses, including auditory, visual, olfactory, gustatory, kinesthetic, and somatic (Bleuler, 1950; Shergill et al., 1998). Studies have shown that there is a relatively high prevalence of hallucinations in schizophrenia spectrum disorders. Auditory hallucinations are the most common at 79%, followed by visual hallucinations at 27%. The prevalence of olfactory hallucinations ranges from 6% to 26%, while gustatory hallucinations occur in 1% to 31% of cases. Somatic/tactile hallucinations have a prevalence of 4% to 19%.

Auditory Hallucinations

Auditory hallucinations are very common in psychotic disorders, occurring in 74% of psychotic patients (Gelder et al., 1998), in nearly 80% of patients with affective psychosis, and close to 90% of patients with a diagnosis of schizophrenia (Ali et al., 2011).

When assessing the presence and nature of auditory hallucinations, it is essential to understand how individuals with psychotic disorders genuinely experience hallucinations (Larøi & Aleman, 2010). According to research, the experience of auditory hallucinations in people with psychotic conditions can be characterized as follows: (1) The individual may hear one or more voices. (2) Most individuals hear the voices of both males and females and can identify who is speaking to them. (3) A person may hear unfamiliar voices, and these voices may be experienced as originating internally or externally. (4) Most people can remember the first time they heard voices. (5) The content of the auditory hallucinations is often negative, accusatory, or distressing (Ohayon, 2000; Larøi et al., 2012; Beavan et al., 2011; McCarthy-Jones et al., 2014; McCarthy-Jones & Resnick, 2014; Resnick & Knoll, 2018).

Furthermore, auditory hallucination may also entail hearing sounds, including sounds of animals. However, typical auditory hallucinations are of voices, including a single voice, more than one voice commenting on a person's behavior, two or more voices conversing about the person, or one or two voices commanding the person to do things.

Command hallucinations, which direct the person toward taking some action, are often experienced by patients as being more negative and more challenging to resist. Command hallucinations have also been associated with more significant illness severity (Mackinnon et al., 2004). The likelihood of acting on command hallucinations increases if the voices are believed to be real, experienced as benevolent, and recognized as being familiar. In addition, delusional interpretations of voices and having limited strategies to deal with voices have been associated with acting on command hallucinations (see Scott & Resnick, 2013).

Some patients may also experience hearing their thoughts spoken out loud. The content of voices can be highly negative – and include derogatory, abusive, and sexual comments. The voices may be of both genders, be those of familiar or unfamiliar persons, or believed to be those of religious figures. They can also be seen as the voices of the Devil, God, spirits, ghosts, or aliens (Larøi et al., 2012; Nayani & David, 1996).

Individuals may experience voices from inside their heads or from external sources. Many clinicians might assume that patients who experience voices stemming from external sources are more severely psychotic; however, the diagnostic significance of hearing voices from external sources has not been established (Aleman & Larøi, 2008; Larøi et al., 2012). Patients can be out of touch with reality even when they experience voices inside their heads. For example, a young man with a diagnosis of schizophrenia reported hearing the voice of the Devil coming from inside his mind because the Devil was residing in him and was speaking to him.

In 2013, Smith et al. conducted an extensive research study on auditory hallucinations, analyzing both normal and psychiatric populations. Their findings identified distinct characteristics of auditory hallucinations that distinguish psychotic individuals from normal. These characteristics include hearing voices speaking in the third person, hearing multiple voices, feeling a lack of control over the voices, experiencing voices frequently and for longer durations (over 30 minutes), hearing voices commenting on the individual, and describing the hallucinations as negative and affecting their daily life.

Visual Hallucinations

Visual hallucinations also occur in patients with schizophrenia and affective psychosis. Approximately 16–70% of patients with schizophrenia and schizoaffective disorders have reported experiencing visual hallucinations. Patients with affective psychosis have also reported visual hallucinations. In psychosis, visual hallucinations almost always occur with auditory hallucinations. The content of visual hallucinations can include images of animals or persons that are both familiar and unfamiliar (Ali et al., 2011).

Olfactory and Gustatory Hallucinations

Olfactory hallucinations have also been reported in patients with schizophrenia-spectrum disorders and affective psychosis. There is some evidence that patients with psychotic depression often perceive a smell stemming from them, whereas patients with schizophrenia may experience the smell coming from external sources. The gustatory hallucinations are not particularly common in psychotic disorders (Ali et al., 2011). However, when they do occur, they may take the form of experiencing a foul taste, with the delusional belief that one is being poisoned.

Tactile and Somatic Hallucinations

Tactile hallucinations involve false sensory experiences on or under the skin; in contrast, somatic hallucinations involve sensory experiences inside the body. In psychosis, tactile hallucinations can take the form of the sensation of being touched (Ali et al., 2011). Somatic hallucinations in psychosis may present as a feeling that one's internal organs are moving or decaying, as well as the sensation of electricity going through one's body. In some cases, the hallucinations can take bizarre forms. For example, one woman felt the sensation of the Devil's penis going through her vagina while she was walking.

From a clinical standpoint, it is essential to note that the phenomenology of hallucinations is not static and can change over time. The fluctuating nature of hallucinations may reflect significant changes in the mental state of patients, which may provide important implications for therapeutic/psychopharmacological interventions (Jones, 2010; Larøi, 2006).

It is important to note a growing movement among some in the mental health community to reframe how hallucinations – typically hearing voices – are understood and worked within a clinical context (Hoffman, 2012). The essence of this orientation is to empower patients, to refrain from pathologizing individuals who have heard voices, and to avoid losing the person while overfocusing on the symptoms.

Multimodal Hallucinations

A comprehensive review of the literature by Montagnese and colleagues (2021) shows that hallucinatory experiences occurring in multiple sensory systems are more common than previously believed. These types of hallucinations, known as multimodal hallucinations, may have a more significant negative impact than unimodal ones, but they have not been studied extensively. The authors conceptualized that a multimodal hallucination could occur in three dimensions: "Time, Relatedness, and Congruence." For instance, a person may experience a visual hallucination of a cat and hear the voice of God a few days later, and these experiences may not be related to each other. They recommend a systematic assessment of hallucination in all sensory modalities.

Delusions

Delusions are false beliefs that are held firmly despite disconfirmation or a lack of evidence. The belief cannot be explained by the person's religion, political beliefs, subculture, or level of intelligence (See Chapters 10 and 15 on distinguishing delusions from cultural beliefs and extreme political beliefs and conspiracy theories). Delusions are conceptualized as a disturbance in thought content and, by definition, a significant impairment in reality testing. As such, the presence of delusions is indicative of a psychotic condition.

Earlier Classification of Delusions

Kraepelin (1896) believed that certain classes of delusions were unique to schizophrenia. He labeled these delusions as "nonsensical." He thought that this nonsensical aspect of delusions was an essential feature in the differential diagnosis of schizophrenia from other disorders with psychosis (Cermolacce et al., 2010). Kraepelin also distinguished paranoia from schizophrenia, indicating that in paranoia, the person has a fixed and systematized delusion. In contrast, in schizophrenia, the individual has hallucinations as well as mental and functional deterioration.

In contrast, Bleuler (1950) gave less weight to delusions as diagnostic indicators of schizophrenia. He conceptualized delusions as secondary symptoms and believed that many different types of delusions occurred in other psychotic disorders. As such, delusions were not considered an essential feature of the differential diagnosis. Instead, Bleuler argued that thought disorders and other classes of symptoms such as ambivalence, autism, and disturbance in affect should be considered as the core features of schizophrenia.

Jaspers (1963), who worked from the phenomenological perspective, identified two different types of delusions and called them *primary* and *secondary*. He argued that the primary, or true, delusions were incomprehensible and that neither the clinician nor the patient could see how the belief was formed. For instance, in the case of a patient who believes that all of the organs in his body have been replaced with a metal plate, it is difficult to understand what sort of experiences led to the formation of this delusional belief. On the other hand, Jaspers believed that secondary delusions are formed from identifiable experiences in a patient's life. For instance, a patient who hears noises coming from his neighbor's apartment may gradually develop a delusion that his neighbor is deliberately making noises to harass him.

Similar to Jaspers' concept of delusions, Schneider (1959) made a distinction between the concepts of "delusional perception" and "delusional belief." He argued that in the case of a delusional belief, there are environmental cues that give rise to the development of delusions. However, with delusional perception, the clinician is unable to see how the patient's perception of environmental cues led to the development of delusions. Schneider believed that specific delusions, just like special types of hallucinations, also had diagnostic specificity for schizophrenia. He labeled these symptoms as "first-rank" symptoms of schizophrenia, which included delusions of thought broadcasting, thought withdrawal, and thought insertion, along with delusions of reference and delusions of being controlled. He separated these delusions from "second-rank" symptoms, which included other types of delusions and hallucinations that were not pathognomonic of schizophrenia.

Contemporary Conceptualization of Delusions

The latest edition of the diagnostic classification system, the DSM-5-TR, defines delusion as:

> A false belief is based on an incorrect inference about external reality that is firmly held despite what everyone else believes and what constitutes incontrovertible and obvious proof or evidence. The belief is not ordinarily accepted by other members of the person's culture or subculture (i.e., it is not an article of one's religious faith).
>
> (American Psychiatric Association, 2022, p. 819)

The above conceptualizations of delusions are consistent with the previous versions of the diagnostic statistical manuals, the DSM-III, DSM-IV, DSM-IV-TR, and DSM-5 (American Psychiatric Association, 1980, 1994, 2000, 2013).

Researchers and clinicians have criticized that many defining aspects of delusions are difficult to assess (see Zapf et al., 2013). For example, clinicians may not know what is ordinarily accepted within a particular subculture or religion (Freeman, 2010). Also, delusion-like beliefs are not uncommon in a normative sample. Two major survey studies with U.S. populations indicated that 16–25% of individuals with no history of a psychiatric illness believed in telepathy, 14% believed that they had seen UFOs, and between 5% and 10% believed that they had contact with ghosts (Gallup & Newport, 1991; Ross & Joshi, 1992).

In addition, no clear guidelines are provided for determining whether an idiosyncratic cultural, religious, or unscientific belief is false enough to meet the threshold for delusions (Oltmanns, 1998; Zapf et al., 2013). Furthermore, evidence from case studies and clinical practice shows that a mental health professional's ability to assess whether a person is making "incorrect inferences from external reality" (American Psychiatric Association, 2022, p. 819) is highly variable and requires clinical judgment and careful exploration. Errors in reasoning are not uncommon in individuals with no mental disorder. Literature from social psychology (Nickerson, 1998) on "confirmation bias" has demonstrated various types of forming ideas and jumping to conclusions based on insufficient facts. More recent examples of these types of errors in reasoning were seen in the various outlandish theories put forth about the disappearance of Malaysian Airlines Flight 370. For example, one explanation was that the two pilots had conspired to kill all the passengers and crew to take the airplane to another country. This theory was formed based on information that the plane had gone well above the altitude at which a loss of oxygen could occur. It was further reasoned that since the pilot's cabin was the only place in the airplane that would have had enough oxygen, the pilots could take control.

Clinicians themselves are not immune from making errors in reasoning. For example, when Ernest Hemingway was hospitalized for depression, he had what appeared to be a paranoid belief that the FBI was following him in a black car. Under the Freedom of Information Act, the FBI file on Hemingway has been made available, and it has become clear that the FBI was following him (see Hotchner, 2011; Mitgang, 1983).

Oltmanns (1998) offers expanded and clinically useful features of delusions, arguing that diagnosis is best achieved by considering delusions' multiple dimensions or characteristics. He indicates that in addition to the degree of conviction and the absence of a shared belief by others, the delusion is "a personal reference" (Oltmanns, 1998, p. 5) rather than an unconventional political, cultural, or scientific belief. Also, he characterizes the person with a delusion as "emotionally committed to the belief" (Oltmanns, 1998, p. 5). The false belief causes significant distress for the person, which potentially impairs functioning. Furthermore, despite experiencing distress, a person with a delusion does not challenge or actively resist the belief.

The following clinical example illustrates Oltmanns' expanded perspective on delusions, in which multiple dimensions or characteristics are considered and assessed.

> The patient is a young woman who gradually became depressed while attending college. One evening, while in the kitchen of her college dormitory, there was a gas leak. Shortly after the leak was repaired, she developed a belief that the odor from the gas had "penetrated" her body. She gradually developed a delusion that she had a foul smell like "gasoline" because any time she walked on campus or entered a classroom, students or faculty either "looked away" or "touched their noses." She believed these cues indicated she must have an odor, although she did not smell the gasoline. She could not entertain an alternative explanation for her experience or consider the possibility that the student's or faculty's actions were unrelated to her. She became so distressed that she dropped out of college, moved to her parent's home, and stopped socializing.

Although friends and family members reassured her that she did not emit a foul odor, she continued with her delusional belief. She indicated that her family and friends were "just being nice" to her. One day, she expressed feelings of hopelessness and suicidal thoughts to her parents, which resulted in admission to an inpatient service. There, she was diagnosed as having major depression with psychotic features and was treated successfully with antidepressant and antipsychotic medications.

In this example, the patient's delusional belief was a personal reference. Her belief that the smell of gas could penetrate her body and remain for weeks was not shared by others. Her delusions caused significant distress and impaired her functioning. Despite experiencing high levels of distress and being confronted with contrary evidence, she was emotionally committed to her belief and did not attempt to resist it or consider different perspectives.

Different Types of Delusions

In the DSM-5 and 5-TR, delusions are classified according to theme or content. One type of delusion that has received special status in clinical practice and differential diagnosis consists of false beliefs that are considered bizarre. In the current and past diagnostic classification system (the DSM-III), bizarre delusions are seen as beliefs that are physically implausible and incompatible with consensual reality and the person's cultural beliefs (i.e., family members are replaced by identical-looking imposters or a person's thoughts are broadcast so others can hear what she is thinking). These delusions are distinguished from non-bizarre delusions, in which false beliefs can conceivably occur in reality (i.e., one's spouse is cheating, or government agents are following the person).

The concept of bizarre delusions is thought to have its roots in the writings of Kraepelin, Jaspers, and Schneider (Cermolacce et al., 2010). Historically, bizarre delusions were regarded as having diagnostic specificity and were commonly present in patients with schizophrenia rather than other psychotic disorders. Similar to certain types of hallucinations, bizarre delusions were given more diagnostic weight than different types of psychotic symptoms. For instance, the presence of one bizarre delusion was sufficient to meet the diagnostic Criteria A of schizophrenia in the DSM-III, DSM-IV, and DSM-IV-TR.

However, the concept and definition of a bizarre delusion have been criticized for various reasons (see Cermolacce et al., 2010). First, clinicians do not reliably agree on what constitutes a bizarre delusion. Specifically, the interrater reliability of establishing the presence of a bizarre delusion has been inadequate (Bell et al., 2006a). Also, the base rate of bizarre delusions remains low, with approximately 4–8% of patients with a first break of schizophrenia having bizarre delusions (Tanenberg-Karant et al., 1995). Finally, empirical studies do not support the idea that the bizarreness of delusions has diagnostic specificity. That is, other psychotic disorders, including affective psychosis, showed evidence of bizarre delusions (Andreasen, 1990). Moreover, others have argued that the concept of bizarreness needs to go beyond just the "content" of a delusion and must also include the "form" and the way the bizarreness is experienced (Cermolacce et al., 2010).

In addition to a distinction between bizarre and non-bizarre, delusions can be classified as being congruent with the predominant mood episode that the patient is experiencing. For example, a patient with major depression and psychosis may believe that his body is decaying. In contrast, another patient with depression with mood incongruence may have a persecutory delusion that the government is trying to kill him (a mood-incongruent psychotic feature).

Specific types of delusions include persecutory, grandiose, erotomanic, guilt, jealousy, reference, and control delusions. Furthermore, patients can also have multiple delusions with no one theme dominating the content. It is important to note that, similar to hallucinations, the content of delusions is not diagnostically specific. For example, although paranoid delusions are typically associated with schizophrenia, many patients presenting with manic psychosis may also demonstrate paranoid delusions. Similarly, while grandiose delusions are often found in bipolar manic conditions, they may also occur in a patient with schizophrenia with grandiose delusions.

Thought Disorder

Thought disorder is among the triumvirate of features most commonly associated with psychosis. Although this term, unlike hallucinations and delusions, has long been a standard part of the clinical lexicon, its precise meaning has proven to be elusive. A lack of conceptual clarity has led to a common misunderstanding regarding the scope of the definition, the underlying mechanisms, and the degree of diagnostic specificity associated with the presence of thought disorder.

More than 100 years ago, both Kraepelin (1896) and Bleuler (1950) identified disturbances in thinking as an important feature in dementia praecox (Kraepelin's term) or schizophrenia (Bleuler's term). Kraepelin focused on the deterioration in intellectual processes that disrupt the ordering of thoughts, thus creating a "derailment" in the course of ideas.

Bleuler viewed a "loosening of associations" between thoughts as one of the fundamental features of schizophrenia. Unfortunately, the terms "derailment" and "loosening of associations" became synonymous with "thought disorder." As generations of mental health practitioners settled for this relatively narrow definition of the term, they overlooked the complex and diverse cognitive and linguistic components of thought disorder among psychotic individuals.

Disturbances of Form versus Disturbances of Content

An early effort to move away from a unitary notion of thought disorder as a disruption in associations was Schilder's (1951) distinction between disturbances in the form and the content of thought. Taylor (1981) sharpened this dichotomy by defining disorders in form as disturbances in rate, fluency, rhythm, flow, filtering, word usage, and associational linkage. In other words, disorders in form involve *how* things are said. Essentially, formal features of thought are dimensions of speech. There is controversy about whether thought disorder is a speech or language disorder (Chaika, 1990; Harvey & Neale, 1983; Johnston & Holzman, 1979) and whether another term should be used to reflect this distinction (Andreasen, 1982). However, the arguments in favor of different terminology have not gained a great deal of traction. Disturbances in the formal characteristics of speech manifest as disorganization, which interferes with coherence and the listener's ability to comprehend what the speaker is trying to say.

In contrast, disorders of content involve *what* the person is talking about. Traditionally, disordered content has been restricted to beliefs such as overvalued ideas, ideas of reference, and delusions. As such, thought disorders of content can be seen as synonymous with delusions and are already represented by this separate symptom concept.

Some have broadened the content category to include ideas and beliefs and how stimuli are interpreted (Grebb & Cancro, 1989). This broader definition of disordered thought content includes not simply *what* the person thinks but *how* he thinks and the reasons behind this thinking (as opposed to *how* things are said, as is the case with disturbances in form). As such, disorders of content subsume capacities to reason logically, form concepts, think abstractly, make inferences, and maintain perceptual and conceptual boundaries.

Weiner's (1966) simple formulation of disturbances in thought processes integrated dimensions of form and content. According to this approach, thinking problems regarding disturbances in focusing, conceptualizing, and reasoning can be analyzed. The first dimension includes problems establishing, maintaining, and shifting attention, which give rise to disturbances in formal features of thought or speech, including scanning, focusing, filtering, pacing, flowing, and associative linkage. The second and third dimensions (concept formation and reasoning) are content-specific variables associated with abstract thinking and inference-making. Concept formation implies the ability to interpret experience at appropriate levels of abstraction and reflects the continuum of concreteness on one end and over-inclusiveness on the other.

Using both various thought disorder scoring systems and clinician and linguist raters, Berenbaum and Barch (1995) expected that two dimensions (disturbed form and content) would account for the range of thought-disorder subtypes. However, the results of their study showed that subtypes of thought disorder could not be simply dichotomized into disorders of form and disorders of content. Instead, their data led them to develop four categories:

1. Disturbances in fluency.
2. Disturbances in discourse coherence.
3. Disturbances in content.
4. Disturbances in social convention.

Disturbances in fluency and discourse coherence included tangentiality, derailment, looseness, grammatical lapses, neologisms, incoherence, and loosely connected associations. Berenbaum and Barch hypothesized that disturbances in fluency and discourse coherence reflect disturbances in the language production system, which relies on attentional and executive resources and is responsible for the planning, monitoring, and editing, as well as the grammatical and phonological encoding, of linguistic information. On the other hand, disturbances of content and social convention reflect problems not in language, per se, but in thinking and "impaired perspective" (Harrow et al., 1989), which demonstrates a failure in one's ability to judge critically the social appropriateness of one's verbal productions. According to Harrow and colleagues, thought-disordered individuals fail to discern whether or not they will sound bizarre or understandable to others.

We think there is a less confusing way to account for the different aspects of thought disorder. Our approach expands the concept of thought disorder beyond the narrow definition of formal thought disorder. Like Berenbaum and Barch, we look at four aspects:

1. *How* things are expressed.
2. *What* is said.
3. *How* conclusions or beliefs are developed.
4. *Who* the information is shared with, and when it is shared.

The *how* dimension refers to the traditional term "formal thought disorder," or disorganized speech or thinking. This is related to *how* individuals express their ideas. Disorders of form are objective data because we hear individuals say their thoughts. Andreasen (1984) referred to this as derailment, disorganization, and disconnectedness of thought processes. Examples include circumstantiality, tangentiality, derailment, flight of ideas, distractible speech, clang associations, and incoherence.

In addition to *how* individuals express their thoughts, there is the *content* of the expressed thoughts. The *what* category encompasses thought disorders of content. Delusions, though classified separately from thought disorders, stem from thought processes. Thus, delusions and unusual ideas are related to what one is thinking.

A definition of thought disorder is incomplete unless we consider how one's beliefs are formulated. We may hear the disjointed way in which individuals express their ideas and the beliefs they hold. However, we are equally interested in the processes of "thinking," "reasoning," and "inference-making," which led to unusual ideas and bizarre beliefs that may or may not be expressed in disjointed ways. Thus, we pay attention to *how* individuals express their thoughts *or ideas, what* those thoughts or ideas are, and *where* they come from in terms of concept formation, logic, and formulation.

Finally, there are the social-pragmatic aspects of thought disorder. These dimensions refer to an awareness of when and with whom individuals express their ideas. The essential issue here is one of timing and appropriate social context.

Positive and Negative Types of Thought Disorder

Just as general features of psychosis can be classified in terms of positive versus negative symptoms, this same distinction can be applied to thought disorder. Positive thought disorder includes formal features of speech, thought content, or underlying reasoning processes that are bizarre, illogical, and confusing to the listener. Harrow and Quinlan (1985) used "bizarre idiosyncratic thinking" to capture the broad category of positive thought disorder manifest in disorganized speech and illogical thinking. Most Schneiderian first-rank symptoms, such as thought broadcasting, thought withdrawal, and thought insertion (Schneider, 1959), are prime examples of positive-thought-disorder content that implicitly reflect underlying illogicality in reasoning processes.

Unlike positive thought disorder, characterized by the presence of bizarre and idiosyncratic forms and content, negative thought disorder is understood as an impoverishment of thought and speech. Here, the absence of normal rate, fluency, rhythm, and flow of thoughts and speech, as well as a constriction in the range of content, defines negative thought disorder. Typical categories are

- Poverty of speech, which includes responses that are brief and unelaborated.
- Poverty of thought content, which reflects empty speech devoid of meaningful information.
- Perseveration of ideas, in which ideas and themes are repeated regardless of changes in circumstances.

In contrast to positive thought disorder, symptoms of negative thought disorder are generally regarded as specific to a subtype of schizophrenia (Andreasen, 1982, 1990) and associated with chronicity and poor outcome (Astrup & Noreik, 1966; Pogue-Geile & Harrow, 1984).

Further contributing to the distinction between positive and negative forms of thought disorder, Liddle and colleagues (Liddle, Ngan, Caissie, et al., 2002) factor-analyzed thought-disorder responses in patients with acute and chronic forms of schizophrenia using their Thought and Language Index (TLI). They found three nearly independent factors that capture characteristics of positive and negative thought disorders:

1. Impoverished thought and language (poverty of speech and speech content).
2. Disorganized thought and language (looseness, peculiar word usage, poor syntax, and logic).
3. Nonspecific dysregulation of thought (perseveration and distractibility).

Continuum of Disordered Thinking

Contrary to Kraepelinian tradition, which viewed thought disorder as a discrete, all-or-none phenomenon, contemporary researchers and practitioners agree that disordered thinking fits along a continuum from normal to psychotic thinking (Andreasen & Grove, 1986a; Harrow & Quinlan, 1977, 1985; Holzman et al., 1986; Johnston & Holzman, 1979; Liddle, Ngan, Caissie, et al., 2002). The distinction between milder forms of thought pathology and more severe levels of thought disorder is widely accepted.

Researchers (Harrow & Quinlan, 1977; Marengo & Harrow, 1985) have demonstrated that mild levels of thought disorder occur frequently, both in patients who have schizophrenia and those who do not. However, the most severe levels of thought disorder occur less regularly among all groups of patients, except for those who are acutely psychotic. Even within the same diagnostic group or individual, there is variability in the degree of thought disorder between individuals and within the same individual, depending on the phase of illness (Harrow & Quinlan, 1977).

If we accept the existence of a continuum of thought disturbances, the term "thought disorder" becomes somewhat misleading in that it implies a distinct and unique entity dichotomous with normal thinking. For this reason, Harrow and Quinlan (1977) proposed that the term "disordered thinking" be substituted for the term "thought disorder." The term "disordered thinking" is consistent with the concept of action language (Harty, 1986; Schafer, 1976) and one that helps avoid the reification of constructs by remaining closer to the raw data of observable behavior.

Cognitive–Neuropsychological Approaches to Thought Disorder

Researchers have increasingly sought to understand disordered thinking from a cognitive neuroscience perspective (Barch, 2005; Elvevag & Goldberg, 2000; Goldberg & Weinberger, 2000; McGhie & Chapman, 1961; Nuechterlein & Dawson, 1984). From this perspective, disturbances in thinking are analyzed in terms of impairment in cognitive functions such as attention, memory, verbal fluency, executive functioning, and processing speed. Both Kraepelin and Bleuler paved the way for later efforts to examine the neurocognitive underpinnings of thought disorder psychologically by highlighting the attentional deficits in schizophrenia. Nuechterlein and Dawson (1984) concluded from their studies that impairments in attention may be more of a "trait" variable for schizophrenic subjects than it is for manic ones. In another series of investigations, Braff and his colleagues demonstrated that individuals with schizophrenia exhibit abnormal information processing when compared to nonpatient controls (Braff & Geyer, 1990; Braff et al., 1992; Braff & Saccuzzo, 1981; Braff et al., 1991). When attention and information-processing functions are impaired, people with schizophrenia may experience increased distractibility in response to a flood of excessive and poorly inhibited internal and external stimuli, leading to cognitive fragmentation and markedly disordered thinking.

Deficits in working memory are related to the attentional vulnerabilities found in patients who have schizophrenia. The working memory system enables a person to hold relevant information in mind while utilizing it to solve problems at hand. Several studies have found a link between working memory deficits and thought and communication disturbances (Goldberg & Weinberger, 2000; Oltmanns & Neale, 1978). Moreover, emotional arousal may further disrupt working memory in vulnerable individuals.

Bentall (2003) pointed out that impairment in semantic memory may disrupt associative links between related ideas. The semantic memory system stores ideas and knowledge and is a complex network of concepts linked by association. Impairment in semantic memory can disrupt associative linkages between ideas, leading to looseness and disconnection between one idea and the next.

Executive functions like self and source monitoring may also contribute to disordered thinking. Self-monitoring relates to individuals' ability to monitor and adjust their speech to their listeners' communication needs and perspectives. The ability to comprehend that others have minds and needs separate from one's own signifies a theory of mind capacity. Thus, deficits in the theory of mind might prevent individuals from recognizing that others might be unable to comprehend what they are trying to say, resulting in an impaired perspective. Deficits in source monitoring (which relates to the older concept of reality testing) may prevent one from identifying the source of a particular stimulus. Individuals may be uncertain whether they *said it* or simply *thought it.* Source-monitoring deficits may make individuals susceptible to missing essential information when speaking to others. In turn, this may make their speech confusing or unintelligible to others. Bentall (2003) hypothesized that an integrated sequence of vulnerabilities consisting of deficits in working memory, semantic memory, self, and source-monitoring could lead to speech that is loose and incomprehensible to others.

Considering thought disorder from various perspectives guards against simple, reductionistic formulations that overlook or exaggerate subtler manifestations of disordered thinking. A more comprehensive definition of thought disorder includes multiple cognitive and language functioning aspects. It addresses the form of thoughts (as expressed through speech), the content of the thoughts, and the conceptual and reasoning processes that give rise to these thoughts. Our definition includes the dimensions of disorganization, impoverishment, and bizarreness, which may manifest in an individual's speech, behavior, or thoughts.

A comprehensive understanding of thought disorder appreciates the links between disorders in thought and communication and disturbances in fundamental cognitive processes governing attention, memory, and self-monitoring. Only with this more comprehensive perspective can we capture the multidimensional nature of disturbances in thought organization. With this in mind, it is vital to distinguish that in contemporary diagnostic and forensic practice, "disorganized thinking" refers to formal thought disorder, assessed by observing how the person talks (i.e., speech).

Disorganized and Bizarre Behavior

Disorganized behavior is a broad concept. There are two categories to consider. The first is odd behavior, which includes strange appearances, unusual attire, and socially inappropriate speech and actions. The second category contains disturbances in motoric behavior. The term "catatonia" refers to different forms of unusual motoric disturbances, thought to reflect an extreme state of agitation. Catatonic behavior can appear as a stupor or intense psychomotor excitement. These motor disturbances can be pronounced and prevent an individual from attending to basic safety and personal-care needs. The classic example of catatonia involves a person who does not move or respond to external stimuli. The catatonic patient may assume bizarre, frozen postures. If someone moves a part of the individual's body, he may remain in that position, no matter how bizarre (known as "waxy flexibility").

The other presentation of catatonia involves a state of psychomotor excitation. In this state, the patient may engage in what appears to be purposeless motor activity to exclude other behaviors. As with catatonic stupor, the individual is unresponsive to external stimuli and may neglect self-care needs.

Negative Symptoms

Apathy, *avolition*, and *anhedonia* reflect a lack of motivation and will and a loss of interest, enthusiasm, and pleasure in activities. *Anergia* refers to passivity and lack of initiation of problem-solving activity. *Alogia* includes impoverished speech production and may manifest as a lack of speech or meaningful content. Flat *affect* describes an absence of visible emotional expressiveness and flexibility.

Negative symptoms are associated with schizophrenia. These include deficits in cognitive functioning, which may persist long after florid signs of psychosis disappear. They are typically less responsive to medication than positive symptoms and may have extrapyramidal side effects that require long-term support and cognitive rehabilitation.

Primary Versus Secondary Negative Symptoms

Researchers have attempted to distinguish between primary and secondary negative symptoms (Carpenter et al., 1988). Carpenter's group viewed primary symptoms as direct manifestations of the illness of schizophrenia, as opposed to those negative symptoms that were secondary to a combination of depression, suspicious withdrawal, psychotic symptoms, and extrapyramidal side effects. They called the first set of factors "primary symptoms." This model held that individuals who have chronic primary negative symptoms formed a subgroup of schizophrenia patients suffering from what was termed a "deficit syndrome."

Kirkpatrick (2014) summarized studies that have shown deficit patients to be less aware of their impairments (including their dyskinetic movements), less depressed and anxious, less suicidal, and more socially isolated. Although deficit patients do not have a less severe pattern of positive symptoms or disorganization, the content of their delusions may reflect less social malevolence and threat. Kirkpatrick and a team of researchers (Kirkpatrick et al., 2011) linked this finding to the lack of social drive associated with patients exhibiting deficit schizophrenia. Deficit patients were also shown to have had greater social dysfunction before the onset of psychosis and a poorer outcome at follow-up. Not surprisingly, deficit patients were found to have greater cognitive and neurological impairment than so-called nondeficit patients.

In addition, Kirkpatrick (2014) described factor-analytic studies that identified two dimensions of negative symptoms (Blanchard & Cohen, 2006). The first is an expressive factor reflecting blunted affect and alogia. The second factor combines anhedonia, avolition, and asociality. Kirkpatrick indicated that preliminary research has suggested that the avolition factor is a more potent predictor of overall dysfunctionality.

Impaired Insight

Perhaps the most common feature of psychosis (Gelder et al., 1998) is poor or impaired insight, which has long been associated with poor treatment compliance, poor treatment outcome, symptom severity, higher relapse rates, lower self-esteem, and impaired psychosocial functioning (Amador & David, 2004; Drake et al., 2000; Francis & Penn, 2001; Kampman et al., 2002; Lacro et al., 2002; Lysaker et al., 2002; Novak-Grubic & Tavcar, 2002). British psychiatrist Aubrey Lewis (1934) defined insight as the correct attitude regarding morbid changes in oneself and the realization that the changes are a result of a mental illness. Jaspers (1963) stated that there is virtually no lasting or complete insight in the presence of psychosis. The International Pilot Study of Schizophrenia conducted by the World Health Organization (1973) confirmed that awareness of emotional illness was absent in 97% of subjects, thus establishing impaired insight as a key feature in schizophrenia. Subsequent studies (Amador et al., 1994; Carpenter et al., 1976; Carpenter et al., 1973) found further evidence that poor insight was a common feature in schizophrenia and other psychotic disorders. Individuals diagnosed as having schizophrenia were found to be significantly less aware of their psychotic symptoms, of having a mental disorder, or of the efficacy of medication than patients diagnosed with schizoaffective disorder or psychotic depression.

Over the past quarter of a century, there has been an explosion of interest in the subject of insight into psychosis. Two major volumes have reviewed contemporary studies that have focused on the concept of insight in patients with psychotic and nonpsychotic disorders

(Amador & David, 1998, 2004; Marková, 2005). As is often the case, different definitions of terminology obscured a more nuanced understanding of the concept of insight in psychosis. Previously understood as a form of defensive denial or evasion, impairments in insight are increasingly conceptualized as a neurocognitive deficit. However, despite interest in the neurocognitive underpinnings of insight (and other psychotic phenomena), the psychological defense model has not been entirely superseded.

Early efforts at understanding insight also focused simplistically on a binary, categorical model, with patients considered to have either intact or impaired insight depending on whether or not they were aware of their symptoms and the need for treatment. However, refinements in definitions and conceptual understanding have led to the development of more sophisticated methods for assessing insight in psychotic individuals. In turn, measurement systems have led to an appreciation of the diverse nature of insight. Insight is no longer understood as an "all or none" or unitary phenomenon but is now treated as a complex, multidimensional concept.

Multidimensional Nature of Insight

David (1990) defined clinical insight in terms of three distinct dimensions:

1. Awareness of illness.
2. Capacity to relabel psychotic experiences as abnormal.
3. Compliance with treatment.

Amador et al. (1991) proposed a more complex multidimensional model, which was eventually narrowed down to two distinct features of insight:

1. Awareness.
2. Attribution or labeling of psychotic symptoms.

This distinction is based on the fact that some patients may be aware of their psychotic experiences but attribute them to reasons other than the presence of a psychotic disorder. Additionally, patients may recognize specific symptoms yet be unaware of others. Marková and Berrios (1992) conceptualized awareness of illness as part of a broader category of self-knowledge rather than as an independent feature of psychotic disturbance. Their concept focuses on changes in the self along a continuum of self-awareness.

In contrast to clinical insight, cognitive insight is a broader psychological construct that refers to evaluating abnormal experiences and recognizing when one's interpretations are incorrect. Cognitive insight seems very similar to the concept of reality testing. Individuals with impaired cognitive insight may be unable to step back from their psychotic experiences and use feedback to test out and correct their conclusions. Beck et al. (2004) distinguished two dimensions of cognitive insight:

1. Self-reflectiveness, which includes the capacity of individuals to observe their mental productions and entertain alternative explanations.
2. Self-certainty or overconfidence in the validity of their beliefs and conclusions.

Insight and Severity of Psychotic Symptoms

Is poor insight a consequence of severe symptoms or dimensions of psychosis, or is it a symptom in its own right? Research has not yielded consistent findings. Some studies using standardized assessment of symptoms have suggested that insight and symptom severity are unrelated (Amador et al., 1993; Bartko et al., 1988; McEvoy et al., 1989). Such studies found no significant correlations between insight and dimensions of psychosis or general measures of symptoms. Confusing matters, other studies found a relationship between impaired insight and measures of symptom severity (Marková & Berrios, 1992; Takai et al., 1992; Young et al., 1993).

Psychosis is currently viewed in terms of dimensions of symptoms, including positive and negative symptoms, disorganization, mania, and depression (Reininghaus et al., 2013; van Os & Kapur, 2009). Studies examining the relationship between insight and dimensions of psychosis have shown several correlations. Mintz et al. (2003) reviewed a large number of studies that examined the relationship between insight and symptom severity in schizophrenia and found a small but significant relationship between lack of insight and both positive and negative symptom severity. Other investigations found an inverse relationship between the presence of insight and disorganization (Amador et al., 1994; Cuesta et al., 1998; Kim et al., 1997; Lysaker & Bell, 1994; Smith et al., 1999; Smith et al., 1998).

Studies have also consistently demonstrated a positive correlation between depression and insight, suggesting that higher levels of awareness of illness and attribution of symptoms are associated with the presence of depression (Smith et al., 2000; Smith et al., 1998). More recently, Reininghaus et al. (2013) found support for many of the above relationships, demonstrating a negative correlation between self-reported insight and the dimensions of positive symptoms and mania, as well as a positive correlation between insight and the depression dimension of psychosis.

In terms of specific symptoms, David et al. (1992) did not find a correlation between insight and hallucinations. Garety and Hemsley (1987) showed that dimensions of delusional beliefs, such as strength of conviction and preoccupation, are also unrelated to insight measures. However, Amador and colleagues (1994) found a modest correlation between delusionality, disorganized behavior, and thought disorder with decreased awareness of the mental disorder; however, the subtle level of the correlation and the existence of methodological shortcomings led the researchers to conclude that level of illness awareness was generally not related to symptom severity. On the other hand, Sanz et al. (1998) indicated that insight scores correlated inversely with the item on the BPRS (Brief Psychiatric Rating Scale) having to do with delusions. Grandiosity has also been shown to be negatively correlated with insight (David et al., 1995; Kemp & Lambert, 1995; Sanz et al., 1998; Van Putten et al., 1976). Finally, Baier et al. (2000) conducted a correlational study between insight and positive and negative symptoms in a sample of patients with schizophrenia and schizoaffective disorder. They found a significant inverse relationship between insight and positive formal thought disorder.

Several researchers (David, 2004; Marková, 2005) attributed the inconsistent findings to different instrumentation and methodology used in studies examining the relationship between insight and dimensions and symptoms of psychosis. Regarding instrumentation, other scales have been developed based on different definitions of insight and different formats (interviews, ratings, and self-report measures). Furthermore, David pointed out that examiner bias might also affect results when ratings of insight and level of pathology are not made blindly and independently. In the end, however, David concluded that although insight is a separate phenomenon, it is modestly influenced by symptom dimensions of psychosis. Specifically, insight is worse in the presence of positive and negative symptoms and psychotic disorganization. Conversely, insight is better in the context of depression.

Differential Diagnosis of Insight

Among major psychotic disorders, schizophrenia has been characterized as having high rates of poor insight. Amador and Kronengold (2004) examined whether poor insight is so uniquely characteristic of schizophrenia that it can be regarded as a differential diagnostic sign. They cited research (Carpenter et al., 1973, 1976), which found poor insight to be a prevalent feature in schizophrenia and a key factor in discriminating it from other psychiatric disorders. Subsequent research efforts by Amador et al. (1994) replicated earlier findings, which showed that the majority of patients with schizophrenia demonstrated moderate to severe unawareness of having a mental illness, including difficulties identifying and correctly attributing symptoms to an illness. Furthermore, in associated field trials using the DSM-IV revised criteria for schizophrenia, 27–87% of patients diagnosed with schizophrenia were unaware of specific symptoms such as delusions, blunted affect, thought disorder, and other aspects of the illness.

More noteworthy, however, was the finding that patients with schizophrenia were significantly less aware of having a mental disorder and of their specific symptoms (e.g., hallucinations, delusions, anhedonia, and asociality) than were patients with schizoaffective disorders and those with psychotic and nonpsychotic major depressive disorders. These findings supported the differential diagnostic significance of poor insight and unawareness of illness/symptoms in schizophrenia compared to other psychotic disorders. Furthermore, the fact that patients with schizophrenia demonstrated less awareness of their illness and symptoms suggested that poor insight was not simply a consequence of psychosis but a unique aspect of schizophrenia.

There was, of course, one important exception. Amador et al. (1994) found that patients with bipolar disorders, whether psychotic or not, demonstrated impaired insight compared to schizoaffective and psychotic depressive groups. Analogous to earlier research, which showed that manic patients demonstrated as much thought disorder as patients with schizophrenia (Pope & Lipinski, 1978), studies of insight in psychosis have shown that manic patients demonstrate levels of poor insight similar to patients with schizophrenia. Thus, based simply on ratings of insight, both patient groups demonstrate high levels of unawareness.

Ghaemi and Rosenquist (2004) reviewed studies that showed significant impairment in insight among acutely manic patients. They cited a group of studies that showed more substantial improvement in insight after recovery from mania than was found in patients with schizophrenia recovering from acute psychotic episodes (Ghaemi et al., 1995; Michalakeas et al., 1994; Peralta & Cuesta, 1998; Swanson et al., 1995). These findings suggested that poor insight in bipolar disorders may be more of a *state-dependent* variable compared to insight in schizophrenia, which has been considered to be *trait-like*. These studies also indicated that poor insight into bipolar disorder was not related to the presence of psychosis. However, nonpsychotic bipolar patients demonstrated insight levels that were comparably impaired as in those who were psychotic.

As previously indicated, depression is associated with better insight. The studies referenced above showed that insight might increase as depression worsens. In patients suffering from major depression with psychotic features, insight is moderately impaired but less than it is in patients with bipolar disorders. Finally, it appears that insight improves significantly in patients recovering from acute episodes of psychotic depression.

Neurocognitive Underpinnings of Insight

Interest in the neurocognitive underpinnings of insight include studies of neuropsychological as well as neural correlates of awareness of illness in psychosis. Morgan and David (2004) reviewed neuropsychological studies. He concluded that there is a weak relationship between insight and general intellectual functioning and a stronger association between insight and nonverbal aspects of cognitive functioning. The most impressive finding has identified a strong relationship between insight and prefrontal lobe executive functions. Impairment in cognitive flexibility, or set-shifting when confronted with evidence that one's beliefs are disconfirmed (e.g., the unreality of delusions), and self-monitoring, specifically error monitoring, contribute to poor insight in psychosis (Aleman et al., 2006; Morgan & David, 2004). Problems with set-shifting and error correction have been compared to the inability to appraise psychotic experiences in the presence of disconfirming evidence correctly.

Neurocognitive investigations have recently included neuroimaging studies to identify brain regions associated with insight (Liemburg et al., 2012; van der Meer et al., 2010). Impaired insight has been linked to self-reflection, which involves awareness of one's thoughts and emotions, as well as decisions about what applies to and what does not apply to the self (David, 1999; Lysaker et al., 2009; van der Meer et al., 2010). Neural correlates of self-reflection involve structures in the prefrontal cortex, the anterior and posterior cingulate, the anterior insula, the inferior frontal gyrus, and the temporoparietal junction/angular gyrus/inferior parietal lobule. In particular, less activation in these regions is associated with problems in self-reflection, which may contribute to impaired insight into one's symptoms and the presence of psychosis.

Insight and Social Cognition

Insight is related to the social cognitive concepts of emotion processing, mentalization, and Theory of Mind (ToM). Insight and accurate self-appraisal are conceptually and neurocognitively associated with understanding other people's minds and mental experiences. ToM involves correct attribution of feelings, knowledge, and intentions to others, whereas cognitive insight involves similar processes about the self. Several studies reported deficits in ToM in schizophrenia (Corcoran et al., 1995; Doody et al., 1998; Drury et al., 1998; Frith, 1992; Langdon et al., 1997; Mazza et al., 2001; Sarfati et al., 1997). Quee and colleagues (2010) concluded that social cognition, specifically deficits in emotional recognition and mentalizing, reduces insight in psychotic subjects. Flashman and Roth (2004) hypothesized that impaired ToM might reduce awareness of one's psychotic symptoms and illness if threatening thoughts and intentions were inappropriately attributed to others.

Deficits in social cognition have been studied primarily in schizophrenia. Recently, Vaskinn et al. (2013) also examined the relationship between insight and social cognition in bipolar patients. Although insight ratings were similar for both the schizophrenia and bipolar groups, they found that clinical insight was more strongly related to social cognition variables in their schizophrenia sample than in their bipolar I sample. In the bipolar I group, impairment in clinical insight was more associated with the presence of positive, negative, manic, and depressive symptoms than with deficits in social cognition.

Deficits in mentalizing capacities also imply that one cannot gauge the social inappropriateness of one's bizarre behavior, delusional beliefs, or inappropriate, thought-disordered speech. Related to unawareness of illness phenomena, psychotic individuals may be similarly unaware of the impact they have on others (which is related to a deficit in self-monitoring) and unaware that others do not understand them or agree with their view of reality. They may demonstrate what Harrow and Quinlan (1985) referred to as an "impaired perspective," an inability to take another person's point of view or see oneself through another's eyes. Thus, both ToM and impaired perspective imply an inability to observe psychological or behavioral phenomena from a distance, whether it be another person's state of mind or one's own experiences, thoughts, and feelings as others experience them.

Ms. G., whom we discuss again in Chapter 5, periodically experienced what she referred to as "broadcast thinking," despite attending therapy regularly and taking antipsychotic medication faithfully. She remained stable because she was aware of her illness and recognized her need for medication to help control her psychotic thinking. Nonetheless, she occasionally reported the recrudescence of her fears that co-workers could hear her thoughts. Typically, she would begin a therapy session with something like, "I know you're going to think I'm crazy, but I thought that the guy on the bus was hearing what I thought because right then, when I thought that, he looked up at me. I know it must sound crazy."

In addition to describing her "broadcast thinking," Ms. G. also used the term "my psychotic problem." Thus, in her words and actions, we hear evidence of different dimensions of insight described by David (1990). Ms. G. was aware that she suffered from an illness, that her symptoms were part of a psychotic disorder, and that she needed to attend therapy and take medications, which she did regularly. Ms. G. also demonstrated an awareness of the other person's perspective by stating that her vignettes about her broadcast thinking must sound crazy to the listener. This capacity for insight, along with effective psychotherapy and the use of medication, helped her function successfully and remain in sustained remission for many years.

Clinical Assessment Points

1. Hallucinations – including auditory, visual, and tactile – are experienced in various contexts in individuals with no history of mental health problems or neurological conditions. As such, the presence of hallucination is in itself not indicative of psychosis.
2. In assessing hallucinations, it is essential to determine the capacity for reality testing. The extent to which a person considers hallucinatory experiences to be true or false has significant diagnostic and treatment implications. Hallucinations are not diagnostic-specific and, as such, are not clinically useful in differential diagnosis.
3. Hallucinations are not static and can change over time. As a result, the assessment of hallucination is best conceptualized as a process in which both the nature of the hallucinations and the person's reaction to the hallucinations may change over time, requiring reassessment.
4. It is recommended to conduct a systematic assessment of hallucinations across all sensory modalities due to the existing literature on multimodal hallucination.
5. Delusions are not diagnostic-specific. The presence of delusions is indicative of psychosis, but patients with schizophrenia-spectrum and affective disorders with psychosis can have similar types of delusions.
6. Delusional-like beliefs are not uncommon in mentally healthy individuals. As such, delusions, similar to hallucinations, are on a continuum with normality.
7. Assessment of delusions is best accomplished by considering multiple characteristics or dimensions, including:

    a. The degree to which ideas are fixed despite contradictory evidence or absence of evidence.
    b. The degree of subjective distress.
    c. The degree of functional impairment.
    d. The degree of convictions and preoccupation with the belief and extent to which the belief deviates from the person's subculture or religion.

8. When conceptualizing *thought disorder*, we need to be aware of four integrated dimensions:

    a. *How* ideas are expressed through speech (expressive component: formal thought disorder).

b. *What* ideas or beliefs are present (content component: delusions, bizarre, and absurd ideas).
c. *How* observations and ideas are put together and formulated (thinking component: errors in reasoning, logic, concept formation).
d. *Where and To Whom* the ideas are expressed (social-pragmatic component: impaired perspective).

9. If one encounters *bizarre behavior* that looks like catatonia, it is essential to think more broadly about the kinds of primary conditions that may include catatonic behavior. Diagnosticians should consider the possibility of psychosis, as well as neurodevelopmental conditions or underlying infectious, metabolic, or neurological disturbances. If psychosis is considered, clinicians need to think beyond the diagnosis of schizophrenia. Whereas catatonia used to be viewed as a behavioral symptom of schizophrenia, it is now understood to occur more frequently in bipolar and depressive psychoses.
10. The challenge for clinicians is to be aware of *negative symptoms* and understand how their lack of diagnostic specificity may lead to misdiagnosis. For example, restrictions in the range of affect, neglect of personal hygiene, and lack of pleasure occur in depression with either psychotic or nonpsychotic features. Likewise, impoverished speech production and verbal fluency may reflect an expressive language disorder. Lack of motivation may be found in individuals with depression or executive dysfunction. In addition, asociality or social withdrawal may be a symptom of depression, anxiety, or a characteristic of an avoidant personality. Patients often do not report negative symptoms, and family members may not recognize negative symptoms as part of a schizophrenia-spectrum disorder. Therefore, assessors must ask the patient and family members about these symptoms.
11. Evaluating dimensions of *insight* in our patients should be a routine part of diagnostic assessment. Clinicians are encouraged to assess their patients' capacity to reflect on their symptoms. When interviewing, ask patients how they understand their symptom experiences and how others might perceive their perceptions, beliefs, and behavior. Furthermore, clinicians need to know whether patients recognize that their symptoms are part of a mental illness and whether they are aware of their need for treatment.

3

ONSET, PHASES, SYMPTOM TRAJECTORIES, AND PROGNOSIS

How does psychosis begin, and how does it progress and resolve? Are there typical patterns of onset, predictable phases, and courses? To address these questions, we review the nature of psychosis onset, phases of symptom development, and typical courses of psychotic conditions. Charting the course of psychosis leads to a discussion about outcome and prognosis.

Onset

The onset of a psychotic episode may be sudden and abrupt or develop gradually over time. Acute onset may be associated with extreme stress and trauma or in the context of peripartum conditions. DSM-5-TR lists both as specifiers associated with criteria for a Brief Psychotic Disorder. In ICD-11, acute onset psychoses are called Acute and Transient Psychotic Disorders (ATPD) but do not include specifiers associated with marked stress or peripartum conditions. Just as these psychotic episodes develop abruptly, they resolve quickly.

Gradual onset may include subtle changes in functioning for weeks to months or longer. The emergence of symptoms may be characterized by changes in concentration, shifts in mood, mental confusion, alterations in the sense of self and reality, and a more insidious, global deterioration in all aspects of psychosocial and adaptive functioning.

Phases

There are similarities between the phases of acute psychosis and those of a traumatic response Cullberg (2006). Whereas crises are typically characterized by an escalation of tension, a turning point, and a recovery phase, psychotic episodes follow a predictable beginning, middle, and endpoint trajectory in which some form of resolution or reconstitution occurs. From the perspective of crisis theory, it is helpful to think about a psychotic episode as a psychological crisis that destabilizes the

DOI: 10.4324/9781003415206-5

individual's orientation to themselves and the reality of the surrounding world and requires adaptation to these disruptive changes.

The progression of the episode includes three or more phases with fluid boundaries; however, psychosis is a heterogeneous phenomenon that does not fit squarely with a prescribed series of phases. Not all individuals will pass through each phase, which may overlap instead of representing a fixed progression.

As described in Chapter 1, psychotic-like experiences (PLEs) may or may not evolve into psychotic episodes. Though not typically considered a phase of psychosis, PLEs may be an early data point in the progression of psychotic phenomena. Prodromal and pre-psychotic phases share similarities as precursors but differ in meaningful ways. Early, middle, late, and post-psychotic phases mark the emergence of positive symptoms and the eventual resolution of psychosis.

The most uncomplicated progression includes three phases: Prodromal, acute, and recovery. In a psychosisnet.com posting, van Os wrote about five stages of psychosis, ranging from early stages to being overwhelmed by acute symptoms of psychosis. These phases are followed by struggling with symptoms, living with psychosis vulnerability, and adjusting to life beyond psychosis. (See link for 5 stages of psychosis and treatment at https://www.psychosisnet.com/psychosis/5-stages-of-psychosis-and-recovery/stage-5-life-after-psychosis/van Os).

Precursors to a psychotic episode may include brief and intermittent PLEs, pre-psychotic, or prodromal phases. The early to middle phases mark the emergence of positive symptoms, and the late-to-resolution phases reflect the stresses associated with post-psychosis recovery. Let us review each point in the evolving process.

Psychotic-like Experiences: A Possible Foreshadowing of Later Psychosis

PLEs are brief and intermittent positive symptoms that may occur without impairment and disruption in adaptive functioning. PLEs may disappear or remain stable over time for many individuals. However, for others, PLEs may reflect a high-risk state and represent the earliest manifestations of a future psychotic episode. PLEs are related to Brief and Limited Psychotic Symptoms, referred to as BLIPS (Yung et al., 1996). BLIPS or PLEs are transitory phenomena analogous to transient ischemic attacks, which often revolve and may never lead to a full-blown stroke.

Prodromal Phase

The term "prodrome" describes a period in which an illness's early signs and symptoms begin to occur before the fully developed illness is present.

Researchers have distinguished between initial prodromes and prodromal periods preceding a relapse (Yung & McGorry, 1996a, 1996b). Typically, a prodromal phase has been viewed as a precursor of psychotic episodes within the schizophrenia spectrum; however, researchers are increasingly exploring whether affective psychoses are preceded by syndrome-specific prodromal phases as well (Correll et al., 2007; Egeland et al., 2000; Mantere et al., 2008; Schothorst et al., 2006; Tillman & Geller, 2003).

The key characteristics of a prodromal phase in schizophrenia are progressive changes in cognitive, somatic–vegetative, emotional, behavioral, and social functioning, which occur over weeks or months, if not longer. Researchers (Yung & McGorry, 1996a, 1996b) have described seven categories in which functioning is gradually deteriorating. Those in the prodromal phase exhibited (1) reduced concentration and attention, thought-blocking, and daydreaming, (2) decreased drive, motivation, and energy, (3) increased anxiety, depression, and irritability, (4) loss of sleep and appetite, (5) increased oddities in behavior and appearance, (6) heightened sensitivity to perceptual stimuli, and (7) progressive alienation, social withdrawal, and suspiciousness. There may also be decreases in hygiene and activities of daily living.

As a result of these symptoms and changes, the ability to study, work, or meet routine demands diminishes. Cullberg (2006) described this phase as combining internal intensity and withdrawal from the outside world. Studies have shown that the length of the prodrome has possible diagnostic and prognostic significance. Furthermore, the longer the prodromal phase, the poorer the schizophrenia prognosis (Chapman et al., 1961; Fenton & McGlashan, 1987; Vaillant, 1962, 1964a, 1964b; Schothorst et al., 2006; Fusar-Poli et al., 2009; Fusar-Poli, Bonoldi et al., 2012). It has been suggested that first-episode prodromes are longer than prodromes preceding relapses. Regarding differential diagnosis, Schothorst and colleagues (2006) described how the prodromal phase is typically longer in adolescents who develop schizophrenia than in those with affective psychoses.

The existence of a prodromal phase in affective psychoses is less studied. Molnar et al. (1988) investigated prodromal symptoms and pre-onset features of bipolar episodes and found that increased activity, elevated mood, decreased need for sleep, racing thoughts, verbosity, increased self-worth, distractibility, and irritability were the frequently reported symptoms leading up to a manic episode. Predictably, a depressed mood, loss of energy and interest, poor concentration, decreased sleep, and morbid thoughts were the most frequently recalled symptoms leading to a depressive episode. Other prospective studies have demonstrated that a long prodromal phase exists before the onset of full-blown bipolar disorder (Egeland et al., 2000). During the prodromal stage, there are three primary syndrome clusters: hypomania/mania symptoms, depressive symptoms, and signs of attention-deficit hyperactivity disorders (Correll et al., 2007; Mantere et al., 2008; Tillman & Geller, 2003).

Prodromal symptoms in schizophrenia and bipolar mania overlap. Although the prodrome in schizophrenia may be slightly longer, a prodromal phase in bipolar mania may also be relatively long and have an insidious onset. Both prodromes have subthreshold symptoms of mood lability, depression, and nonspecific psychopathology. Despite overlapping symptoms, a schizophrenia prodrome has been found to include more social isolation and strange or unusual ideas (53.3% compared to 18% in bipolar prodrome) Correll et al. (2007).

Pre-psychotic Phase

In describing the onset of an active period of psychosis, Cullberg (2006) distinguished prodromal from pre-psychotic phases, noting that each occurred in roughly half of the people who become psychotic. Those individuals who become psychotic without progressing through a lengthier prodromal phase may experience what Cullberg (2006) called a "pre-psychotic stage." Unlike the slow incubation of a prodromal phase in which there is a gradual erosion in biopsychosocial and adaptive functioning, the pre-psychotic stage is characterized by a much more rapid onset of psychotic symptomatology. In this shorter period, before psychotic symptoms appear, the individual may experience the world as more frightening and dangerous. Others may appear hostile and threatening, and what they say may make less sense. Increased internal tension and anxiety may cause one to withdraw from others who seem to have become less trustworthy. Increased anxiety and social alienation may lead to clashes with others, including uncharacteristic outbursts of anger. The motives and intentions of others may become suspect as the person imagines that they are talking about or making references to him. In addition, there may be the experience of hearing voices. An inability to sleep may lower one's tolerance, disrupt cognitive functioning, and exacerbate anxiety that something ominous occurs. The person may suddenly worry that he is losing it and is about to go crazy.

Early to Middle Phase

The strange and frightening nature of the pre-psychotic or prodromal phase shifts when one becomes actively psychotic. To lower the intolerable anxiety that she is going mad, the individual may search for explanations for what seems threatening and inexplicable. The progression of unexplainable changes in the external world and the alterations within the individual's perceptual and emotional experiences take on a meaning that begins to cohere and provide a rationale for what has been happening. At some point, the individual may develop an explanation for the voices and other changes she has experienced. Previously hidden meanings, messages, and signs are increasingly apparent, leading the psychotic individual to formulate an understanding of all that has occurred. Discovering hidden meanings diminishes the anxiety of losing one's mind, and a sense of coherence may return.

Chapter 1 showed compelling examples of Humpston's "desperate search for explanations and understanding." We also saw how Nick's anxious search for hidden clues and codes on the Internet was finally resolved in one clarifying memory when he heard words from a song that provided the elusive explanation for his intolerable experiences and sense of perplexity.

However, this restorative process comes at the expense of a severe sacrifice of reality testing and insight. Delusional formulations become unshakable and provide order and meaning for what had previously felt murky, incomprehensible, and frightening. With paranoid or persecutory delusions, the enemy responsible for the threat and torment can now be identified and held in check.

Late Phase and Resolution

It is usually with the institution of stabilizing treatments and medication that the florid symptoms of psychosis begin to abate. Slowly, the hallucinatory phenomena begin to clear as delusional thoughts fluctuate regarding their dominance. Gradually, delusional explanations play a lesser role as the individual can question her reality. Some may feel a sense of relief as their connection with the world and reality is restored. However, this process may take time and not proceed linearly.

The experience of having been through a psychotic denial of reality is a profoundly disruptive and traumatizing event that the individual will need to integrate. Furthermore, the difficulties that occurred before the onset of the psychotic episode often have not disappeared, and those that occurred because of it must be faced and managed. This process can increase one's sense of loss and despair. Being hospitalized and diagnosed with a significant mental illness can be an enormously painful, life-altering experience that can cause many to give way to despair and shame. Humpston and Chadwick's words about recovering their sanity are haunting. Using her own experiences to understand the psychotic process, Humpston (2014) wrote:

> In an instinctive search for meaning in the face of the confusion with which he meets the world and others, he loses insight into one's mentality. Once he regains insight, he must confront the cold "reality" that his reality has not been real.
>
> (p. 241)

For Chadwick (2014), whose grandiose paranoid delusions had placed him at the center of a massive persecutory plot, recovery was exquisitely painful: "Reflecting on this post-psychosis is particularly sickening, embarrassing, and humiliating" (p. 484).

Jeffries (1977) described the trauma of being psychotic and noted that this was a neglected aspect of treatment. Riedesser (2004) wrote about how the experience of acute psychosis and subsequent recovery is associated with traumatic stress. The loss of one's sense of reality, relationships, and, ultimately, one's sense of self, not to mention possible terrors of persecution, fit a definition of trauma. Riedesser quoted a patient who reflected on the traumatic effects of his psychosis.

> The traumatic aspect of the disease was that it controlled me every single moment. I constantly had delusions without being able to do anything about them. Every psychotic thought increased my psychic injury. All relationships grown over time broke up. At the worst time of my distorted perception of reality, I even feared that my mother could poison me. . . . My psychosis has left a deep scar on my soul.
>
> (p. 64)

Course

Cullberg (2006) described three courses that a first-episode psychosis might take. He referred to these as Types A, B, and C, representing roughly one-third of first-episode psychoses. Type A refers to discrete, single-episode "breaks," whereas Type B may include repeated episodes interspersed with periods of adequate functioning. In contrast, Type-C psychoses include chronic, life- and personality-altering illnesses that continue throughout life.

Type A: Sudden Onset Psychotic Episode

Type A is characterized by an isolated episode that comes suddenly (often in response to an identifiable stressor), includes significant positive features, and resolves quickly, with or without medication and therapy. Symptomatically, these patients may be indistinguishable from those with other kinds of psychotic conditions but typically include significant emotional turmoil and lability, confusion, and impairment in functioning.

In DSM-5-TR, Type A psychosis is classified as a Brief Psychotic Disorder (BPD) based on at least one positive symptom (specifically hallucinations, delusions, or disorganized speech). The criteria also indicate that there will be a return to a premorbid level of functioning. Specifiers designate whether the episode occurred as a reaction to marked stressors, which would define the episode as a "brief reactive psychosis." However, because it is not assumed that extreme stress or trauma will always be a precipitant, Brief Psychotic Disorders also include the specifier "without marked stressor(s)." A third specifier related to onset in the context of peripartum conditions. BPDs may occur across the lifespan and be more common in women (Fusar-Poli et al., 2022). They represent a minority of first-onset psychotic disorders (2–7% according to DSM-5-TR, 2022). Regarding the likelihood of relapse, DSM-5-TR places this rate at greater than 50%. However, the possibility of relapse does not change or reduce the individual's overall social functioning.

In ICD-11, Type A psychoses are called Acute and transient psychotic disorders (ATPD) and can have a longer duration (up to three months versus the one-month criterion in DSM-5-TR for Brief Psychotic Episodes), resulting in a low diagnostic overlap between the two diagnostic classification systems. Several specifiers with ATPD include positive, negative, manic, psychomotor, and depressive symptoms; however, marked stress is not listed as a possible precipitant.

Although many Type A psychoses occur in the context of specific triggering events (e.g., stress, trauma, or peripartum conditions), they may also result from drug-induced or acute medical disorders. The onset and course may be similar; however, such conditions would not be diagnosed as BPD or ATPD. Instead, they are designated as Substance/Medication-Induced Psychotic Disorder, Psychotic Disorder Due to Another Medical Condition (DSM-5-TR).

Type B: Episodic Psychoses

The distinction between the Type A group and episodic psychoses has to do with the predictable recurrence of psychotic episodes in the future. There remains a heightened vulnerability for relapse over time, with therapy and antipsychotic medications employed preventively.

As with Type A psychotic states, environmental stressors can be precipitants of episodic psychoses, tipping the balance and leading to the development of core psychotic symptoms. However, unlike Type A single-episode psychotic states, Type B episodic states may develop in the context of genetic vulnerability and childhood stresses. Relapses may be sudden when they occur, appearing with comparatively minor provocation or stress. Subsequent relapses may even lower the threshold for additional relapses in the future.

However, during the periods between their psychotic states, individuals in the Type B group may return to their premorbid levels of personality functioning.

Type C: Enduring or Chronic Psychoses

There are different ways to characterize this final group of individuals with psychosis. Although it is tempting to attach familiar diagnostic labels to this group, it is helpful to think about the process and not get ahead of ourselves with specific diagnoses for this discussion. *Enduring psychosis* is a term selected to identify a chronic and relatively fixed set of symptoms. This is not to suggest that the patients in this group remain chronically and entirely out of touch with reality, as the more florid symptoms of the psychotic state may remit with medication and stabilizing treatment. Nonetheless, these individuals never entirely return to their premorbid level of functioning. Instead, there is a gradual erosion of aspects of personality functioning, often reflected by social, occupational, and cognitive changes. During the periods between florid manifestations of psychotic functioning, the individual with Type C psychosis may exhibit residual psychotic phenomena manifested in idiosyncratic speech and thinking, odd behavior, social withdrawal, and increasing signs of impairment in aspects of memory and executive functioning.

Onset may be gradual, ushered in by a prodromal period of adverse changes in cognition, social participation, sleep-wake cycles, grooming, and behavior that precede the eruption of more florid symptoms of psychosis. Finally, following the acute phase's resolution, negative symptoms still compromise the individual's functional adaptation.

Furthering the notion of "psychosis as trauma" and recovery from psychosis as a post-traumatic response, Riedesser posited whether residual negative symptomatology might be considered psychic numbing to avoid intrusive recollections of the traumatic psychotic events. Like any post-traumatic state, individuals seek to avoid thinking, feeling, and speaking about their experiences to avoid the risk of becoming retraumatized.

The concept of psychosis as a traumatic event and recovery from psychosis as a post-traumatic syndrome makes intuitive clinical sense. Indeed, first-person accounts of the recovery process suggest that recovery involves integrating enormously traumatic experiences. Thus, despite the challenge, early detection and psychosis prevention efforts might prevent two debilitating mental-health disorders – psychosis and subsequent post-traumatic stress disorder (PTSD).

Separating the clinic course into brief/transient, episodic, or chronic/continuous is a crude and static attempt to capture the highly variable nature of psychosis. A more current effort to re-examine the course of psychotic disorders used follow-up data on over 300 patients over ten years to identify different symptom trajectories (Morgan et al., 2022).

The data yielded four symptom patterns with the percentage of patients in each group:

1. Remitting/improving (with shorter and less frequent relapses, 58.5%).
2. Late improvement (initially persistent symptoms with remissions later, 5.4%).
3. Late decline (initial remission followed by more persistent symptoms, 5.6%).
4. Persistent (prolonged periods of continuous presence of symptoms throughout, 30.6%).

A strikingly high 73% of the remitting group had recovered at follow-up, whereas none of the persistent group had. The remitting group also showed shorter and less frequent relapses than the other groups. Predictably, there was a strong relationship between symptom trajectory and social outcome, with the remitting group functioning at a higher level. Despite admitted methodological limitations, Morgan et al. found that individuals in the persistent group were over-represented by urban Black men of Caribbean descent with lower levels of premorbid education and IQ They were more isolated, socially disadvantaged, exhibited fewer affective symptoms, had extended periods of untreated psychosis, and most likely suffered more severe health-related problems. Those in the late decline group resembled the profile of the persistent group. The late remitting group showed more improvement around three years post-onset of psychosis. The duration of their untreated psychosis was much shorter, and they were more likely to meet the criteria for a substance abuse disorder.

Prognosis

The prognosis for recovery, with fewer or no relapses, is better for individuals diagnosed with brief psychotic episodes than for schizophrenia. Individuals whose psychotic symptoms have remitted within three months have half the risk of relapse compared with those diagnosed with schizophrenia whose symptoms have remitted, which is considered a positive prognostic sign within the schizophrenia spectrum. Additionally, affective symptoms, a sudden versus gradual onset, and a lack of social isolation are associated with more favorable outcomes. In contrast, an urban environment, lower premorbid cognitive functioning, and education characterize those with less favorable outcomes. Time spent in a prodrome and the duration of untreated psychosis may also predict a poorer outcome.

Clinical Assessment Points

1. Brief psychotic episodes are not always precipitated by stress. In such cases, assessing underlying personality functioning and genetic vulnerability is important.
2. Given the heterogeneity of symptom trajectories, primarily when improvement occurs much later, it is essential to continue monitoring symptoms in patients who initially do not appear to improve.
3. When the clinical presentation is complex and unclear, psychological testing may be instrumental in establishing a differential diagnosis, determining comorbidity, and contributing to an individualized treatment plan.
4. In addition to interviews, family history, and testing data, talking with collateral sources may help clarify the nature of the onset and severity of psychotic symptomatology. However, because of the traumatic nature of the first psychotic episode, family members may be traumatized. As such, immediate family members may not always be able to provide the most reliable information.
5. As we shall see, a trauma history can be viewed as a risk factor for the subsequent onset of psychosis. Therefore, practitioners should inquire about trauma histories in patients they evaluate for psychosis.

Part II

DIAGNOSTIC CONCEPTS

4

DIAGNOSTIC CLASSIFICATION

Past and Present

Evolving Diagnostic Concepts of Psychosis

Understanding the diagnostic classification of psychotic disorders requires a review of historical changes in psychiatric nosological systems. In reviewing these changes, there are multiple factors that we need to consider. These include:

- Tracing the conceptual changes in how psychosis has been understood over time.
- Noting how affective symptoms have been understood in the diagnosis of psychotic conditions.
- Being aware of key empirical studies in differential diagnosis.
- Understanding the impact of new psychotropic medications on diagnostic practice.

Finally, it is essential to realize how, with the advent of the DSM-III, the shift in emphasis to interrater reliability began to shape current diagnostic practices for all conditions, including psychoses.

Kraepelin's Concept

Kraepelin (1896) distinguished two psychiatric conditions, dementia praecox and manic-depressive illness. He separated the two conditions based on the course of the illness and indicated that both conditions had similar symptoms, such as delusions and hallucinations. However, those patients with dementia praecox tended to have a poorer prognosis and showed an earlier chronic course with significant deterioration of functioning. In contrast, manic patients had a better prognosis, showed more remissions, and did not exhibit substantial deterioration of functioning. Kraepelin considered schizophrenia as a fundamental brain disease in which the nature of its etiology needed further understanding and study (Kendell, 1986). He thought of the course and outcome of the illness as

DOI: 10.4324/9781003415206-7

the most important defining and discriminating features of the two illnesses (Andreasen, 1983a).

Bleuler's Concept

In 1911, Eugene Bleuler published his classic book, *Dementia Praecox and the Group of Schizophrenias*. Bleuler accepted Kraepelin's classification but emphasized the importance of assessing certain classes of psychological symptoms. He was influenced by Freud's psychoanalytical theory and thought that dementia praecox was psychological in origin and could best be characterized by the splitting of the essential functions of personality. Bleuler used the Greek words "schizo" (to split) and "phren" (mind) to rename dementia praecox "schizophrenia" (Bleuler, 1950; Kendell, 1986).

Bleuler's now-famous four classes of diagnostic signs of schizophrenia, which became known as "Bleuler's 4 As," included:

1. Autism.
2. Association (loosening of associations).
3. Affect (disturbance and incongruity).
4. Ambivalence.

In particular, he believed that some aspect of thought disorder, which took the form of loosening of associations, was present in every schizophrenic patient and that other symptoms, such as delusions and hallucinations, were secondary to the illness. In contrast to Kraepelin's narrow definition of schizophrenia, Bleuler broadened the concept by emphasizing specific symptoms as more characteristic and vital than the course and the outcome of the illness (Andreasen, 1983a). Furthermore, Bleuler's conceptualization of schizophrenia as a psychological disorder rather than a brain disease also contributed to broadening the definition of schizophrenia. As a result, this new characterization soon began to resonate with American psychiatry, which at the time had been heavily influenced by psychoanalytic theory (Kendell, 1986).

Schneider's Concept

German psychiatrist Kurt Schneider (1950) was influenced by Kraepelin's concept that schizophrenia had a non-psychological origin (Kendell, 1986). Schneider believed that certain classes of symptoms had diagnostic specificity for schizophrenia. He subsequently labeled these as "first-rank symptoms." These symptoms included delusions of thought broadcasting, thought withdrawal, thought insertion, specific auditory hallucinations in which voices have a running commentary on one's behavior, and delusions of reference. He considered these symptoms to be pathognomonic of schizophrenia and separated them from "second-rank symptoms," which included thought disorder and other types of hallucinations and delusions.

Schneider's approach to diagnosing schizophrenia was like Bleuler's in that he emphasized a cross-sectional examination of symptoms, which de-emphasized the clinical course of the illness (Andreasen, 1987). However, as an approach to diagnosing schizophrenia in contrast to Bleuler's 4 As, the Schneiderinan first-rank symptoms were more easily identified and reliably assessed (Kendell, 1986). Schneider's concepts became influential in American psychiatry (Andreasen, 1983a; Sussman & Cancro, 1988). In both the DSM-I and DSM-II editions, the types of schizophrenia were defined broadly and were characterized by the Schneiderian symptoms unique to each. Significant psychotic symptoms were underemphasized in the diagnosis of manic-depressive illness; instead, mania was described as a disorder that was episodic and characterized by irritability, elation, and flight of ideas (Sussman & Cancro, 1988). In short, for decades, the diagnostic classification of a psychotic disorder was defined by a mixture of Bleulerian and Schneiderian conceptualization (Kendler, 1990).

The Role of Affective Symptoms

Kraepelin (1921) recognized that individuals with affective psychosis had a different clinical course that was not consistent with his conceptualization of dementia praecox. Others also had begun to describe patients with varying patterns of recovery. Kasanin (1933) described a group of patients who had psychotic episodes characterized by a short duration of one week to a few months, followed by a full recovery. He labeled this group as having "acute schizoaffective psychosis."

Other researchers (Vaillant, 1962; Langfeldt, 1960) also became interested in the study of these patients and identified several factors that they thought contributed to their quick recovery. These factors were acute onset, presence of confusion, absence of schizoid premorbid adjustment, and, most importantly, the presence of affective symptoms and a genetic predisposition for affective illness. Vaillant and others (Stephens et al., 1966) considered these patients a subgroup of schizophrenia patients who had good prognostic signs, which included having affective symptoms.

Empirical Studies in Differential Diagnosis

In the early 1970s, several significant studies compared diagnostic practices in the international community with those in the U.S.A. In these studies, psychiatrists from different countries evaluated patients interviewed on videotape. These studies pointed out that compared to psychiatrists from the international community, American psychiatrists had a narrow concept of mania and an overly broad concept of schizophrenia. The result of this tilt was an underdiagnosis of manic depression, on the one hand, and an overdiagnosis of schizophrenia, on the other (Andreasen, 1983a).

Pope and Lipinski (1978) supported the broader definition of mania by demonstrating that the first-rank Schneiderian symptoms were not pathognomonic of schizophrenia. They showed that 20–50% of patients with manic-depressive illness reported similar kinds of psychotic symptoms. Similarly, Carpenter and Strauss (1973) said that the 11 Schneiderian first-rank symptoms were found in 23% of affective-disorder patients and were even found in small numbers of character-disorder patients. Carpenter and Strauss also showed that these symptoms had no relationship to outcome. In another study, Harrow et al. (1968) noted that nearly 70% of a group of patients diagnosed with mania had hallucinations and delusions, compared with 100% of a group diagnosed with schizophrenia. Carlson and Goodwin (1973) showed that 70% of manic-depressive patients, in the absence of any medication, manifested clear-cut schizophrenia symptoms, including loosening of associations, bizarre delusions, and bizarre psychomotor activity. In short, these studies provided compelling evidence that Schneiderian symptoms previously thought to be pathognomonic of schizophrenia were common in manic patients with psychotic features.

Development of Lithium

In the 1970s, lithium carbonate was used successfully in the treatment of manic-depressive illness and gradually became recognized and widely used as the treatment of choice for mania (Andreasen, 1983a). Many clinicians also began to use lithium with schizoaffective patients, and many of these patients responded well. In addition, the clinicians began to observe that neuroleptic medication, which was the treatment of choice for schizophrenia, produced a severe side effect called tardive dyskinesia (Andreasen, 1983a). Tardive dyskinesia is a permanent physical deformity marked by rapid and stereotypic movement of the jaw, lips, and tongue (Kane & Smith, 1982). The risk of producing tardive dyskinesia motivated many clinicians to change their diagnostic practices and, when in doubt, consider affective diagnosis (Andreasen, 1983a). As a result, the notion of differential diagnosis of schizophrenia versus affective disorder and the concept of schizoaffective disorder drew increased interest, which resulted in attempts to narrow the diagnosis of schizophrenia and broaden the diagnosis of affective disorder (Andreasen, 1987).

Development of the DSM-III

All the previously mentioned factors have led to changes in the diagnostic classification of schizophrenia. In 1972, Feighner and his colleagues published the St. Louis criteria, which were highly Kraepelinian and emphasized the course of the illness, duration, and clusters of symptoms. The St. Louis criteria were later modified to the Research Diagnostic Criteria (RDC) (Spitzer et al., 1978). Both the RDC and the St. Louis criteria narrowed the concept of schizophrenia by limiting the duration of the illness to six months. They broadened the definition of affective disorder by recognizing that many so-called schizophrenic symptoms were also present in mania.

The American Psychiatric Association's diagnostic classification systems – DSM-III (1980), DSM-III-R (1987), DSM-IV (1994), and DSM-IV-TR (2000) – adopted the exclusionary clause of the St. Louis criteria and the RDC; that is, the diagnosis of schizophrenia should be made only when a patient showed psychotic symptoms either actively or predominantly for six months. That earlier system also accepted the notion that psychotic symptoms that were once considered to be pathognomonic *only of* schizophrenia could be seen in other psychotic and mood disorders.

Concerning schizoaffective disorder, the DSM-II and DSM-III-R did not give specific criteria and no longer considered schizoaffective as a subtype of schizophrenia. Instead, the diagnosis of schizoaffective disorder was made when the patient showed a mixture of mood and psychotic symptomatology (Spitzer et al., 1978).

In summary, the diagnosis of schizophrenia has gone from being overly narrow (Kraepelinian) to excessively broad (Bleulerian) and from an emphasis on course to an emphasis on symptoms. Starting with the publication of DSM-III in 1980, the diagnosis of schizophrenia again returned to a narrower definition. In contrast, the definition of manic affective disorder has been expanded. And schizoaffective disorder, once a subtype of schizophrenia, has become a separate diagnosis (Andreasen, 1983a, 1987; Sussman & Cancro, 1988).

Development of the DSM-5 and DSM-5-TR

Both the DSM-IV and DSM-IV-TR continued with the same classification of psychotic disorders and affective disorders. In contrast, the newest version of the DSM introduces changes in diagnostic criteria for psychotic disorders and schizoaffective disorders. Although the changes are not substantial (Paris, 2013), they do follow the historical trend of de-emphasizing cross-sectional evaluation of specific symptoms and putting greater emphasis on the duration of psychiatric symptoms, stressing the importance of mood symptoms and the temporal relationship between psychotic symptoms and mood symptoms.

Furthermore, in the DSM-5 and the DSM-5-TR, the importance of using bizarre symptoms (i.e., Schneiderian symptoms) as diagnostic indicators has been removed. Thus, in contrast to the DSM-III, DSM-IV, and DSM-IV-TR, delusional disorder and all other psychotic disorders can have bizarre delusions. The bizarre delusions and Schneiderian-type hallucinations are not given any diagnostic weight in schizophrenia since the research has indicated that these symptoms are by no means pathognomonic of schizophrenia and, as such, may occur in affective disorders with psychotic features.

The subtypes of schizophrenia have also been removed from the new diagnostic classification system because of a lack of research on their validity. Although previous research indicates that paranoid schizophrenia has substantial differences in age of onset, course of hospitalization, severity of symptoms, premorbid social adjustment, and cognitive style (see Margaro, 1981; Meissner, 1981; Zigler & Glick, 1984 for review), the newer research does not support these previous findings (Tandon et al., 2008; Paris, 2013).

The International Classification of Disorders

(ICD-11)

The World Health Organization (WHO) revised the previous International Classification Disorder (ICD-10). Gaebel (2012) reviewed and critically examined the significant changes in the ICD-11 related to the classification of psychological disorders. They outline the following changes:

1. The new ICD-11 renamed major non-affective psychotic disorders as "Schizophrenia spectrum and other primary psychotic disorders." It includes schizophrenia, schizoaffective disorder, acute and transient psychotic disorder, schizotypal disorder, delusional disorder, other primary psychotic disorders, and unspecified primary psychotic disorders.
2. Psychoses occurring in the context of manic or depressive episodes are now classified as affective disorders, and other psychoses due to medical or drugs are considered non-primary disorders.
3. Regarding the diagnosis of schizoaffective disorder, the criteria for diagnosis of schizophrenia and a mood disorder must be met simultaneously or within a few days of each other. Gaebel (2012) points

out that in contrast to DSM-5 and -TR, the ICD diagnosis of SA disorder is cross-sectional and does not include a longitudinal criterion.

4. Like the DSM-5 and -TR, the ICD-11 also does not allow the diagnosis of attenuated psychosis syndrome,
5. The ICD-11 added specifiers to record the symptoms' presence, absence, and severity. Valle (2020) explains that the use of specifiers adds dimensionality to the assessment of psychotic disorder and allows for a more compressive and accurate assessment of psychotic signs and symptoms along a dimension of severity. It is very similar to the DSM-5 specifiers and includes positive symptoms, negative symptoms, and depressive symptoms: manic symptoms, psychomotor symptoms, and cognitive impairments.
6. While both the DSM-5, -TR, and ICD-11 maintain a categorical conceptualization of the diagnosis of schizophrenia spectrum disorder, they also include a dimensional approach that takes into account the existence of a gradual and quantitative variation at the level of signs and symptoms between different mental disorders (Valle, 2020). The dimensional approach has altered the previously held belief that schizophrenia is entirely a separate disorder from the affective disorder with psychotic features and has changed the diagnostic hierarchy for schizophrenia. One can now diagnose bipolar disorder with schizophrenia (see First, 2014).

Clinical Assessment Points

1. The diagnostic classification of psychotic disorders continues to be more in line with Kraepelinian tradition than with Bleuler, emphasizing the duration of illness and placing less diagnostic weight in the cross-sectional assessment for differential diagnosis. Neither formal thought disorder nor bizarre delusions or Schneiderian-type hallucinations are given special status in diagnostic classification.
2. Although positive symptoms of psychosis, including hallucination, delusions, and disordered thinking, are essential in establishing a diagnosis of psychotic disorder, they play a less important role in diagnostic classification. Instead, severe or moderate mood episodes and duration of illness are necessary features in separating various diagnostic classifications.
3. Paranoid schizophrenia, which was an essential diagnosis in clinical practice, has been removed, along with other subtypes of schizophrenia.
4. The diagnostic conceptualization of schizophrenia spectrum disorders remains categorical, but the dimensional aspect of signs and symptoms of the disorder is emphasized in both DSM-5, -TR, and ICD-11.

5

PSYCHOSIS CATEGORIES, DIMENSIONS, CONTINUA, AND SPECTRA

When assessing psychosis, clinicians confront an array of descriptive terms, which may clarify and sometimes confuse essential concepts. For example, *underlying psychosis, psychotic continuum, psychotic syndromes, psychotic spectrum, subthreshold psychosis, psychotic proneness, psychotic dimensions, psychotic states,* and *psychotic experiences* may be used interchangeably or to represent different aspects of psychotic phenomena. Seiler et al. (2020) reviewed seven psychosis-related terms representing points along the continuum of psychosis and noted confusion and inconsistencies in how the terms are used. Defining and organizing terminological diversity will help clinicians understand conceptual similarities and distinctions and sharpen diagnostic decision-making.

Diagnostic assessment follows four overlapping approaches by grouping psychotic phenomena into categories, dimensions, spectra, and continua. *Categories* describe discrete syndromes with specific symptoms, etiologies, courses, and fixed boundaries that separate them from other disorders. *Dimensions* refer to symptoms that occur trans diagnostically and blur the boundaries between traditional diagnostic categories. A spectrum refers to conditions linked by similar symptoms and underlying causal mechanisms. Spectra also captures the heterogeneity within a defined diagnostic category. Finally, symptom dimensions exist along a *continuum* of severity, ranging from milder expressions in nonpsychotic, "normal" individuals to severe manifestations in acute and chronic psychoses.

Unfortunately, clinicians may use these terms interchangeably, which creates confusion, obscures meaning, and reduces diagnostic clarity. We review each term to sharpen our clinical vocabulary, increase diagnostic accuracy, and improve communication when assessing psychosis.

Categorical Approach

Historically, the diagnosis of psychoses was based on Kraepelin's (1896) categorical model. Kraepelin's system of classifying psychoses employed a

DOI: 10.4324/9781003415206-8

qualitative approach that viewed psychotic disorders as discrete, natural disease entities with clearly defined boundaries, distinct etiologies, symptom profiles, courses, and responses to treatment. Throughout much of the twentieth century, Neo-Kraepelinian thinking dominated psychiatry and formed the basis for classifying psychotic disorders worldwide. However, some began to criticize the dogmatic and rigid application of Kraepelin's nosology, which some called "hyperkraepelianism" (Michels, 1984), because it reified categories of mental disorders while ignoring fluid boundaries and shared symptomatology. Over the last 25 years, the scientific basis of categorical diagnoses has been increasingly questioned. Concerns about the fuzzy borders between categorical diagnoses, the heterogeneity of symptoms between individuals who share the same diagnosis, and the high degree of comorbidity have collectively challenged the validity of the categorical approach.

While diagnostic categories became an easy target for critics promoting an empirical dimensional alternative, some argue that it is premature to scrap categorical approaches entirely (Paris, 2013; David, 2010; Lawrie et al., 2010). They note that while discrete diagnostic categories may not fit neatly with the messiness of clinical realities (best demonstrated in a dimensional approach), they continue to offer advantages over strictly dimensional approaches to diagnosis. Specifically, categorical diagnoses provide familiarity and clinical utility and enhance clinician communication. Finally, some have expressed practical concerns about a strictly dimensional approach to diagnosis (Paris, 2013). Dimensions focus on symptom categories, which must be collated to aid clinicians in making differential diagnoses for treatment planning. While psychosis symptom dimensions can be placed on a continuum of severity, there still needs to be a threshold to help determine when a symptom reaches a psychotic level. As discussed in Chapter 2, distinguishing between the sense of reality, on the one hand, and reality testing, on the other, helps answer the threshold question. Thus, the marker for determining the presence of an active psychotic state is typically the loss of reality testing or insight, typically found in delusions.

Dimensional Approach

As indicated previously, researchers have long criticized the empirical underpinnings of categorical diagnoses and instead proposed a quantitative, dimensional approach to understanding psychosis (Andrews et al., 2009; Bentall, 2003; Carpenter et al., 2009). A dimensional approach is based on empirical support for the finding that psychotic symptomatology is best explained by several symptom dimensions, which occur both trans diagnostically and, in milder degrees, among nonpsychotic individuals in the general population. Proponents of a dimensional concept believe that traditional diagnostic categories do not capture the degree of variability, comorbidity, and continuity of psychotic symptoms, regardless of standard diagnostic classification. Advocates of a dimensional approach charge that Kraepelinian taxonomists are acting much like the League of Nations – said to have overlooked or ignored great historical, tribal, ethnic, and religious diversity and imposed arbitrary boundaries on vast territories of the Middle East to create nation-states – by artificially constructing and then reifying discrete diagnostic syndromes of psychoses. Their argument is that by creating arbitrary categories, traditional diagnostic systems have ignored the symptomatic realities of individuals with psychoses.

Historically, researchers used factor-analytic techniques to identify multiple symptom dimensions that characterize psychosis. Using a neurological model from the nineteenth-century British neurologist Hughlings Jackson, Crow (1980) suggested two subtypes of schizophrenia based on the presence of positive or negative symptoms. The main symptoms in positive, or Type I schizophrenia, included hallucinations and delusions, whereas Type II, or negative schizophrenia, was characterized by emotional flatness, apathy, and social withdrawal. Liddle (1987) tested this two-factor model and identified a third cluster of psychotic symptomologies characterized by cognitive disorganization, which included focusing and filtering problems associated with disturbed language.

Attempts to identify dimensions underlying the psychopathology in psychosis have alternated between a singular-dimensional model, or unitary psychosis factor (Berrios & Beer, 1994), a five-factor model (Demjaha et al., 2009; Emsley et al., 2003; van Os et al., 1999; van Os & Kapur, 2009), or an eight-dimensional model (Barch et al., 2013).

Proponents of the singular-dimensional approach propose a general psychosis factor that subsumes all of the symptom dimensions in affective and nonaffective psychosis. There were even proposals to deconstruct the diagnosis of psychosis in the DSM-5 by eliminating different categories and replacing them with a single dimension of general psychosis (First, 2006).

Reininghaus and colleagues identified a general psychosis factor and five specific factors in samples of individuals with early onset and enduring psychosis (Reininghaus et al., 2013). Advocates of the five-dimension approach based their pentagonal model on factor-analytic studies of the PANSS (Positive and Negative Syndrome Scale), which yielded the following symptom clusters: (1) positive symptoms, (2) negative symptoms, (3) cognitive disorganization, (4) manic excitement, and (5) depression. According to this model, symptoms on the *positive dimension* include hallucinations, delusions, grandiosity, suspiciousness, unusual thought content, and lack of judgment and insight. The *negative symptom dimension* comprises blunted affect, emotional withdrawal, poor rapport, passive and active forms of social withdrawal, lack of spontaneity, motor retardation, and disturbance of volition. *Disorganization* includes difficulties with conceptual and abstract thinking, stereotyped thinking, poor attention, preoccupation, disorientation, odd mannerisms, and posturing. The *mania dimension* consists of symptoms of excitement, hostility, uncooperativeness, and poor impulse control. Finally, the *depression dimension* includes preoccupation with somatic concerns, anxiety, guilt, tension, and depression.

Reininghaus et al. correlated different dimensions with traditional diagnostic categories and levels of acuity. Not surprisingly, their findings showed that patients with chronic or enduring psychoses had more negative and fewer positive and manic-like symptoms than patients in the early group. Both groups of patients shared equal amounts of cognitive disorganization. However, when examined by diagnosis, patients with schizophrenia scored higher on dimensions of negative symptoms, positive symptoms, and disorganization. In contrast, patients diagnosed with bipolar disorders scored higher on the positive and manic dimensions. Other interesting findings included the negative correlations between insight, on the one hand, and positive and manic excitement, on the other. Similarly, higher scores on the depression dimension correlated with insight.

The DSM-5 and -TR define psychosis by five symptom domains: Delusions, hallucinations, disorganized thinking (speech), grossly disorganized or abnormal motor behavior (including catatonia), and negative symptoms. However, an expanded eight-factor dimensional model forms the basis of the Clinician-Rated Dimensions of Psychosis Symptom Severity scale found in Section III of the DSM-5-TR. This expanded dimensional model is consistent with the work of the DSM-5 Psychotic Disorder Work Group (Barch et al., 2013; (Heckers et al., 2013). The approach conceptualizes eight domains assessed in patients with psychotic symptoms. These domains are (1) hallucinations, (2) delusions, (3) disorganized speech, (4) abnormal psychomotor behavior, (5) negative symptoms (restricted emotional expressiveness and avolition), (6) impaired cognition, (7) depression, and (8) mania. The Psychosis Work Group expanded the list of symptom dimensions to capture variation in severity and to assist in treatment planning. Whereas the five-factor model by Reininghaus et al. (2013) collapses hallucinations and delusions into a positive-symptom dimension, the DSM-5 committee chose to separate them because of their differential presence in some patients versus others and the different approaches used to treat each.

Additionally, with increased interest in catatonia, they pulled abnormal psychomotor behavior out of the negative symptom dimension and made this a separate domain. The negative domain reflects the two subdomains of symptoms described in Chapter 2: restricted emotional expression and avolitionality. Although there was empirical support for separating these two sets of symptoms, the group decided to keep them as two aspects of the negative domain.

The group also introduced a domain of cognitive impairment in response to studies showing that a high number of individuals with psychotic disorders demonstrate impairments in cognitive functions (Reichenberg et al., 2009), which are predictive of functional disability (Cervellione et al., 2007; Heinrichs et al., 2008; McClure, Bowie, Leung et al., 2007; McClure, Bowie, Patterson et al., 2007). Finally, the group moved away from the "disorganized thought" concept and focused more on observable speech. Thus, their dimension of "disorganized speech" focuses more narrowly on speech cohesiveness and coherence and does not address underlying problems in logic, which are reflected by impairments in conceptual and abstract thinking.

Recognizing the heterogeneity of symptoms in schizophrenia, including the prevalence of obsessive-compulsive features, researchers factor analyzed the PANSS, incorporating data from a broader range of scales, including the Yale-Brown Obsessive Compulsive Scale (YBOCS, Grover et al., 2018). Their results yielded seven factors (positive, depressive, negative, mania, anxiety, and two sets of obsessive-compulsive factors).

Hybrid Approaches

The DSM and ICD were built on categorical assumptions that each diagnostic syndrome is a distinct entity with fixed boundaries that separate it from other disorders. However, DSM-5-TR (APA, 2022) authors acknowledged that while adopting a categorical approach to classifying mental disorders, a dimensional approach may increase reliability and better represent the lack of clear boundaries between and the continuous nature of symptom severity within diagnostic syndromes. At the same time, they noted the limitations of dimensional descriptions, which are less useful and less familiar to clinicians seeking to make differential diagnoses for treatment planning purposes (suggesting that clinicians often favor categories).

Due to shifting views about categories vs dimensions, DSM-5 and -TR offer a hybrid model opting for the coexistence of categories and dimensions.

> For reasons of both clinical utility and compatibility with the categorical ICD classification required for coding, DSM-5 continues to be a primarily categorical classification with dimensional elements that divide mental disorders into types based on criteria sets with defining features.
>
> (APA, 2022, p. 15)

Thus, both diagnostic systems opted for a hybrid approach, retaining categories but incorporating dimensions, continua, and spectra into the diagnostic model.

Before DSM-5, several researchers tried to establish hybrid models to not throw out the convenience and utility of the categorical baby with the invalidity of the bath water. Proponents of utilizing both dimensional and categorical approaches argued that, despite their limited validity, categorical approaches to understanding psychoses have clinical utility (van Os et al., 1999; van Os & Kapur, 2009). Esterberg and Compton (2009) also argued for a hybrid approach, presenting the advantages of categorical and dimensional approaches to diagnostic understanding. They emphasized that the categorical approach is more reliable because it contributes to better communication about the treatment of patients in clinical settings, whereas the dimensional approach, based on empirical underpinnings, provides improved validity.

Despite their advocacy of a dimensional approach to diagnosis, both the Reininghaus study and the DSM-5 Psychosis Work Group moved in a direction that combines dimensional and categorical approaches. Reininghaus proposed that DSM-5 categories be associated with different dimensions. Essentially, all DSM-5 categories of psychosis would reflect the general psychosis dimension. Schizophrenia-spectrum and other psychotic disorders and bipolar disorders would reflect the presence of positive symptoms, whereas only schizophrenia-spectrum/other psychotic disorders would include negative symptoms. Disorganization can be found in the schizophrenia spectrum and other psychotic disorders. The mania dimension would weigh heavily in bipolar and related disorders with psychotic features, and depression would be associated with diagnosing psychotic features in major depression and bipolar depression. The latest editions of the DSM reflect the importance of thinking and assessing dimensionally while retaining diagnostic categories.

Not all dimensional approaches support a hybrid approach combining dimensionality with traditional diagnostic categories. The Hierarchical Taxonomy of Psychopathology (HiTOP) is a contemporary factor analytic approach to diagnosis rooted in a hierarchical dimensional model (Kotov et al., 2017, 2022). The model begins with a general psychopathology, or p factor, yielding three Superspectra (Psychosis, Emotional Dysfunction, and Externalizing). The Psychosis Superspectra subsumes two spectra, Psychoticism (Thought Disorder) and Detachment, each including sets of maladaptive traits and symptom components (See Exhibit 1). Psychoticism (Thought Disorder) and Detachment Spectra reflect the positive and negative factors of psychosis.

Exhibit 1

Psychosis Super Spectra

Spectra	Psychoticism (Thought Disorder)	Detachment
Maladaptive Traits	Fantasy Proneness/Unusual Experiences/Unusual Belief/Peculiarity	Emotional Detachment Social Withdrawal/Anhedonia/Romantic Disinterest
Symptom Components	Mania/Dissociation/Reality Distortion/Disorganization	Inexpressivity/Avolition

Work with HiTOP is ongoing, but the consortium researchers demonstrated advantages over traditional categorical approaches when assessing the level of functioning and other outcome-related variables. The HiTOP consortium has advanced our understanding of psychopathology and the structure of psychosis. However, despite its potential for classifying psychotic phenomena, critics have raised methodological and conceptual concerns that suggest the model, in its current form, is neither ready for clinical use nor a replacement for DSM and ICD categorical models (Haeffel et al., 2022).

Problems with terminology conflate factors with symptoms. HiTOP researchers chose the term "Thought Disorder" for the Spectra, representing positive symptoms. Confusingly, they try to distinguish this from the familiar term "Formal Thought Disorder," which they also call "Disorganization." Mihura and colleagues (2023) pointed out the inconsistency in terminology, which may lead to confusion. In recent publications, HiTOP researchers have used the term "Psychoticism" for the positive Spectra; however, they include "Thought Disorder" in parentheses. The term "thought disorder" has been problematic enough, and the use of it on a Spectra level in HiTOP further muddies the waters.

Psychosis Spectrum and Continuum

The terms "spectrum" and "continuum" are often confused, and their meaning varies according to the context. Technically, a spectrum is a range of values between two endpoints, and a continuum defines the quantitative range of values. Spectra address diversity within diagnostic categories, while continua relate to symptom dimension severity across a broader population.

Psychosis Spectrum

Diagnostic spectrums typically refer to groupings or "families" of related conditions that share certain features and underlying mechanisms but differ in symptom presentation and severity. The spectrum concept is meant to capture heterogeneity within categories. Some use the term broadly to describe a *spectrum of psychotic disorders* (Fuji & Ahmed, 2007) to identify the universe of diagnosable psychotic conditions without necessarily including the concept of severity and dysfunctionality. Conversely, psychosis categories are often conceived as spectra, as in the case of the schizophrenia spectrum in DSM-5 and -TR.

In contrast, Sbrana and colleagues (2005) employed the term *psychotic spectrum* to identify a full continuum of subthreshold symptoms, personality traits, "soft signs," as well as full-scale major psychoses. In this context, Sbrana et al. developed a continuum model to highlight various domains of psychotic-like symptoms in a broader range of patients not diagnosed as actively psychotic. The term "spectrum" here is used interchangeably with a continuum of symptom severity, creating some semantic confusion.

Vas Os and Reininghaus (2016) proposed a "transdiagnostic psychosis spectrum" ranging from affective to nonaffective psychosis. Their model incorporates genetic predisposition and five symptom domains (positive and negative symptoms, disorganization, mania, and depression), with varying degrees of environmental factors (e.g., childhood trauma, urbanization, cannabis use) to assign different levels of risk for transition to psychosis. According to van Os and Reininghaus, the transdiagnostic psychosis phenotype underlies schizophrenia and bipolar disorder and has continuity across subclinical and clinically significant symptom levels.

Psychosis Continuum

The psychosis continuum embodies a full range of psychotic symptom expressions from normal range to subsyndromal to clinically significant (DeRosse & Karlsgodt, 2015). A continuum is inherent in dimensional and spectrum approaches to conceptualizing and classifying psychotic phenomena. As mentioned earlier, symptom dimensions occur both trans diagnostically and along a continuum of severity. The Clinician-Rated Dimensions of Psychosis Symptom Severity matrix in the Assessment Measures section of DSM-5-TR is a prime example of the relationships between dimensions and continua, or levels of severity.

Conditions within a spectrum also vary in severity. Here, the continuum is for intra-spectrum disorders, not individual symptom dimensions. For example, schizotypal personality disorder and schizophrenia belong in the same diagnostic spectrum but vary along a continuum of symptom severity.

Viewing psychotic phenomena along a continuum from sub-threshold symptoms, on the one hand, to full-blown threshold disorders, on the other, allows one to use a dimensional approach while preserving the utility of differential diagnostic categories. Core symptom features of psychosis may occur along a continuum of severity without reaching the threshold required for considering a patient psychotic. However, as noted previously, the threshold for separating subthreshold from threshold psychotic symptoms is not always clear. The assessment tool provided in the DSM-5 to rate the severity of symptom dimensions was intended to be a helpful aid in making this determination, but it still leaves diagnostic decision-making up to the clinician.

The prevalence of subthreshold psychotic-like experiences (PLEs) is roughly 7% in the general population (Linscott & van Os, 2013). PLEs are high but transitory developmental phenomena in children and adolescents, but they do not continue in 80% of individuals. Persistent subthreshold psychotic experiences persist in only 20%, and an even smaller portion of individuals (7%) develop psychotic disorders. The prevalence of psychotic experiences led Linscott and van Os to establish a proneness-persistence-impairment model of psychosis (2013) and vas Os and Reininghaus (2016) to propose an extended and transdiagnostic psychosis phenotype in the general population.

In addition to situations where a patient presents with isolated, subthreshold core features of psychosis, there is a broader range of patients and nonpatients who demonstrate low-grade or softer signs of core psychotic symptomatology. There is abundant literature dealing with the concept of "proneness to psychosis." Early researchers developed psychometric scales to identify constructs such as "psychoticism," a dimensional aspect of personality functioning (Eysenck, 1952; Eysenck & Eysenck, 1976), and "schizotypy," a multidimensional concept related to psychosis proneness (Bentall et al., 1989; Claridge et al., 1996; Meehl, 1962).

Other researchers have developed measures to identify "softer" manifestations of core psychotic symptoms in the nonpsychotic and general population. The Magical Ideation Scale (Eckblad & Chapman, 1983), Peters Delusional Inventory (PDI) (Peters et al., 1999, 2004), Perceptual Aberration Scale (Chapman et al., 1978), and CAPE (Stefanis et al., 2002) were developed to measure a continuum of core features of psychosis (i.e., disorganized thinking, delusions, hallucinations, and negative symptoms) that occur in the general population and may help detect individuals at high risk for developing psychosis.

To be more specific, dimensional approaches identify the following examples of psychotic phenomena that exist along a continuum from the nonclinical, at the low end, to the psychotic extremes. These include feelings or beliefs that:

- You are being watched or talked about.
- You can read other people's minds.
- Other people can read your mind.
- Words have hidden meanings.
- People are making secret agreements behind your back.
- Things in magazines or on TV are written especially for you.
- You are being contaminated.
- People think you are odd because of your beliefs.
- You understand things that others do not.

It also includes perceptions that:

- Voices are talking about you or your actions when no one is there.
- You can hear noises or sounds that others do not hear.
- You feel someone is touching you when no one else is around.
- Your body is changing or has changed shape.
- You hear your own thoughts spoken aloud in your head and worry that someone near may be able to hear them.
- You see something that no one else can see.
- You smell or taste something that no one else can smell or taste.

We can also capture soft signs of psychotic phenomena by using traditional psychiatric terms and concepts such as:

- Overvalued ideas.
- Fixed ideas.
- Ideas of reference.
- Concrete thinking.
- Magical thinking.
- Vague speech.

Diagnostically, we may also think of subthreshold psychotic phenomena as characteristic of certain nonpsychotic disorders – specifically borderline and schizotypal personality disorders. Traditionally, these stable, nonpsychotic personality disorders have included psychotic-like features that may surface in the context of specific stressors. Moreover, the presence of psychotic phenomena in a given nonpsychotic individual may be viewed as a vulnerability factor that increases the risk that the person may develop a psychotic disorder.

Thus, within the category of experiences we call "subthreshold psychotic phenomena," we could have (1) nonpatients who acknowledge softer, low-grade manifestations of psychotic symptoms, (2) patients with severe personality disorders who experience milder, transient psychotic symptoms, or (3) individuals with isolated psychotic symptoms who are at risk for developing a full-blown psychotic disorder.

Despite the value of a dimensional continuum, there are several concerns about the scientific basis, conceptual soundness, and clinical utility of the full continuum model and the existence of a transdiagnostic psychosis phenotype in the general population (Lawrie, 2016). The finding that PLEs are frequent in the general population may reflect how psychotic phenomena are assessed (David, 2010). For example, self-report scales may yield false positives (people reporting PLEs that are not verified with follow-up questions), which may, in turn, artificially inflate estimates of the prevalence of psychotic phenomena in the general population.

Additionally, the nature of the continuum itself has been questioned. While it is one thing to assume a quantitative continuity of psychotic-like symptoms in the population, it is another to assume that psychotic disorders are not qualitatively distinct and occur on a continuum with normal experience (Lawrie, 2016). The point is that there are not just quantitative differences between "normal" individuals and those suffering from psychosis; the differences are also qualitative in nature.

Additionally, David argued that psychopathological continua are complex and multidimensional (2010). He distinguished between two types of continua: Type I continua involve traits or symptoms that occur on a population level, whereas Type II continua may occur within individuals diagnosed with a psychotic disorder. For example, a Type I continuum may apply to a range of hallucinatory and delusional experiences across the population. Such experiences may vary in severity according to frequency, intensity, and level of distress and conviction associated with the hallucination or delusion. However, David argued that there is a qualitative difference between the nature of these subthreshold symptoms that may occur in some so-called "normal" people and those occurring during a psychotic state or disorder. In essence, David suggested that continua are, at best, discontinuous quasi-continua.

Another question about a full continuum model is where one establishes cut-offs that separate normal range, subthreshold PLEs from the onset of a psychotic episode. Again, subdimensions like frequency of symptoms, level of distress, conviction, and preoccupation may pertain to overall severity, but at what point on the continuum does an individual become psychotic?

We emphasized in Chapter 1 that delusions or hallucinations with impaired reality testing, which results in a loss of reality testing, are the necessary criterion for diagnosing psychosis. However, even these hardcore symptoms may exist in isolation or an attenuated form below the threshold for diagnosing a psychotic disorder. For example, Tricia, in Chapter 1, was experiencing hallucinations yet demonstrated preserved reality-testing; she did not think they were real. Although we concluded that she was not actively psychotic, she clearly presented with a symptom typically associated with psychosis. Similarly, some patients demonstrate severely disordered and illogical reasoning in their responses on psychological tests, but they do not exhibit clinical signs of psychosis (e.g., hallucinations and/or delusions with impaired insight). Although they may be demonstrating a symptom associated with psychosis, they fall beneath the threshold for making a clinical diagnosis of psychosis.

However, as much as we would like to erect firm boundaries between the psychotic and the quasi-, pseudo-, or almost psychotic, some individuals appear to have dual citizenships that enable them to traverse the border from our shared reality to their private psychotic realities. We might ask ourselves how firmly and tenaciously individuals must hold to their delusional beliefs and how impaired their insight must be for us to determine that they are currently psychotic.

In this regard, consider the experiences of Ms. G., an attorney who has been treated for many years for heightened anxiety that colleagues are removing things from her desk and "listening" to her thoughts. Ms. G. used the term "broadcast thinking" to describe this experience. She had been diagnosed with a schizoaffective disorder controlled with antipsychotic and mood-stabilizing medication and psychotherapy. Thus, there was the documented presence of a diagnosable psychotic disorder, which was in remission and controlled by her treatment. Yet, despite her sustained involvement in psychotherapy and regular use of antipsychotic medications, Ms. G. remained vulnerable to fleeting moments of delusional thinking. For example, when traveling alone on a bus, in administrative meetings, or seated in a crowded theater, Ms. G. sometimes became convinced that others must be able to hear her vile thoughts. At such moments, there was no question that these frightening experiences (perceptions that others were staring at her, grinning, or laughing under their breath, which represented alterations in her sense of reality) and conclusions (based on her interpretations of these experiences) were real for her. She took random glances or eye contact from strangers to prove her beliefs were real and that others could hear her thoughts. At such times, she could not test reality, step outside her immediate terror, encapsulate delusional explanations for what she was experiencing, and discriminate what Bromberg (2011, p. 390) called "the real from the really real." She could talk about such experiences afterward in therapy, where she would report, "It happened again; I had more psychotic thinking."

Despite the delusional level of her fleeting beliefs, Ms. G. had not been hospitalized for over 30 years. Her regimen of weekly individual psychotherapy and antipsychotic medication had been stabilizing factors. In addition to the beneficial effects of her treatment and other restorative influences in her life, Ms. G.'s stability can be tied to her recognition that her delusional thinking is a symptom of a disorder effectively reduced by compliance with prescribed medications and ongoing psychotherapy. However, during the incidents in question, she experienced a sudden collapse of mental space or reflective capacity, leaving her feeling porous and terrified. Ms. G. was correct that in those fully medicated moments, she became fleetingly but actively psychotic.

Ms. G. could achieve enough distance and doubt to regain a degree of insight that her "broadcast thinking" may not have occurred after all. In this context, the word "may" highlights her uncertainty about what was real for her and "really real" or possible by conventional standards. While she may have lacked the unassailable conviction of someone with a fixed, unalterable delusion, she was not entirely ready to dismiss her experiences as false. Thus, a woman lived in the interstices between the psychotic and not psychotic. Ms. G. had some capacity for insight into her symptoms. She was able to function at work and in the community. Her chronic psychotic disorder was, for the most part, successfully controlled by her ongoing treatment. However, despite her relative stability, she continued to demonstrate a "double awareness" and persistent delusional belief, which, at times, would cross the pencil-thin line that separates psychotic-like phenomena from actual psychotic states.

Clinical Assessment Points

1. We agree that avoiding a zero-sum approach to this issue provides diagnosticians the best of both worlds. Becoming aware of empirically derived factors or dimensions that exist – to one extent or another – across a range of psychotic conditions increases our conceptual understanding, while grouping dimensions into distinct diagnostic categories is useful in our clinical work. The dialectic between a dimensional approach, on the one hand, and a categorical diagnostic approach, on the other, is like Weiner's distinction (1977) between representational inferences, which are closely tied to our observations and data, and higher-order symbolic or diagnostic inferences, which are based on a clustering of representational inferences.
2. Distinguishing between points on the continuum of psychotic phenomena is challenging. Psychometric instruments and performance testing are sensitive to psychotic phenomena; however, relying on test scores to determine whether an individual is psychotic, at imminent risk, prone to psychosis, or stably schizotypal often does not provide the precision we require to make clinical decisions. Therefore, in keeping with this book's theme, assessing psychotic phenomena requires a multi-method approach that incorporates skilled clinical interviewing, a thorough review of history, reliance on collateral sources of information, and the use of a range of testing instruments.

6

DIFFERENTIAL DIAGNOSIS OF PSYCHOTIC DISORDERS

Psychosis profoundly impacts the level of insight and degree of trust and, in some cases, impairs the patient's ability to communicate coherently or rationally. As a result, the differential diagnosis of psychotic disorders is a challenging task (Fuji & Ahmed, 2007; Skodol, 1989). In this chapter, we place advances in the most recent version of the Diagnostic Statistical Manual DSM-5-TR (APA, 2022) at the center of our review. First, we examine the conceptual issues related to the differential diagnosis of psychosis. Then, we introduce a modified approach for the differential diagnosis of a psychotic disorder. Finally, we discuss differential diagnosis by examining the core diagnostic features of relevant disorders and the challenges one encounters in arriving at accurate diagnoses in clinical practice.

In the DSM-5-TR, three conceptual issues are essential in making a differential diagnosis of psychotic disorders. They are as follows:

1. The principle of diagnostic hierarchy.
2. The importance of mood episodes.
3. The duration of the disturbance.

We review each issue separately.

The Principle of Diagnostic Hierarchy

Since the appearance of the DSM-III, diagnostic classification systems in psychiatry have emphasized the diagnostic hierarchy in differential diagnosis. Although clinicians are encouraged to assign multiple diagnoses, some take precedence over others. As a result, certain diagnostic combinations cannot occur together. For example, if a patient's psychotic symptoms are directly due to a general medical illness, then other psychotic disorders cannot be diagnosed. Similarly, if a patient presents with severe depression with psychotic features but has a history of past manic episodes, the diagnosis of major depression with psychotic features cannot

DOI: 10.4324/9781003415206-9

be made. In this case, the patient will either have a diagnosis of bipolar disorder, with the most recent episode of depression with psychotic features, or schizoaffective disorder, bipolar type.

A critical conceptual change in the DSM-5 is that the diagnostic hierarchy for schizophrenia has been changed. One may now diagnose bipolar disorder *with* schizophrenia (see First, 2014). An example would be a patient who meets the criteria for schizophrenia and has a history of a full-manic episode of one week's duration. In this case, the patient cannot be given a diagnosis of schizoaffective disorder because the duration of the manic episode has been too brief. Neither can the patient be diagnosed as having a bipolar disorder with psychotic features because the psychotic symptoms do not occur exclusively during mood symptoms, and the duration of psychotic illness is six months or more.

Importance of Mood Episodes

In the DSM-5-TR, there is considerable symptom overlap in psychotic disorders. Patients with different psychotic conditions can have similar clinical presentations. For example, hallucinations, delusions, thought disorders, and even bizarre types of delusions can occur in patients with schizophrenia, schizoaffective disorder, and mood disorders with psychotic features. As noted in Chapter 2, the long-held belief that Schneider (1959) advocates that different types of delusions or hallucinations can be helpful in differential diagnosis is no longer supported by the literature on differential diagnosis. As such, the focus of the differential diagnosis has shifted from a cross-sectional assessment of various psychotic symptoms to an evaluation of the unique core diagnostic features of each disorder (Black & Grant, 2014). In the case of psychotic disorders, the presence of prominent mood symptoms and the type of mood episodes are the essential diagnostic distinguishing features (First, 2014). For example, since the development of the DSM-III, schizophrenia, schizophreniform, and brief reactive disorders are all differentiated from mood disorders with psychotic features by the relative absence of mood episodes rather than types of psychotic signs and symptoms.

Duration of Illness

Starting with the DSM-III, increased emphasis has been placed on the course, duration of illness, and duration of specific symptoms in the conceptualization of psychotic disorders. In some psychotic disorders, the duration of illness is the only core diagnostic criterion that differentiates one disorder from another. For example, in the DSM-5-TR, the diagnostic criteria for schizophrenia, schizophreniform, and brief reactive psychotic disorder are almost identical, except for symptom duration and illness course. Similarly, in mood disorders with psychotic features, the temporal relationship between the onset of psychotic symptoms versus mood symptoms and the total duration of mood symptoms is essential in establishing an accurate diagnosis.

In short, according to the DSM-5-TR, after establishing the presence of psychotic symptoms, clinicians must be mindful of diagnostic hierarchy, focus their clinical attention on the presence and history of significant mood depressive or manic episodes, and carefully assess the onset and duration of illness. We cannot establish an accurate diagnosis according to current standards without considering these principles.

Current Approach to Differential Diagnosis

The DSM-5-TR, similar to the DSM-IV, DSM-IV-TR, and DSM-5, advocates using a decision tree in which the clinician systematically arrives at the differential diagnosis by considering relevant diagnoses using specific criteria (First, 2014). The first step is to rule out whether the psychosis is caused by substance use or a general medical condition. Only after ruling out these two conditions can the clinician go on to the specific psychotic-disorder decision tree and systematically consider all possible psychotic disorders, including mood disorders with psychotic features.

However, we propose a slightly different approach when it comes to the differential diagnosis of psychotic disorder. We believe clinicians should first consider whether the patient's clinical presentation and expressed symptoms occur in the context of psychosis *before* questioning the etiology of the symptoms.

Modified Approach to Differential Diagnosis of a Psychotic Disorder

In our modified approach, the clinician first determines whether the patient's presenting symptoms meet the threshold for a diagnosis of psychosis. For example, with a patient who presents in the emergency room with violent ideation, the clinician should first consider if there is any evidence that the patient's violent thoughts occur in the context of psychosis. Similarly, if a patient presents in an outpatient setting with complaints of anxiety, we suggest first considering the possibility that anxiety symptoms may be a response to delusions or hallucinations.

There are several rationales for this modified approach. First, we believe it is crucial not to miss the diagnosis of a psychotic disorder; thus, by considering it first for every clinical presentation, one can ensure that it is sufficiently explored. We believe failure to diagnose a psychotic disorder accurately can potentially have a detrimental impact on the patient by possibly delaying treatment. For example, patients with first-episode psychosis have a poorer outcome the longer their symptoms go untreated (Marshall et al., 2005). Furthermore, untreated psychosis can potentially place patients at risk for violence (Keers et al., 2014). Finally, psychosis requires immediate clinical attention, irrespective of its etiology. At a minimum, a period of observation is needed, and in most cases, treatment with antipsychotic medication is warranted.

Second, there is also evidence in the literature that patients' cross-sectional presentations unduly influence clinicians, and, as a result, clinicians may not sufficiently explore other psychiatric disorders. For example, studies show that when clinicians use unstructured clinical interviews, they are more likely to miss other comorbid diagnoses (Zimmerman, 2008). Additionally, clinicians often do not sufficiently explore manic and hypomanic episodes in patients presenting with major depression (see Bowden, 2001).

Third, almost every clinical presentation could occur in the context of psychosis.

Many nonpsychotic symptoms, such as anxiety, depression, social withdrawal, and agitation, are often present in psychotic conditions, and these symptoms can potentially mask an underlying psychotic etiology. For example, a patient who presents with symptoms of agoraphobia could be psychotic, and their reason for not leaving home may be due to paranoid delusions rather than anxiety.

Finally, the practice of considering psychosis first in the differential diagnosis has been recommended in other clinical presentations. For example, a review of suicidal ideation and the associated behavioral decision tree (see First, 2014, p. 69) shows that the first aspect of the decision tree is whether suicidal ideation or behavior is related to psychotic symptoms.

After determining the presence of psychotic symptoms, the clinician then goes through the recommended steps in the DSM-5-TR differential diagnosis and considers whether psychosis is due directly to the influence of drugs or a medical condition. If these conditions are ruled out, the next step would be to assess whether the patient is experiencing, or has ever experienced, any significant mood symptoms. In the final step, if there are no mood symptoms, the clinician can proceed with the psychotic decision tree and evaluate specific criteria for nonaffective psychotic disorders.

Core Diagnostic Features of DSM-5-TR Psychotic Disorders

In discussing the differential diagnosis of psychotic conditions, it is essential to understand the core diagnostic characteristics of mental disorders that may either have psychosis as a feature or have clinical presentations that may appear similar to psychotic symptoms. What follows is a list of diagnoses and their core features according to the DSM-5-TR.

Substance-Induced Psychotic Disorder

Substance use, including either illicit or prescribed medications, must be determined as a *direct cause* of the psychotic symptoms and not simply as a worsening of the pre-existing psychotic condition. Psychotic symptoms typically occur only during intoxication, withdrawal, or its immediate aftermath. For instance, if a patient with a diagnosis of schizoaffective disorder uses cocaine and experiences active psychotic symptoms, he would not be diagnosed as having substance-induced psychotic disorder because cocaine use has exacerbated his primary psychotic disorder. In this example, the patient would be given a diagnosis of schizoaffective disorder and cocaine abuse. Drug use can also trigger psychosis in individuals who never had a primary psychotic disorder but have a genetic predisposition to one. In such cases, the patient is given a diagnosis of substance-induced psychotic disorder with a rule-out of a primary psychotic disorder. These patients may need at least four weeks of being drug-free before finalizing a non-substance-induced diagnosis. However, the recommended four-week drug-free period may not be sufficient for some classes of drugs since the effects of substance use can last longer.

Illicit Drugs and Psychosis

It is a widely accepted fact that the consumption of alcohol and many illegal substances can lead to psychotic symptoms (DSM-5-TR). However, the impact of cannabis and methamphetamine on the development, progression, and manifestation of psychosis is more complex and nuanced (Fiorentini et al., 2021; Shah et al., 2017). Therefore, they are discussed in detail in what follows.

Cannabis Use and Psychosis

Cannabis is widely used illegally, with 6–7% of Europeans and 15.3% of Americans using it yearly (World Drug Report, 2019). The use of cannabis can result in psychoactive effects that may cause psychotic symptoms such as paranoia and hallucinations. It can also lead to negative symptoms, feelings of disinhibition or dreaminess, and heightened awareness of music, sounds, colors, and tastes. Studies show that acute episodes of cannabis-induced psychosis can last from a few days to several months (Curran et al., 2016). More importantly, cannabis users have the highest conversion rate for substance-induced psychoses to either schizophrenia or bipolar disorder (Shah et al., 2017).

Ksir and Hart (2016) conducted a review of studies that investigated the relationship between cannabis use and psychosis, both in individuals with a diagnosis of schizophrenia and those experiencing first-episode psychosis. They concluded that cannabis is not the direct cause of psychosis, but rather, individuals with pre-existing vulnerability to psychosis are more likely to engage in early and heavy cannabis use. The researchers emphasized the importance of identifying early and heavy cannabis use as a potential warning sign, along with other non-drug-related behaviors such as poor academic performance and early or heavy use of cigarettes or alcohol.

On the other hand, Murray et al. (2017) reviewed experimental studies of cannabis on normal individuals and prospective epidemiological research. They concluded that cannabis use can cause dose-related psychotic symptoms and other cognitive, behavioral, and psychophysiological effects in a person without a genetic predisposition for schizophrenia spectrum disorders. The authors of the review study concluded that there are consistent findings that cannabis use is associated with an increased risk of psychotic symptoms, with the highest risk associated with early onset and daily use of high-potency cannabis and synthetic marijuana.

Methamphetamine Use and Psychosis

Methamphetamine is a highly addictive psychostimulant that can be consumed in various ways, such as ingestion, injection, inhalation, or smoking. It can induce a variety of positive psychotic symptoms depending on the dose (Acklin, 2017).

More recently, Fiorentini and colleagues (2021) conducted a comprehensive review of all major studies on meth-induced psychosis. They noted that in various studies, the percentage of meth-induced psychosis cases ranges from 37.1% to 17%. Persistent psychosis that lasts for more than a month, even after abstaining from meth for more than a month, is experienced by about 25% of people, according to some studies. They also found that persecutory delusions were the most prevalent post-symptom reported in 84% of studies, followed by auditory (69%) and visual (65%) hallucinations, hostility (53%), conceptual disorganization (36%), and depression (31%). Negative symptoms were less common (6–19%). The lifetime prevalence of MIP was 42.7%, and the rates were higher for those who only used meth (43.3%). Although there is a significant overlap between meth-induced psychosis and schizophrenia, acute meth-induced psychosis is associated with visual and tactile hallucinations. In contrast, schizophrenia is characterized by pronounced thought disorder and negative symptoms.

Fiorentini et al. (2021) concluded that the available data on the persistence of psychosis after acute intoxication and withdrawal are limited to studied substances such as cannabis, cocaine, and methamphetamines. Even when a diagnosis of substance-induced psychosis is made, the conversion rate varies significantly across different substances and studies, influenced by factors such as subsequent abstinence and individual vulnerability. The authors argued that substance abuse at a young age increases the risk of a more probable conversion to a severe condition.

Prescription Drugs and Psychosis

Many prescription medications can also directly cause psychotic symptoms. Some of the common medications include corticosteroids, cardiac medications, and anti-parkinsonian agents. In addition to causing hallucinations, paranoia, and delusions, they can also induce nonpsychotic symptoms such as delirium, cognitive impairment, and mood-related symptoms (see Ambizas, 2014).

Psychotic Disorder Due to Another Medical Condition

As with substance use, medical illness must directly cause the psychotic symptoms, not simply exacerbate the pre-existing psychotic condition. Late onset of psychotic/manic symptoms, visual and olfactory hallucinations, presence of confusion, or marked memory changes should alert the clinician to a possible medical illness directly causing the psychosis (First, 2014; Ali et al., 2011; Fuji & Ahmed, 2007).

Schizophrenia Disorder

The patient must show evidence of active psychotic symptoms for one month, and the duration of total disturbance must be six or more months. The diagnosis cannot be made based solely on negative symptoms or gross disorganized behavior. That is, the patient must present with at least one positive symptom, such as hallucinations, delusions, or disorganized thinking, plus one more symptom. In addition, the level of functioning must be markedly below that level achieved prior to the onset of the disorder.

Schizophreniform Disorder

The patient's clinical presentation is identical to the diagnostic criteria for schizophrenia, except that the duration of symptoms is less than six months.

Brief Reactive Psychotic Disorder

The patient presents with symptoms like schizophrenia, but the duration of symptoms is less than one month. Also, in contrast to schizophrenia, brief reactive disorder does not include negative symptoms as diagnostic criteria. The presence of stressors as a trigger for the development of psychotic symptoms is no longer necessary.

Delusional Disorder

The patient's clinical presentation is limited to the presence of delusions. There is a relative absence of hallucinations, or if hallucinations are present, they are not as pervasive and are often related to the presenting delusion. The patient shows no evidence of disorganized speech or behavior. In past diagnostic classification systems, a patient with delusional disorder could only have non-bizarre delusions. This has now changed. In the DSM-5, the presence of bizarre delusions does not exclude the diagnosis of delusional disorder.

Schizoaffective Disorder

The diagnostic criteria for schizoaffective disorder were changed in DSM-5 to improve inter-rater reliability (Black & Grant, 2014), and no further changes were made in DSM-5 TR. In this disorder, there must be an uninterrupted period of illness during which the person presents concurrently with both psychotic and mood episodes. For psychotic episodes, the person must meet Criteria A symptoms of schizophrenia, which include the presence of two psychotic symptoms, one of which must be hallucinations, delusions, or disorganized speech. For mood episodes, if there is a major depressive episode, the criteria A1 (depressed mood) must be met. The person must then have at least one core psychotic symptom for two weeks or more in the absence of mood episodes. Finally, mood episodes must be present for more than 50 % of the lifetime duration of the illness.

Bipolar I Disorder with Psychotic Features

The clinical presentation must include at least one lifetime manic episode, but a history of depressive episodes is not necessary. In Bipolar I disorder, psychotic symptoms must only occur when the person is manic, depressed, or experiencing a mixed episode. In contrast to schizoaffective disorder, psychotic symptoms in bipolar disorder can only occur concurrently with mood symptoms, which may be mood congruent or mood incongruent (See Kleiger & Weiner, 2023). Also, psychotic symptoms cannot occur during hypomanic episodes.

Major Depression with Psychotic Features

The clinical presentation must include a history of at least one depressive episode, characterized by either a persistent depressed mood or loss of pleasure for most of the day for at least two weeks. Similar to bipolar disorder, psychotic symptoms can only occur concurrently with mood symptoms. In addition, individuals with major depressive disorder can have both mood-congruent or mood-incongruent delusions and hallucinations.

Other Specified Schizophrenia-Spectrum Disorders and Other Psychotic Disorders

The clinical presentation includes the presence of some psychotic symptoms but does not meet the full criteria for any psychotic disorder. The difference between other specified schizophrenia-spectrum disorders and other psychotic disorders depends on whether the clinician chooses to specify features of the diagnosis that were present in the patient. For example, a patient with a two-day history of hallucinations without any impairment, followed by remission of symptoms, will be diagnosed as having another psychotic disorder.

Schizotypal Personality Disorder

The symptoms do not meet the threshold for psychotic conditions, and the person has not had a psychotic episode in her lifetime. In addition, symptoms such as magical thinking, suspiciousness, and social isolation do not occur during schizophrenia or other psychotic and mood disorders. Sometimes, patients with residual symptoms of schizophrenia may appear symptomatically, like those with schizotypal personality disorder. However, since they have had a full-blown psychotic episode, they cannot be diagnosed as having a schizotypal personality disorder.

Paranoid Personality Disorder

The paranoia in this personality disorder is limited to paranoid ideation, pervasive suspiciousness, and lack of trust in others; however, these symptoms do not reach the threshold for psychotic conditions. Furthermore, similar to schizotypal personality disorder, the patient has never had a full-blown psychotic episode. In addition, the paranoid symptoms do not occur during schizophrenia, delusional disorder, or other psychotic and mood disorders.

Body Dysmorphic Disorder with Absence of Insight/ Delusional Beliefs

The DSM-5 and 5-TR have recognized that there are patients who hold a delusional belief that defects they perceive in their appearance are real. In previous editions of the DSM, these patients were diagnosed as having a delusional disorder. However, in the DSM-5 and -TR, they are diagnosed as having body dysmorphic disorder, absent insight/delusional beliefs.

Obsessive-Compulsive Disorder with Absence of Insight/ Delusional Beliefs

Similarly, patients with obsessive-compulsive disorder can have false beliefs that reach a delusional level. For example, a patient may believe that touching the surface of objects will contaminate him and, as a result, must wash his hands repeatedly. He may hold on to this belief with a high level of conviction that impairs his reality-testing ability. In the past diagnostic classification systems, these patients were also diagnosed as having a delusional disorder. However, in the DSM-5, they are now diagnosed as having a variant of obsessive-compulsive disorder. Patients with such clinical presentation would be diagnosed with obsessive-compulsive disorder, absent insight/delusional beliefs.

Post-Traumatic Stress Disorder

The core features of Post-Traumatic Stress Disorder (PTSD) include experiencing, witnessing, or hearing about a traumatic event that meets the criteria A definition of trauma. The symptoms of flashbacks, traumatic thought intrusions, paranoia, hypervigilance, avoidance, depersonalization, and derealization might be confused as psychotic symptoms. However, in PTSD, reality testing is often maintained, and hallucinations (flashbacks), paranoia, and hypervigilance are, at least in part, trauma-related.

In some cases, both diagnoses of PTSD and psychosis are warranted. For example, an individual with PTSD can have transient psychotic symptoms or comorbid psychotic disorder, or a person with a psychotic disorder can have PTSD, including dissociative symptoms.

In short, there can be a complex interplay of trauma and psychosis (Hardy & Mueser, 2017). In our experience, we have identified the following presentations: (1) A reaction to a traumatic event directly causes psychotic disorder. (2) PTSD symptoms can cause transient impairment in reality testing. (3) PTSD symptoms can exacerbate an already existing psychotic disorder. (4) A psychotic disorder is unrelated to trauma or PTSD. Finally, (5) a reported trauma could be false and based on a delusional belief.

Challenges in the Differential Diagnosis of Psychotic Disorder in Clinical Practice

As discussed previously, the core features in the differential diagnosis of psychotic disorders are duration, prominence of mood disorder, a temporal relationship between the onset of drug use, or the presence of a medical etiology. However, in actual clinical practice, assessing the onset and duration of a psychiatric disturbance is challenging. It requires the patient or their family to accurately recall the onset and duration of illness and the presence of mood-related symptoms. Additionally, the temporal relationship between the onset of drug use and the development of psychotic symptoms may be complicated to determine based on symptom presentation or the patient's responses to interview questions. Although a small number of studies have suggested that symptom presentation in individuals with substance-induced disorder can be differentiated from those with a primary psychotic disorder, the findings have not been replicated (see Caton et al., 2000).

Several other factors make it particularly difficult to assess the role of substance usage in determining psychotic symptoms. The first challenge is that substance-abusing patients may be in denial about their drug use. Second, many patients coming to the psychiatric emergency room with psychotic features may not agree to or be able to provide urine to obtain toxicology results (First, 2014). As a result, clinicians may not know the extent or type of substances used. Third, some new forms of drugs, such as Ecstasy or K-2, are not routinely tested and may not appear in standard toxicology screening. Fourth, a period of drug-free observation is often needed to determine if substance use was the direct cause of a patient's psychosis. The DSM-5-TR recommends an observation period of up to four weeks. Patients are discharged well before four weeks in many clinical settings, making accurate diagnosis difficult. Moreover, chronic use of drugs such as methamphetamine can induce psychotic symptoms that can last six months, even after a period of being drug-free (Sato et al., 1992).

Earlier studies examining patients with primary psychotic disorder and substance misuse have demonstrated that misdiagnosis is relatively common (Addington & Addington, 1998). One study (Shaner et al., 1998) with a sample of 165 male patients with chronic psychosis and cocaine use took a multi-method approach, including structured clinical interviews, collateral information, medical records, and toxicology. The researchers could make a definite diagnosis in only 25% of the sample. This study found that among the factors contributing to inaccurate diagnosis were poor recollection of the duration of drug use concerning psychotic symptoms, inconsistent reporting, and an insufficient period of absence from drugs. Additionally, drug-induced psychosis, such as that caused by methamphetamine, can persist beyond the recommended four weeks after cessation of use.

A careful assessment of mood episodes is needed in the differential diagnosis of nonaffective psychotic disorders versus mood disorders with psychotic features. Moreover, this requires that patients, family members, and, in some cases, providers be able to identify whether mood symptoms were present at the onset or began after the onset of psychosis. Relying on patients who are having psychotic experiences to determine the onset of their illness and its relationship to mood symptoms with psychosis is indeed challenging. Family members also may not be good historians regarding the patient's clinical presentation. Skodol (1989) presented evidence from studies showing that even in cases where there was a documented history of psychosis and manic episodes, both patients and their family members had difficulty recalling them. He argued that the stigma associated with mental illness, the bizarre nature of some symptoms, the lack of insight related to psychosis, and the active suppression or denial of illness resulted in an under-reporting of symptoms by patients and family members. As a result, relying on patients' and family members' recollections to help clinicians identify and describe past episodes of psychosis has less value than many would think. Therefore, it is not surprising that a diagnosis such as schizoaffective disorder has had such poor interrater reliability, necessitating changes in the diagnostic criteria in the DSM-5 (Black & Grant, 2014).

Furthermore, there are studies demonstrating that clinicians often have difficulty eliciting past manic and hypomanic episodes (Bowden, 2001). Surprisingly, a diagnosis of major depressive disorder had very low interrater reliability in the DSM-5 field trials (Regier et al., 2013). The authors of the field trials attributed the low interrater reliability to the heterogeneity of diagnosis of major depression, as well as to the presence of comorbidity with other disorders.

All of this indicates that establishing mood episodes and determining their relation to the onset of psychotic symptoms remains challenging. Given these challenges, multiple collateral sources are often needed to confirm an accurate diagnosis (Skodol, 1989). Whenever possible, the use of structured interviews or screening measures with unstructured clinical examination has been shown to enhance the accuracy of diagnosis (Zimmerman, 2008).

Finally, residual psychotic symptoms may be confused with personality disorder features. Similarly, subthreshold symptoms in partially treated patients may be confused with another disorder. For example, an inpatient with schizophrenia who is not taking his medication may respond to the therapeutic structure of an inpatient unit and become more organized, revealing only paranoid ideations. In the absence of any collateral history of psychosis, the patient can be seen as having paranoid personality disorder.

Clinical Assessment Points

1. We advocate that when evaluating patients, clinicians should consider the presence of psychotic symptoms in any clinical presentation. In this modified approach, the clinician can potentially ensure that psychotic symptoms are sufficiently explored, which may reduce the possibility of inaccurate diagnosis.
2. There is considerable symptom overlap among different psychotic disorders. The focus of the differential diagnosis of psychotic disorders centers on the duration of illness, the presence of mood disorder, and the temporal relationship of mood, substance use, or medical illness to the onset of psychotic symptoms.
3. Given the comorbidity of substance use with psychosis, careful assessment of onset, duration, frequency, amount, and method of use is essential in differential diagnosis.
4. The challenges in differential diagnosis of psychosis include accurately identifying the duration of the illness and determining the temporal relationship between mood, substance use, and onset of psychotic symptoms. As a result, a multi-method assessment – including direct clinical interview of patients, review of mental-health records, and collateral contact with the patient's family and providers – is essential more in the differential diagnosis of psychosis than in other conditions.

Part III

ASSESSING PSYCHOSIS

7

ASSESSING PSYCHOTIC DIMENSIONS WITH CLINICAL INTERVIEWING

A clinical interview is the primary and most essential assessment method for evaluating psychotic disorders (Shea, 2016). It offers the most flexibility in exploring symptoms and allows the clinician to observe signs of psychosis, such as thought disorder, negative symptoms, and disorganized behavior. In this chapter, we will discuss what we consider to be the most effective clinical interview techniques and questions in assessing psychosis. Consistent with the dimensional perspective of psychosis, we will evaluate eight symptom domains proposed by Barch et al. (2013). These include:

1. Hallucinations.
2. Delusions.
3. Disorganized speech.
4. Bizarre and abnormal psychomotor behavior.
5. Negative symptoms.
6. Cognitive impairment.
7. Depression.
8. Mania.

During the clinical interview, we advocate a collaborative, culturally sensitive, and empathic attitude toward the patient. The clinician focuses on understanding the phenomenological aspect of the patient's symptoms, experiences, subjective meaning of their experiences, and beliefs, including their reasoning. A skilled and thoughtful clinical interview is analogous to the physical exam for the physician. It is our necessary starting point. Before referring a potentially psychotic individual for further diagnostic assessment, we begin with a careful interview assessment of the symptom dimensions characteristic of psychosis.

DOI: 10.4324/9781003415206-11

Hallucinations

The first step in assessing hallucinations is to accurately establish that the person is or has, in fact, experienced hallucinations. The best method for evaluating hallucinations is to ask a patient directly (Khadivi, 2021). It should be noted that allowing patients to talk about their hallucinations is often experienced in a positive way (Stephane et al., 2003) and may have therapeutic implications (Larøi & Aleman, 2010).

Suppose the patient does not report hallucinations as a problem during the interview. In that case, we find that it is best to normalize the experience of hallucinations by providing a context for the patient to explain if he has ever experienced hallucinations. We begin by asking a general question: "Sometimes, when people are experiencing stress [*include the patient's description of the problem*], they have unusual experiences, such as hearing voices or seeing things when there is nothing to hear or see." If the patient has active substance use, we will ask about hallucinations in the context of drug or alcohol use before asking if she has had similar hallucinatory experiences without the use of substances.

If the clinician wants to be more direct, we found the following question most helpful: "Do you ever hear or see things when there is nothing to see or hear?" We prefer to ask this instead of questions that compare the patient's experience with that of others, such as, "Do you ever hear or see things that others do not hear or see?" Although these questions help assess hallucinations for many patients, some patients do not respond favorably to being compared to others. Furthermore, some patient responses to these questions do not clarify whether they are experiencing hallucinations. For instance, some patients respond, "I do not know what others can hear or see, but I was hearing people talking." Other responses include, "If people were there, they could also hear (or see) what I saw."

The experience of hallucinations must be distinguished from illusions, which are misinterpretations of actual stimuli (Aleman & Larøi, 2008). Consider the following example. During a clinical interview, a patient with a diagnosis of schizophrenia said, "I hear them calling me a 'faggot.'" Staff members on the ward could be heard talking in the background, and she misinterpreted a word. The patient thought she listened to the word "faggot" in their actual conversation. This is an example of an auditory illusion, not a hallucination.

Hallucinations can also be confused with ideas of reference, in which individuals interpret events in the external environment as directed at them (Skodol, 1989). For example, sometimes patients insist that people are talking about them. However, when you inquire further, it becomes clear that they are not actually hearing voices but, instead, are seeing people having conversations that they falsely infer are about them.

Since hallucinations can occur in all sensory modalities, we find it easier to assess olfactory and gustatory hallucinations together, as well as separately from tactical and somatic hallucinations. Here are some examples of how one might begin to explore these experiences:

- Have you ever smelled or tasted anything unusual or strange?
- Have you ever felt something unusual, weird, or frightening on your skin or inside your body?

If the patient answers yes, we will ask them to explain further or give examples.

If the patient reports hearing voices, we explore to learn if the voices are commenting, commanding, or conversing (the three Cs of auditory hallucination). In addition to assessing the content of hallucinations, it is helpful to ask whether the person hears more than one voice and whether the voices talk to each other or about the person. For example, we would ask:

- Do you ever hear more than one voice at the same time?
- Do the voices ever talk about you?
- Have the voices talked to each other about you?
- Do they ever make comments about what you do?
- Have you ever heard a voice or voices speaking your thoughts out loud?

In the case of command hallucinations, we found the following questions most helpful:

- Whose voice do you hear?
- Do you ever hear the voices of people you are familiar with?
- Have you ever heard the voice of the Devil (or God) speaking to you?
- Do the voices ever tell you to do something?
- If yes, what do they tell you to do?
- Do the voices ever tell you to harm yourself and others?
- How often do you follow what the voices tell you to do?

If the patient has followed the command hallucinations, explore what actions he has taken in response to the voices they hear. If he has not, ask, "How do you manage not to follow what the voices say?"

After assessing the type and the content of hallucinations, it is essential to determine the frequency, degree of insight, perceived control, time of day, emotion, and the level of distress (if any) associated with hallucinations. However, the most essential aspect of the assessment of hallucinations is the patient's capacity to test the reality of her hallucinatory experiences.

Therefore, clinicians must assess the following two aspects of hallucinations: first, the presence of a false sensory experience, and second, the interpretation of that experience by the person. Clinicians may wish to avoid placing the patient in a position where they have to justify their hallucinations. However, knowing the degree of insight present when the patient hallucinates is essential. Using auditory hallucinations as an example, we tactfully inquire:

- How do you explain that you hear voices?
- Do you think someone is talking to you?
- What makes you so convinced that the voices are real?
- What else might explain hearing voices?
- How is it possible to hear voices if no one is around?

Berrios and Brook (1984) make an important distinction between what they call "spontaneous" versus "assisted insight." This clinical distinction suggests that insight or the ability to test reality exists along a continuum and that whether the patient can arrive at insight unassisted or with the help of the examiner can have implications for therapeutic intervention. For example, the patient who demonstrates spontaneous insight may be more amenable to forming a therapeutic alliance and more receptive to examining the nature and extent of his psychotic experiences.

Concerning the emotional impact of hallucinations, if the patient is not visibly distressed, it is a good idea to ask how troubled she is by her hallucinations. In addition to assessing the level of distress, it is important to inquire about what emotions are triggered or are associated with the experience of hallucinations. Finally, explore the degree of control and any coping strategies that the patient might employ to manage her hallucinations.

Delusions

Similar to assessing hallucinations, the first task in evaluating delusions is to establish accurately that the patient has ideas that meet the threshold for delusions. The DSM-5 committee working on schizophrenia-spectrum disorders changed the definition of delusions: "from erroneous beliefs to fixed beliefs that are not amenable to change in light of conflicting evidence" (Heckers et al., 2013, p. 2). The committee's rationale was based on earlier criticism of the DSM definition of delusions (Spitzer, 1990). They pointed out that, with some exceptions, clinicians cannot be entirely sure that a given belief coincides with reality. For example, suppose an individual indicates that the government is monitoring him. In that case, the only way to determine whether his belief meets the threshold of a delusion is to assess his reasoning, the evidence he presents as the basis for his belief, and how fixedly he holds his belief.

The best techniques for assessing delusions are open-ended questioning, detailed exploration, focusing on the patient's reasoning, and understanding the basis of his belief (Khadivi, 2021). In addition, the interviewer must assess the firmness of the beliefs in light of the evidence and the patient's capacity to consider alternative explanations.

In clinical practice, one is often faced with three types of presentation by the patient regarding delusions. In the first type, the patient has overt delusional thinking. Here is an example. A patient was brought to the hospital after she broke the back of her family's large television set and tried to get into it to "travel back in time."

Interviewer: What happened at home when you ended up in the hospital?

Patient: I am the inventor of a time-traveling machine, and I was planning to travel back in time. I told my mother, but she is not educated. She freaked out when I broke the TV and called the ambulance.

The second type of patient discusses ideas or says something during the interview that requires further inquiry to establish the presence of delusions. The following exchange exemplifies this type of presentation:

Interviewer: We have been talking for 20 minutes, and I am struck that you do not mention any people in your life.

Patient: I stay away from them.

Interviewer: You must have your reasons.

Patient: People are controlling.

Interviewer: I'm not sure what you mean by controlling.

Patient: They control everything that I do.

Interviewer: How do they manage to control everything that you do?

Patient: With a chip that they put in my teeth.

Interviewer: How do you know a chip was placed in your teeth?

Patient: The dentist looked suspicious to me. I don't think he is a dentist. He also covered my mouth when he was fixing my teeth.

The third type of patient reveals no overt delusional or unusual beliefs spontaneously and does so only in response to specific questions assessing delusional thinking. Since delusions of reference and persecutory delusions are the most common psychotic presentations (see Freeman &

Garety, 2006), we routinely evaluate them using a modified question that was introduced to assess violent thoughts in suicidal patients (see APA, 2003). We have found that the following question often elicits concerns about others, some of which might be non-delusional. But it offers an opening and allows a transition so the clinician can inquire about persecutory delusions and other types of delusions: "Are there people out there who are responsible for your suffering [*for your problem/for your being hospitalized*]?" If this question is affirmative, we explore the paranoia and probe for delusions of perception, control, and grandeur. If no paranoia or other delusions are elicited, we still screen for those delusions. We use questions modified from the SCID-I (First et al., 2002) to do this:

- Have you ever experienced receiving specific messages from other people or your surroundings?
- Have you ever thought that the TV or social media were sending you specific messages only to you?
- Do you ever feel that someone or something controls your thoughts or actions?
- Do you ever think that people are following you or planning to harm you?
- Do you have special talents that others do not know about? How about any special powers to do things?

To assess whether a belief reaches the threshold of delusion, one must consider multiple aspects of the belief. Appelbaum and colleagues (2000) demonstrated the importance of going beyond the content of delusions to evaluate the dimensional aspects of delusions. They used the McArthur–Maudsley Delusions Assessment Schedule (Taylor et al., 1994), which assesses six dimensions of delusions. Consistent with that approach, it is essential to explore:

1. The degree of conviction.
2. The pervasiveness of the belief.
3. The emotions associated with the belief.
4. The actions taken or not taken in response to the belief.
5. The degree of preoccupation with the belief.
6. The extent to which the belief changes during the clinical interview and expands and incorporates others.

In addition, following Oltmanns' perspective on delusions (1998), it is essential to assess the degree to which the delusion is distressing and to which it is causing impairment in functioning.

Disorganized Speech

Disorganized speech, or formal thought disorder, is challenging to assess, and studies have demonstrated that attempts to evaluate it can be highly unreliable (Skodol, 1989; Khadivi, 2021). Furthermore, disorganized speech in isolation and the absence of other accompanying symptoms of psychosis may occur in normal individuals. Frances (2013) has argued that formal thought disorder is not subtle and must be evident from the patient's speech. He correctly argues that focusing too heavily on mild signs of formal thought disorder can result in overdiagnosis of psychosis. In DSM-5, disorganized speech must be severe and easily recognizable by the clinician (see First et al., 2016).

As indicated in Chapter 2, Andreasen (1979) developed a scale for assessment of Thought and Language Communication (TLC) for clinical practice. In this scale, she expanded and refined the definition of various types of formal thought disorders, which increased interrater reliability. Her precise definitions of formal thought disorders and her TLC scale are easily adapted to the clinical interview.

The first task is to assess the forms of thought disorder the patient demonstrates. Andreasen (1979) distinguished two types of formal thought disorder. The first, referred to as positive thought disorder, is characterized by derailment, disorganization, and disconnectedness of the thought process. It includes circumstantial thinking, tangentiality, derailment, distractible speech, clang association, and incoherence. Andreasen advocates using the term "derailment" to capture the disorganization of thought processes and replacing the terms "loosening of associations" and "flight of ideas." She defines *derailment* as:

> A pattern of spontaneous speech in which the ideas slip off the track onto another that is clearly but obliquely related or onto one completely unrelated. Things may be said in juxtaposition that lack a meaningful relationship, or the patient may shift idiosyncratically from one frame of reference to another. At times, there may be a vague connection between the ideas, and at other times, none will be apparent. This pattern of speech is characterized as sounding disjointed.
>
> (Andreasen & Black, 2006, pp. 39–40)

Andreasen also redefined flight of ideas as a derailment with pressured speech (a pattern of speech that is highly productive and difficult to interrupt). Similarly, tangentiality is conceptualized as a form of derailment in which the patient answers the question tangentially or obliquely. The response may be only indirectly related to the question or completely irrelevant (Andreasen & Black, 2006). Additionally, the tangential speaker may simply not answer the question at all. Note how the patient fails to respond to the question asked:

Clinician: How is it that you are in a psychiatric hospital?
Patient: I let people shine their darkness onto me; darkness needs to leave them, and I do not mind if it falls on me. In some way, I am a messenger, but I do not want to be one. I was in college before coming here. Being educated is important to my mother.

Finally, distractible speech, most often seen in patients during manic episodes, describes how the person becomes distracted by external stimuli (an object on an examiner's desk, an article of the examiner's clothing), which can result in the patient abruptly moving to a different topic area, thus getting off the track of what they were saying before.

Clinician: Good morning. I've heard that you are not too happy to be here today.
Patient: That's right, doctor, I have been telling the staff that I don't belong here – Oh, my God! Are those pictures of little animals on your tie? They are so cute! I love animals. Are you a vegetarian?

The second type of formal thought disorder (negative thought disorder) is characterized by a peculiar and restricted thought process that includes neologisms, thought-blocking, illogicality, poverty of speech, and poverty of speech content. In these types of thought disorders, the patient's speech is either characterized by highly idiosyncratic or markedly improvised thinking. The poverty of speech is characterized by restriction in the amount of spontaneous speech. The individual does not elaborate, and her replies to questions are brief, contracted, and concrete, requiring frequent prompting from the interviewer.

Interviewer: How was your childhood?
Patient: Okay.
Interviewer: What was your relationship like with your parents?
Patient: Bad.
Interviewer: Could you say more?
Patient: No, not really. It was okay, I guess.

In contrast, poverty of content of speech reflects an adequate amount of speech that conveys little information. Responses to interviewer questions tend to be vague or repetitive.

Interviewer: What made you decide to take an overdose of your pills?

Patient: The pills were the ones prescribed by Dr. E., you know, because they're supposed to be taken, and I was, you know, looking for them in the morning when my mother came home, you know. She works, and was talking to me about my pills, which she picked up, you know. They were in the cabinet, and I was looking for them when my mother came home.

The best interview technique to assess formal thought disorder involves open-ended questions that allow the patient to talk uninterrupted for at least five minutes, alternating simple questions with more complex ones (Andreasen & Black, 2006). Sometimes, asking open-ended questions from different aspects of a patient's life might be necessary.

Proverb interpretation can also be used to assess thought disorder. Since culture and education can impact proverb interpretation, we recommend using them only with patients who are native English-speaking and have at least a high-school education. We usually begin by asking about a familiar proverb to introduce the task. For example, we might ask, "Do you know what proverbs are? They are sayings that have a specific meaning. For example, can you tell me what it means when people say, 'Do not cry over spilled milk'?"

If the person can interpret abstractly, we go forward with others. We want to ask about proverbs that vary in difficulty level and are not overly familiar. Here are some of the common ones we ask about:

- People who live in glass houses should not throw stones.
- The tongue is the enemy of the neck.
- The good is the enemy of the best.

One of our patients, who had her first episode of psychosis, responded as follows to a proverb:

Interviewer: Can you tell me what this saying means? "People who live in glass houses should not throw stones."

Patient: Doctor, who is watering the plants?

In this example, most likely, the patient association went from *glass houses* to *greenhouses*.

Finally, interviewers can assess the patient's underlying conceptual abilities by asking simple questions about how two ideas are alike or what they have in common. Here, we are looking for the patient's ability to identify conventional concepts. Examples of such questions include:

- In what way are a nose and a tongue alike?
- In what way are milk and water alike?
- How are revenge and forgiveness alike?

Abnormal Psychomotor Activity and Disorganized Behavior

Observation is the best method for assessing abnormal psychomotor behavior. We want to attend to the patient's manner of dress, hygiene, gait, fluidity of movement, posture, flexibility in establishing eye contact, and volume and prosodic qualities of speech.

Negative Symptoms

In the clinical interview, we want to observe evidence of two distinct aspects of unfavorable symptoms, as noted in Chapter 2 (see Barch et al., 2013):

1. Restricted emotional range.
2. Avolition.

In the most severe form of emotional restriction, the patient shows a flat affect marked by reduced facial expressions or gestures. In avolition, the patient demonstrates diminished – or, in severe cases, a marked absence of – self-initiated activity. Differentiating negative symptoms from depressive symptoms can be challenging. However, patients with prominent negative symptoms generally do not have cognitive characteristics of depression, such as hopelessness, pessimism, guilt, or self-deprecation. In addition, unlike depression, the course of negative symptoms is not episodic.

Cognitive Impairment

Individuals with psychosis can have multiple cognitive deficits in attention, concentration, memory, abstract ability, speed of processing, and executive functions (Green et al., 2004; Reichenberg et al., 2009). In addition to conducting a clinical interview, we recommend systematically assessing these domains using established cognitive screening tests. Traditional mental status examinations may not be sensitive enough to capture deficits in psychotic patients with higher premorbid cognitive functioning, nor are they comprehensive enough to capture essential aspects of cognitive domains. In addition, patients with limited premorbid cognitive functioning show global deficits across the board on traditional mental status examinations. Ideally, clinicians can use well-validated and comprehensive neuropsychological screening tools (Gold et al., 1999; Hobart et al., 1999). However, these are typically not practical for use during the psychiatric interview. Instead, we use the Montreal Cognitive Assessment (MOCA; Nasreddine et al., 2005), a brief screening tool for cognitive deficits that can easily be incorporated into an interview.

Depression

Depressive syndrome typically has three clinically useful domains as the assessment focus (Moran & Lambert, 1983). The first domain is cognitive and includes self-deprecating thoughts, hopelessness, pessimism, guilt, and suicidal thoughts. The second domain encompasses mood – including depressed mood – constricted affect, loss of pleasure, and diminished interest. The third domain involves neurovegetative signs and symptoms, including reduced sleep, appetite, insomnia, or hypersomnia. All three domains should be assessed during the interview. It is essential to clarify the persistence of a depressed mood and listen for indications of diminished pleasure.

Mania

Assessing active manic symptoms during the interview is less challenging than retrospective evaluation of past manic episodes (Khadivi, 2023). There are studies indicating that clinicians have difficulty accurately diagnosing past manic episodes when the patient presents as depressed (see Bowden, 2001). Similarly, there has been an increase in the diagnosis of bipolar disorder, suggesting that clinicians are prematurely attributing mood lability and other symptoms to mania (see Paris, 2013; Kleiger & Weiner, 2023). These findings have resulted in changes in the diagnostic criteria for mania in the DSM-5 to increase specificity and make it easier to assess past manic or hypomanic episodes (Black & Grant, 2014).

In assessing mania, the clinician must establish two criteria:

1. A mood disturbance that is persistently irritable, elevated, or expansive.
2. A persistent increase in goal-directed activity or energy.

The interviewer must also assess the presence of other core manic symptoms such as inflated self-esteem, grandiosity, and diminished need for sleep (Khadivi, 2023). We found questions from the Structured Clinical

Interview for DSM-5-Clinical Version (SCID-5-CV; First et al., 2002) to be the most effective approach to assessing a manic mood disturbance. These questions evaluate both the episodic nature of the manic episodes and the elevated, expansive, or irritable quality of the mood. For example, we would ask, "Has there ever been a period of time when you were feeling so good, high, excited, or hyper that other people felt that you were not your normal self or you got into trouble?" If the patient answers affirmatively, she is asked to describe this episode. If the answer is no, we query further: "What about a period of time when you were so irritable that you found yourself shouting at people or starting fights or arguments?" We follow up by asking about the duration of episodes and whether this led to hospitalization: "How long did that last? Did you have to go to the hospital?" After establishing a mood disturbance, assessing whether the patient experienced increased energy or goal-directed activity is best.

Clinicians must be careful with some of the questions they ask. We always need to consider the life circumstances of the patients we interview. For example, questions about overspending money may be less pertinent to patients from economically disadvantaged backgrounds who may not have credit cards or disposable income. Furthermore, questions regarding distractibility often are nonspecific and may be difficult for a patient to answer. In contrast, the other core manic symptoms – including diminished need for sleep without feeling tired, racing thoughts, and grandiosity – are vital diagnostic signs and, as such, are essential to assess. Patients can be asked directly about their diminished need for sleep without experiencing fatigue. We listen for evidence of racing thoughts and distractibility in how patients communicate during the interview. An inflated self-concept and grandiosity are also evident in how the individual describes himself, whether in talking about his delusional beliefs regarding his superpowers or special status or in his descriptions of his expansive plans, ambitions, and accomplishments.

Challenges Interviewing Actively Psychotic Individuals

Conducting a clinical interview with individuals experiencing psychotic symptoms can be quite challenging. Acutely manic and psychotic individuals may elicit unique common reactions from clinicians (Sullivan, 1947; Khadivi, 2023). For instance, patients with severe disorganized speech may make it difficult for the clinician to collect relevant clinical information. Patients with paranoia and hostility may evoke anxiety and make it challenging to develop an assessment alliance, and those with negative symptoms may find it difficult to engage. In navigating these challenges, it is essential to realize that actively psychotic individuals are doing the best they can (Schlesinger, 2003) and that psychosis may serve as a self-protective mechanism against further psychological disintegration. As such, clinicians should aspire to cultivate a compassionate, understanding attitude "with no desire to change the patient" (D. Shapiro, personal communication, March 4, 2020). This kind of empathic mindset can potentially foster the alliance and enhance the diagnostic interview process. In this regard, it is important to remember Harry Stack Sullivan's (1947) perspective that all psychopathology is fundamentally interpersonal. As such, interviewers seek to understand the meaning and impact of symptoms on the individual's relationships (see Evans III, 2024).

Regarding techniques of clinical interviewing, we recommend the following:

- Use close-ended questions with a person who has severe disorganized speech.
- Be formal, transparent, and not overly friendly with an acutely paranoid person. Also, avoid using the "high valence" empathic statement, which aims to offer a deep understanding of emotions not fully articulated by the patient (Shea, 2016).
- When the person is guarded or has delusions of control or persecution, use the technique of asking permission ("Would be okay with you if . . .") or use selective interpersonal self-disclosure ("For me to understand your perspective, I would need to ask you questions, but I also sense that asking questions may be experienced as intrusive, how do you want me to proceed?").
- With a person with negative symptoms, one often experiences the person as "moving away" (Havens, 1996) from the interviewer. Because of that, using empathic, validating, and observational statements is often more effective than questions in engaging the person before transitioning into the information-gathering phase of a clinical interview.

Clinical Assessment Points

1. The best interview method to assess hallucinations is to ask about them directly.
2. We assess delusions through a detailed exploration of the patient's reasoning and understanding of the basis for forming his beliefs and by assessing the degree of the patient's conviction in his beliefs in the light of conflicting evidence.
3. In assessing disorganized speech or formal thought disorder, we ask simple and complex open-ended questions that allow the patient to talk uninterrupted for at least five minutes. Because many patients might oppose a request to tape-record their responses, the clinician

should consider whether it is worth asking the patient to do this. If you feel that the question might jeopardize rapport or contribute to the patient's uneasiness, suspicion, or mistrust, then dispense with such a request – do not tape record.

4. Careful observation is the best interview method for assessing abnormal and disorganized behavior.
5. Negative symptoms are best assessed by focusing on the two subcategories of adverse symptomatology: restricted emotional range and avolition. Here, again, we carefully observe the patient's flexibility and range of affect, as well as her ability to initiate and engage in reciprocal communication.
6. Assessing cognitive deficits is the domain of performance testing. The best interview method for assessing cognitive impairment is to use standardized cognitive screening measures.
7. In assessing the degree of depression, the interviewer listens for evidence of a persistently depressed mood and anhedonia. As noted previously, distinguishing depression from negative symptoms and cognitive impairment can be tricky. Unlike negative symptoms, depression typically includes more dysphoric ideation and emotions such as pessimism, hopelessness, guilt, or self-deprecation.
8. In assessing the past episodes of mania and hypomania, the interviewer must focus on the presence of mood episodes in combination with a heightened energy level and a persistent increase in goal-directed activity.
9. Clinicians should adopt a respectful, compassionate, and understanding attitude – neither acting overly friendly nor reserved – with no desire to change the patient.

8

ASSESSING PSYCHOTIC PHENOMENA WITH PSYCHOLOGICAL TESTS

Testing also affords a good view of psychological functioning because it requires patients to "display" a variety of ego functions, not merely to "describe" ego functioning as they might do during interviews (Miller, 1987, p. 507). Readers are directed to a comprehensive review of the psychological assessment of disordered thinking and perception, which is a key component of assessing psychosis (Weiner & Kleiger, 2021).

At this point, readers might ask, "Why test?" We have seen how the clinical interview can be an incisive diagnostic instrument. When symptom dimensions are understood conceptually, we can tailor our interview questions more specifically to assess and elicit psychotic symptoms. So, under what conditions should patients be referred for psychological testing, and with which patients might it be most useful? In other words, what can testing tell us that we cannot discern from a skilled clinical interview? To answer these questions, it is necessary to begin with a discussion about the nature, purpose, and methods of psychodiagnostic or psychological assessment.

The Nature and Purpose of Psychodiagnostic Testing

Psychodiagnostic assessment is inherently multi-methodological. Multi-method assessment is critical in the assessment of disordered thinking and perceptual anomalies (Bornstein, 2021; Mihura & Starin, 2023). For example, in addition to conducting a clinical interview, assessors administer a range of reliable and valid measures to a patient in response to identified referral questions. Testing is most effective when used to address specific questions related to diagnostic understanding and treatment planning. Diagnostic understanding may extend far beyond diagnostic labeling to include formulations about the structure and dynamics of the individual's personality. This perspective has been recently amplified in Bram and Peebles' excellent work on the value of psychological testing (2014).

DOI: 10.4324/9781003415206-12

Three response dimensions are important to consider when conducting a psychological assessment. First, we pay particular attention to formal test scores. Formal scores are objective, quantifiable representations of test performance that can be compared to appropriate normative groups. Second, we listen not just for the content of a patient's responses but also for the themes that are conveyed in their responses. Finally, as examiners, we understand that the unfolding nature of the relationship between the patient and examiner can be a rich source of qualitative information about the intersubjective and interpersonal dimensions of personality functioning.

Selecting a range of instruments, as opposed to just one test, to assess an individual with psychotic features remains the first task of the assessing clinician. It goes without saying that we must utilize empirically valid instruments with proven psychometric characteristics that have been based on samples not unlike the patients we are evaluating. The next step involves deciding which instruments to include in our battery: neurocognitive instruments, objective tests, self-report measures, personality inventories, or performance and projective techniques.

Psychological or Neuropsychological Assessment?

Should a patient presenting with psychotic features receive a psychological or neuropsychological evaluation? The answer depends on what we are seeking to learn about the patient. Psychological evaluations focus on affect and mood, representations of self and others, relational style, perception, judgment, reality-testing, concept formation, abstract thinking, reasoning, and insight. Psychological assessment can address basic questions concerning whether the patient might be vulnerable to psychosis, the severity of his symptoms, and under what conditions his thinking and reality-testing might be most compromised. Additionally, we can determine tolerance of affect, capacities to establish meaningful relationships, and the extent to which he is able to form a therapeutic alliance. A skilled psychological assessment can contribute to a differential diagnosis; however, without sufficient history and information about the duration of symptoms, it may not be able to establish a DSM-5 diagnosis of a specific psychotic disorder.

In contrast, neuropsychological testing assesses cognitive functions such as working and semantic memory, attention, executive functioning, processing speed, verbal fluency, and social cognition, to name but a few (Yalof, 2021). As noted in Chapter 5, neuropsychological evaluations help identify the degree of cognitive impairment associated with psychotic symptoms and assist with planning for treatment and cognitive rehabilitation (Reichenberg et al., 2009).

Both types of evaluations have their place in the assessment of psychosis. In a broad sense, psychological assessment may tell us more about the person with the psychosis, whereas the neuropsychological evaluation may provide more detailed information about the degree of impairment in specific areas of cognitive functioning.

Self-Report Measures: Multi-Scale Personality Inventories

Personality inventories provide a systematic way for a patient to present her symptom complaints, depict key aspects of her behavioral, social, and emotional functioning, and respond to questions about her thinking, beliefs, and perceptions. However, with the patient who may be experiencing psychotic symptoms, self-report instruments have limitations. Psychosis may interfere with the abilities of some patients to focus and concentrate sufficiently in order to read and comprehend test items.

Personality inventories such as the MMPI-2 (Butcher et al., 1989; Nichols, 2021; Tarescavage & Selbom, 2021), the MMPI-3 (Ben-Porath & Tellegen, 2020), and PAI (Morey, 1991; McCredie et al., 2021) are among the most popular instruments used in the context of clinical diagnostic assessment with patients referred for evaluation of psychosis. Each instrument has multiple scales and subscales designed to assess psychotic phenomena. Not only do these multi-scale inventories yield a great deal of information about symptom and personality functioning, but, unlike most symptom-based rating scales, they include a set of validity scales designed to assess response variables that may affect validity. Validity scales help the examiner identify test-taking characteristics such as symptom exaggeration, excessive denial, or inconsistent and random responding, which may affect the validity of the results.

Examination of validity scales is particularly important in the assessment of patients referred for evaluation of psychosis. It is not uncommon for patients to remain guarded about, or patently deny, their hallucinations or delusions for fear they will be hospitalized without the possibility of discharge if they endorse their psychotic symptoms in clinical interviews or on self-report inventories. In such cases, the patient may not endorse any items suggestive of psychopathology, not to mention psychotic symptoms, on personality inventories. We may, however, view elevations on validity scales as an indication that the patient is under-reporting or denying his symptoms. This finding will alert the treatment team to obtain collateral information before making a clinical decision.

Performance Measures: Direct Assessment of Functioning

Unlike objective testing measures, performance-based methods reflect what an individual does rather than what she, or a third-party rater, can or decides to tell us. Miller (1987) compared methods of inquiry and noted that when individuals respond to the performance requirements of the testing situation, they display their ego-functioning, behavioral, and response potentials. We are interested in what patients, their family members, and other raters tell us; however, comprehensive assessment remains incomplete without an assessment of functioning based on actual performance measures. In essence, performance testing tells us what a patient cannot.

Performance measures include a wide range of testing procedures in which what the patient does is as important, if not more so, than what he says. For example, it is one thing to ask someone about his memory, reality-testing, and ability to think in an organized manner and form mature concepts; it is another matter to assess these functions directly by having the person engage in a performance task constructed to measure these variables. In some performance tasks, the instructions given to the individual are clear, and the object of the task is apparent. Nearly all neurocognitive instruments are based on a standard and explicit set of instructions that specify what the person must do to perform the task. Thus, the individual is provided with a structured problem-solving task, which is presented with clear-cut directions and expectations. Other sets of performance measures are based on briefer, open-ended, and more opaque instructions. Typically referred to as "projective tests," these instruments present individuals with an ambiguous stimulus and, with little direction, ask them to respond. "Projective testing" is no longer the preferred term because it is thought to minimize the cognitive and perceptual problem-solving aspects of these procedures.

Although a variety of performance-based and projective procedures may be useful in assessing aspects of psychosis (Kleiger, 2003), the best example of a projective performance test for addressing questions about the potential for psychotic functioning is the Rorschach Inkblot Method. The patient is handed ten inkblots, one at a time, and asked little more than "What might this be?" Due to its unstructured and ambiguous nature, the Rorschach is uniquely suited for assessing a patient's thought organization and reality testing. It has a long history of use as a psychodiagnostic instrument in the assessment of psychosis and thought disorder (in particular, Rorschach, 1921/1942; Rapaport et al., 1946; Johnston & Holzman, 1979; Solovay et al., 1987; Holzman et al., 2005; Kleiger,

1999, 2017; Kleiger & Mihura, 2021; Weiner, 2021; Meyer & Mihura, 2021). Rorschach himself had a great deal of experience working with psychotic patients and identified response patterns that were characteristic of these patients. Rapaport and his colleagues elaborated on ways in which the Rorschach could identify disturbances in thinking as evidenced by the patient's verbalizations on the test. Holzman and his group (Johnston & Holzman, 1979; Solovay et al., 1987; Holzman et al., 2005) operationalized Rapaport's Rorschach measures of disturbed thinking and developed a psychometrically robust instrument – the Thought Disorder Index (TDI) – that not only advanced the assessment of thought disorder but contributed to an understanding of the nature of thought disorder and its differential manifestations in different psychotic groups of adults and children (Holzman et al., 2005).

Mihura demonstrated in her meta-analysis of Rorschach research that the Rorschach indicators of psychosis, particularly thought disorder and impaired reality testing, were extremely robust (Mihura et al., 2013). Finally, even those who have been staunch critics of the Rorschach have acknowledged the solid empirical basis for using the Rorschach to assess psychotic phenomena (Wood et al., 2003). According to this group of stalwart Rorschach critics, who called for a moratorium on the clinical use of the test, "A few Rorschach scores are useful for the evaluation of thought disorder . . . For this reason, they can provide useful information for the diagnosis of schizophrenia, bipolar disorder, borderline personality disorder and schizotypal personality disorder" (Wood et al., 2003, p. 259).

Two studies compared composites from the Comprehensive System (CS) and R-PAS for assessing disordered thinking and perception in international samples (Taiwan and Serbia) of psychotic individuals (Dzamonja-Ignjatovic et al., 2013; Su et al., 2015). Both studies demonstrated that R-PAS performed better than the CS in measuring key aspects of disordered thinking and perception. Additionally, these studies showed the adaptability of R-PAS in a multi-cultural, international setting.

The Value of Testing Psychotic Patients

We now turn to the questions of when to test and whom to test, addressing them from three different perspectives:

- Testing to provide clarity in cases of diagnostic ambiguity.
- Testing to tell us what a patient cannot.
- Testing to help establish a baseline of functioning in first-episode psychoses.

Testing to Address Diagnostic Ambiguity: Am I Missing Something?

Consider the following patient, referred by his psychiatrist, who had been treating him for social anxiety and OCD:

Mark had shared his intrusive thoughts about violent sexual assaults, which entered his mind in an unbidden manner, causing a great deal of distress and prompting him to engage in ritualistic washing to manage his intrusive ideas. The therapist understood these symptoms as manifestations of severe OCD. However, when Mark began talking about how his body was filled with "cloudy vapors" and about his urge to "cut them out" of him, his psychiatrist became concerned that something else might be going on and questioned if Mark might be psychotic.

This vignette is typical of the patients we see in our diagnostic consultations, individuals being treated by competent colleagues for conditions they thought they had understood diagnostically. However, the patient's puzzling behavior and lack of response to treatment often raise new questions about the diagnosis.

In some cases, psychological testing provides a more sensitive measure of an individual's difficulties than can be determined from a face-to-face interview. For example, we may know from therapy sessions that our patient is somewhat guarded and suspicious; however, testing may be a more finely tuned measure of the extent of her suspiciousness and the conditions under which her suspicions become more clearly paranoid, potentially jeopardizing the treatment alliance.

Testing to Tell Us Things that the Patient Cannot

Although a clinical interview may be a more direct way to assess the presence of hallucinations and delusions, testing methods have been shown to be powerful tools for assessing a patient's thought organization, reality testing, and cognitive functioning. These are implicit aspects of functioning that are more difficult for us to observe and for patients to talk about themselves in objective and quantifiable ways. Disorganized speech might be apparent from our clinical interviews, but errors in reasoning, concept formation, and abstract thinking most often need to be demonstrated in an individual's task performance. Similarly, aspects of executive functioning such as verbal fluency, processing speed, working memory, and cognitive flexibility are best captured by an individual's performance on testing procedures. Ratings of an individual's processing and executive functioning by parents and teachers are invaluable; however, they are not substitutes for direct assessment of these functions on cognitive–neuropsychological tests.

Testing to Establish a Baseline in First-Episode Psychosis

Establishing a baseline of cognitive and psychological functioning after an individual has suffered his first psychotic episode may not be able to provide a definitive differential diagnosis, but it can yield important information for developing treatment and rehabilitation plans. For example, testing can delineate intellectual strengths and weaknesses, ego functions such as reality-testing, self-reflection, synthetic capacities, fluid reasoning, and capacities to empathize and mentalize, which are relevant to treatment planning.

Likewise, neuropsychological testing after the psychotic symptoms have been effectively treated can highlight areas of residual cognitive impairment that might affect prognosis and social and occupational adaptation. In fact, the DSM-5 Psychosis Work Group recommended neuropsychological assessment for psychotic patients in order to understand the extent of cognitive impairment for treatment planning and rehabilitative efforts. They emphasized that clinical interviews and self-report methods are less sensitive to the types of impairment observed in patients who have schizophrenia. When a full neuropsychological evaluation cannot be obtained, Barch and colleagues (2013) recommend using briefer batteries of tests for cognitive impairment. The RBANS (Gold et al., 1999; Hobart et al., 1999) is one such screening, which has been shown to be a useful measure for assessing cognitive status and prognosis in patients with schizophrenia.

The Effects of Medication on Testing Indices of Psychosis

Mental health professionals considering referring a potentially psychotic patient for psychological testing often ask whether the individual should be tested when off medication. Clearly, the need to begin an acutely psychotic and agitated patient on medication trumps the value of waiting until the person can be scheduled for testing. However, just as neuroleptic medication has an effect on reducing positive symptoms, so does it reduce indications of more florid signs of thought disorder on psychological testing. Several studies found that thought disorder scores on the Rorschach, as measured by the TDI, decreased over the course of treatment with antipsychotic medication (Hurt et al., 1983; Spohn et al., 1986). The most severe signs of thought disorder and gross distortions of reality were most likely to be reduced or eliminated; however, residual, less dramatic indications of thought pathology were found to persist (Gold & Hurt, 1990).

Contrary to these findings, a team of Italian researchers demonstrated that Rorschach composites sensitive to disordered thinking and perception (reality testing) were not significantly affected by antipsychotic medication (Biagiarelli et al., 2015). Thus, the data are somewhat contradictory. The TDI and Italian studies showed that essential markers of disordered thinking and perception were not appreciatively affected when subjects were tested on antipsychotics, while other research indicated a decrease in the severity of coding for such markers.

Psychodiagnostic Assessment of Dimensions of Psychosis

We focus now on the psychological testing methods that are useful for assessing psychotic phenomena. Instead of cataloging various testing instruments, we follow a similar format to the one established in Chapter 7 and organize recommended testing procedures according to the different symptom dimensions described by both the DSM-5 group (Barch et al., 2013; Heckers et al., 2013) and the Reininghaus et al. (2013) study. Although this organizational format establishes a link to the preceding chapter on interviewing, it differs somewhat from the eight dimensions described in Chapter 7. The slight variation is a product of the inherent differences in the nature of clinical interviewing and psychological testing. For example, whereas it makes sense to assess hallucinations and delusions separately in the process of a clinical interview, it makes more sense to collapse them into a single positive-symptom dimension for psychological testing, as the Reininghaus study did. Additionally, while the dimension of disorganized speech is a relevant target for interview assessment, we broaden this dimension for the purposes of psychological assessment to *cognitive disorganization*, which will allow us to examine underlying conceptual problems and errors in reasoning. The resulting list of seven domains for presenting test findings includes the assessment of:

- Positive symptoms
- Cognitive disorganization and errors in reasoning
- Disorganized and abnormal psychomotor behavior
- Negative symptoms
- Cognitive impairment
- Depression
- Mania

In addition, we include a discussion of the assessment of insight, self-reflection, and aspects of social cognition. Although not considered an independent dimension or factor of psychosis, insight is an important variable that has treatment and prognostic implications.

For those readers interested in more specific details about which test scales and indices are associated with symptom dimensions, we have prepared a series of tables in Appendix A. The information in the tables includes the names or symbols for the scales and subscales that have been empirically or conceptually linked with the dimensions under consideration. The list is not intended to be exhaustive nor to promote a sign approach to test interpretation. Instead, we offer it as a starting point for clinicians to organize and think conceptually about psychological testing variables according to the empirically derived dimensions of psychotic symptomatology.

Before presenting test variables associated with different dimensions of psychotic experience, it is important to state that no single scale, subscale, or scoring variable is pathognomic of general psychosis or any particular symptom or dimension of psychosis. Although all of the scoring variables presented in the following sections are empirically valid measures, many testing scores and scales are associated with multiple dimensions. For example, the MMPI-3 Scale *PSYC-R* (Psychoticism-Revised) may be an indicator of general psychosis, the presence of positive symptoms, or simply a proneness to psychosis in an individual who is currently not psychotic. Furthermore, many of the scoring variables described here might suggest the presence of actual psychotic symptoms when they reach a certain level of severity or psychotic-like phenomena in other personality disorders when they occur at lower levels of severity. The essential point is that multiple sources of data (i.e., history, interview material, and multiple test variables from inventories and performance measures) are necessary for making diagnostic inferences. Multiple methods of assessment, yielding convergent data points, are the standard of practice for competent psychodiagnostic inference-making.

Positive Symptoms

We focus on testing variables that provide support for the presence of two prominent dimensions of positive symptomatology:

- Hallucinations
- Delusions

Hallucinations

Psychological testing instruments may be less useful in the assessment of hallucinatory experiences. Although patients may acknowledge hallucinations on personality inventories such as the MMPI-2, MMPI-2-RF, MMPI-3. and PAI, affirmative responses are binary in nature and do not allow for assessment of the patient's capacity to test the reality of their reported hallucinatory experiences. As with affirmative responses on critical items pertaining to delusional beliefs, we encourage evaluators to ask follow-up questions about the various aspects of the patient's endorsement of hallucinations. In this regard, the clinician can follow the guidelines laid out in the previous chapter on clinical interviewing to gain a more detailed understanding of the nature and characteristics of the reported hallucinatory experience.

Although the Rorschach is a test of thinking and perception, there are no empirically based indices for identifying hallucinations. At best, the Rorschach may reveal a perceptual predisposition for hallucinatory experience. For example, a high number of Form Quality minus (FQ–) responses could be a test equivalent of pseudo perceptions. Form-level percentage, considered an index of reality-testing, refers to the perceptual fit or how well the patient's responses match the reality of the inkblot contours and conform to what other people typically see. Thus, when someone gives an FQ– response, she is seeing something that has little or no basis in reference to the actual form features or reality of the inkblot. FQ– responses indicate that the individual is distorting her interpretation of the stimulus – in effect, seeing something that is not there. The problem is that FQ– responses are not specific to psychosis and certainly are not indicative of hallucinatory experience. These responses occur in a broad range of nonpsychotic conditions, signaling lapses in judgment and accuracy of impressions. However, when the FQ– percentage is extremely elevated, and other psychotic features are present, it is reasonable to infer that the individual may demonstrate positive symptoms that may conceivably include hallucinations.

Delusions

The MMPI-3, MMPI-2-RF, and PAI all have scales, subscales, and critical items pertaining to delusional thinking. Most of the items on these scales contain explicit questions regarding the subject's direct experience of delusional beliefs. Although these items do not capture all types of delusion, the advantage of self-report items is that they may provide an opportunity for the psychotic patient to endorse a delusional belief. When patients endorse items suggestive of delusions, it is important to inquire, after the fact, what they meant by this endorsement. As advocated in Chapter 7, we maintain a curious and respectful stance and ask open-ended questions, encouraging the patient to "tell us more" about his response. A brief inquiry into positive responses is critical in determining how the patient interpreted the item and what he meant by his response. For example, consider this example: Mr. P. endorsed a critical item from a personality inventory pertaining to the experience that someone was controlling his thoughts. When asked to say more about this, he explained how his mother was always trying to convince him to change his attitude about his schoolwork and spend more time studying.

The Rorschach cannot directly assess the presence of delusional beliefs. However, it can provide indirect information about the patient's cognitive–perceptual style of processing information, his preoccupations and possible fears, and his errors in reasoning that may, under certain conditions, give rise to delusional beliefs. For example, an excessive focus on small and unusual details of the inkblot may reflect an idiosyncratic perceptual style in which the individual hyper-attends or searches for difficult-to-see aspects of the stimulus. Various combinations of scoring variables constitute a composite measure of suspiciousness, guardedness, and possible paranoia. Response content reflecting themes of danger, protection, scrutiny, judgment, and external control may also suggest a high degree of suspiciousness or paranoia.

Additionally, individuals who use an incidental detail of the inkblot to justify an entire response, regardless of the adequacy of perceptual fit with the contours of the inkblot, are engaging in an ideational process called *jumping to conclusions*, described by Garety et al. (2011). According to these authors, substantial research exists that demonstrates a response bias that underlies the presence of delusional beliefs. Thus, when a subject looks at Card III of the Rorschach and responds, "It must be a heart because it's on the right side of the blot," the patient is justifying this response on the basis of a single, incidental detail. In jumping to conclusions, she is also ignoring other possibilities (e.g., additional details on the right side of the inkblot, the many other things the detail on which she focused could have been, as well as other aspects of the inkblot that do not fit with her percept of a heart). Furthermore, there is the inappropriate conviction and certainty with which she responded that "it must be a heart." In this single response, we have the cognitive underpinnings for the formation of a delusional belief. This is not to say that this type of response indicates the presence of a delusion. It is nothing more than a marker of a particular kind of reasoning process that, under sufficient stress, may produce a delusional belief.

Cognitive Disorganization

As we have indicated, psychological assessment lends itself to a broader definition of the dimension that the DSM-5 Psychosis Work Group labeled "Disorganized Speech." In their factor-analytic study of the PANSS, the Reininghaus group (2013) study found that PANSS items loading high on their Disorganization Dimension had to do with

- Conceptual disorganization
- Difficulties in abstract thinking

- Stereotyped thinking
- Mannerisms and posturing
- Disorientation
- Poor attention
- Preoccupation

This broader definition of cognitive disorganization is consistent with our discussion of thought disorder in Chapter 2.

To simplify matters and adapt research findings to the process of psychological testing, we group symptoms of cognitive disorganization into two domains:

- Disorganized speech resulting from impaired focusing and filtering.
- Errors in conceptual thinking and reasoning.

Disorganized Speech: Focusing, Filtering, and Self-Monitoring Problems

Impairment in focusing and attention has long been studied by psychosis researchers (Braff, 1993). Difficulties with attentional focusing, controlling and filtering irrelevant associations, working memory, and self-monitoring may make one's speech loose and disorganized. Failure to monitor whether sufficient cohesion between one's ideas interferes with discourse organization and disrupts coherence. The results are the kinds of formal thought disorder that Andreasen (1979) described as derailment, tangentiality, and distractible speech.

Although personality inventories include scales and subscales constructed to address thought disorder, we believe this is a complex and multifaceted symptom that does not lend itself well to assessment by self-report. Nonetheless, in Appendix A, we list some of the scales and subscales from personality inventories purported to measure aspects of cognitive disorganization.

A broad range of neuropsychological measures are available to assess components of attentional focusing, working memory, and self-monitoring that may pertain to disorganized, derailed, and distractible speech. Tests of attention should include measures of focusing and screening out irrelevant internal and external distractions, as well as sustaining and controlling attention. Tests of working memory provide measures of how well an individual can hold relevant topic information in mind as he engages in conversational discourse. Finally, the assessment of self-monitoring gauges how aware an individual is of his behavior, including what he is saying and doing.

For the Rorschach and other performance tests, we focus on responses that reveal disruptions in focusing and filtering that might result in the emergence of off-track and inappropriate verbalizations (Kleiger, 1999, 2017; Kleiger & Mihura, 2021; Mihura & Starin, 2023). Focusing and filtering problems on the Rorschach may take the form of intrusive or loose associations that stray from the individual's response to an inkblot. The instructions on the Rorschach are to respond to the question "What might this be?" and not to associate freely with the blot. Thus, the object of the task is to remain focused on the inkblot stimulus and not stray from it. The following example shows an individual's difficulty in maintaining focus and an appropriate cognitive filter, which results in a loose, rambling response that leads the subject away from the task. Response to Card V:

> This looks like a bat . . . My uncle shot one in his backyard. I really hate bats, but I'm told they are good for the environment, which has all sorts of problems with air pollution. The government really needs to do something about all of this stuff. The leaking of all these classified documents is what happens when the government loses control over what is put in the air.

In wandering away from the task and his initial response, the respondent demonstrated an abrupt derailment in his thinking as he loosely hopped the rails from his initial response of a "bat" to his "uncle" to the "environment," "air pollution," and then abruptly to the "leaking of classified documents." Remember, this patient's wandering response was prompted by the simple question of "What might this be?" when handed Card V. In this example of disorganized speech, the patient had great difficulty staying focused, maintaining a task-specific response set, filtering out information that was highly irrelevant to the task, and monitoring the inappropriateness of his response to the instructions.

Listening for oddities in verbalization in subjects' responses to Wechsler subtests is another useful way to assess thought organization and verbalization. For example, administering the comprehension subtest in current editions of the WAIS-IV and WISC-IV often yields mini-speech samples, which may reveal problems in focusing, filtering, and discourse coherence. Here, the test-taker is invited to respond to an open-ended question that assesses common sense, judgment, and attunement to social reality and also determines the ability to screen out irrelevancies and organize one's verbalizations. The following example illustrates how the respondent struggled to stay focused and organized while screening out competing ideas when asked a question about the importance of keeping a promise: "Promising is between two people who vow to uphold a contract, like when you get married and pick out rings for each other. And when you plan a wedding, you commit to invite the same people." Clearly, peripheral, less relevant associations to the word "promise" resulted in a highly discursive and confusing verbalization that moved the person far away from the question, which was never really answered.

Errors in Reasoning: Conceptual and Abstract Thinking Problems

As with disorganized speech, self-report inventories are less suited for identifying specific idiosyncrasies in reasoning and abstract thinking. At best, the MMPI-2, MMPI-3, and PAI may provide crude measures of errors in reasoning and confusion. However, to understand the underpinnings of an individual's capacity to reason in appropriate and realistic ways, we need to utilize performance measures that provide an opportunity for the person to show us how he reasons. The Rorschach is a wonderful technique for eliciting errors in thinking and reasoning. Subjects may reveal their errors in reasoning by inappropriately generalizing, combining details and concepts, or basing their conclusions on irrelevant details (Weiner, 1966). In some cases, their responses to the inkblots will be overly vague and inappropriately abstract and, in others, too concrete.

Some individuals reveal their erroneous reasoning on the Rorschach by infusing their responses with an inappropriate level of detail and elaboration. In this case, the subject does not *wander away* from the inkblot task, as does the tangential or distractible patient, but, instead, becomes *immersed* in it. For example, 16-year-old Eddie saw Card VII this way:

> It looks like two women from different cultures. They are the same but different. You can tell that they come from the same background but have gone their separate ways. Their looks and postures indicate that they have hostile intentions, plotting revenge against each other. Or maybe both are trying to get the same man who they fell in love with. But he probably chose one or the other, and now they are trying to settle the score.

In responding to the Rorschach instructions, Eddie engaged in excessive and inappropriate elaboration. He overinterpreted and drew inferences that could not be supported by any of the objective features of the inkblot itself. This form of reasoning error is commonly referred to as *confabulation* because the subject adds an inappropriate amount of detail and an unjustifiable degree of specificity that extends far beyond anything evident in the reality of the stimulus.

Failure to maintain boundaries between different concepts may appear as an incompatible combination of images that violate the constraints of reality. In some cases, separate concepts are inappropriately combined, while each concept retains its separate identity. For example, the response *people with bird heads* inappropriately integrates two concepts (people and bird heads) into a single response. Bizarre combinations of images (e.g., *a bat with landing gear*) or images and actions (e.g., *a man shedding his skin*) are so peculiar that they suggest underlying psychotic-level reasoning.

In other cases, the collapse of conceptual boundaries is more extreme, resulting in a confusing condensation. An example of this more severe collapse of conceptual boundaries would be the response, "It all looks like an island, but this looks like a spot of blood. So it could be bloody islands where all the wars have been." The collapse of conceptual boundaries in this example is between an island and a spot of blood. In this response, the subject has merged two separate concepts into a single area of the inkblot. This kind of response, referred to as *contamination*, is viewed as a serious sign of disordered thinking.

Some Rorschach responses may also be inappropriately abstract or distant from the stimulus features of the inkblot. For example, here is what one respondent said that Card VIII looked like: "This is the creation of the world. The colors symbolize creation, sky, earth, and hell. Evolution of the species from the primordial ooze to the upright form of modern mankind." Those familiar with the Rorschach know that Card VIII looks nothing like this. The subject responsible for this response has used the card as a stimulus for concepts that are inappropriately abstract and removed from the reality of the stimulus.

Projective storytelling tests such as the Thematic Apperception Test (TAT) and Children's Apperception Test (CAT) can elicit both focusing and filtering problems, as well as inappropriate reasoning and inference-making (Teglasi, 2021; Jenkins, 2023). For example, nine-year-old Shelly, referred because her teachers were concerned about her behavior with other students, told the following story about the first card of the CAT, which shows three little children sitting at a table. Shelly said that the children were hungry and looking for food. They left their house and found a big apple walking toward them:

> The apple said, "Hi, my name is Ronnie." One of the kids asked if he could eat him, and the apple said, "No, but I'll show you where there is a cave." In the cave, they found a purple frog and a big green, red, and golden bird, and an orange toad that were shooting blue dots at the cave, which made blotches all around the wall. The snow was coming in, and it was summertime. The baby ran outside and said, "What is wrong? Why is it snowing?" Then, he saw the frog, bird, and toad costumes on the ground, so he said they were all just faking. They all went looking for them and found a weird girl named "Lockbeard." The baby then tried to pull off her face, and she said, "What are you doing?" The children apologized and returned to her house, where they saw

> pictures of frogs shooting blue darts, which they didn't like. So, they all ran home.

Although the instructions for the TAT and CAT ask the respondent to "make up a story with a beginning, middle, and ending," Shelly went well beyond the task instructions and told a story that was highly embellished, illogical, and mildly incoherent. She introduced fantastic, unseen characters (a talking apple and colored animals), which were engaged in odd actions ("shooting blue dots at the cave"). She abruptly shifted to seemingly unrelated ideas (snowing and finding animal costumes that implied that they were all faking) and finally introduced another random unseen character named Lockbeard, whose face one of the original characters tried to pull off.

Researchers and clinicians have used other psychodiagnostic instruments to measure concept formation and verbal reasoning. Object-sorting tests (Vygotsky, 1962; Goldstein, 1939; Goldstein & Scheerer, 1941; Hanfmann & Kasanin, 1942) and proverbs tests (Benjamin, 1944; Gorham, 1956) have been used to measure concreteness and overinclusion, two of the early concepts that were viewed as central deficits in schizophrenic thought disorder. Marengo et al. (1986) constructed a comprehensive measure of bizarre–idiosyncratic thinking based on two brief verbal tests, the Gorham Proverbs Test (Gorham, 1956) and the comprehension subtest of the WAIS (Wechsler, 1955), which were shown to be reliable measures of the presence, severity, and type of disordered thinking.

Abnormal Psychomotor Behavior

Bizarre and abnormal psychomotor behavior are best assessed through observation of the patient during the process of testing. As noted in Chapter 7, we pay close attention to how the patient looks, dresses, walks, behaves, and interacts during the testing process. Thus, hygiene, attire, gait, eye contact, posture, and movement are all sources of observational data that will inform our assessment.

In addition to these parameters of behavior, we observe how a patient handles and responds to the testing instructions and the testing materials. For example, when instructed to begin a test, does the patient readily comply, or does he sit motionless and stare at you? Or, when given a Rorschach card, does the patient take and hold it as instructed, or does she remain mute and unresponsive when you prompt her to take the card? Additionally, does the patient do anything bizarre or unusual with the testing stimuli? For example, one patient accepted Card II, stared at it, and promptly sniffed it. Similarly, when handed Card I, another patient abruptly jumped out of his chair because he saw a bat flying directly toward him.

Negative Symptoms

Recall from Chapter 2 how, in their reviews of factor-analytic studies of negative symptoms, both the DSM-5 Psychosis Work Group (Barch et al., 2013) and Kirkpatrick (2014) summarized findings that identified two distinct domains of negative symptoms:

- Restricted emotional expression
- Avolition, asociality, and anhedonia

In keeping with this distinction, we organize psychological tests, scales, and scoring variables according to these two components of the negative symptoms dimension.

Flat and Diminished Expression of Affect

While flat affect is an observable aspect of the patient's mental status, personality inventories offer a variety of scales and subscales that assess aspects of flat affect and emotional withdrawal. On the Rorschach, reduced affectivity may be represented in terms of an absence of color as a determining factor in one's responses. How an individual attends to and uses – as opposed to ignores – color on the inkblots is associated with the processing of emotional stimuli. Thus, the absence of color in a Rorschach record suggests a lack of emotional spontaneity and a general avoidance of the emotional aspects of experience.

Avolition, Asociality, and Anhedonia

The MMPI-2, MMPI-2-RF, MMPI-3, and PAI also have scales and subscales pertaining to this subdomain of negative symptomatology. Thus, specific scales reflect anhedonia, apathy, and lack of initiative and will. Additional scales focus on social avoidance, indifference, withdrawal, and detachment.

Manifestations of avolition on the performance measures may include test responses that reflect impoverished verbalization, including short and contracted answers with minimal elaboration. One might also detect longer, rambling responses that reflect a poverty of meaning. For example, on the Rorschach, subjects may become overly vague when describing what they see in the card or express a sense of confusion or perplexity as they try to make sense out of the inkblot in response to the standard instruction, "What might this be?" Simple, linear responses that ignore possible relationships between aspects of the inkblot may reflect diminished mental energy and a lack of engagement with the complexity of the inkblot. Such simple responses to single aspects of the blot may reflect limited synthetic capacity or interest in the interactive nature of experience.

Finally, the absence of human content among one's responses on the Rorschach may suggest asociality or a diminished interest in people, oneself, or relationships. Thus, an absence of human representation can be taken as a possible sign of social disengagement or avoidance.

Cognitive Impairment

Assessing cognitive impairment is a core function of neuropsychological testing. Deficits in intellectual and executive functioning, verbal learning, fluency, processing speed, concept formation, and flexibility may be associated with psychosis. Intellectual functioning is best assessed with Wechsler tests of intelligence, including the WISC-V (Wechsler, 2014) and WAIS-IV (Wechsler, 2008), which have sub-tests measuring processing speed and working memory. The Woodcock-Johnson-IV Tests of Cognitive Abilities (Schrank et al., 2014) also include a range of subtests measuring verbal fluency and working memory. Earlier in the chapter, we mentioned the RBANS (Gold et al., 1999; Hobart et al., 1999), a battery that screens for cognitive impairment in schizophrenia.

Concreteness, being stimulus-bound, perseveration, stereotyped responses, and cognitive rigidity are all characteristics of impaired cognition, which can be evident through many testing procedures. Patients may exhibit concrete thinking, rigidity, and perseveration on measures of concept formation and abstract thinking. Patients who offer the same response (e.g., "It's a bug") to each of the Rorschach inkblots may be demonstrating a rigid, inflexible cognitive set, which leads to response perseveration. Perseverative responses on the Rorschach may reflect rigidity and problems relinquishing a particular idea. Patients who give perseverated responses such as "It's a bug" or something similar for many of the cards often are unable to shift sets and respond to the cognitive demands of the task.

Although perseverative responses may reflect defensiveness and resistance to engage in the test, they can also be products of deficits in one's ability to think in a representational manner. The Rorschach is a representational task. When handed the blots, the subjects must make a symbolic interpretation. Hence, the instruction given to the patient is always, "What might this be?" rather than "What is this a picture of?". Individuals who demonstrate cognitive deficits do not grasp the interpretative nature of the task. Instead, they respond to the task in a more concrete manner. Concrete responses on the Rorschach are described as "stimulus-bound," as subjects take the inkblot as a literal stimulus to be recognized as opposed to a symbolic stimulus to interpreted. Concrete responses reflect what has been termed a "loss of abstract attitude" (Goldstein & Scheerer, 1941). Examples of overly concrete responses include the following:

Card II. "Looks like it could be a fly, but it is way too big to be a fly. It is about the size of a sparrow."
Card VII. "This must be the North Pole up here because it is on the top of the card."

Depression

Personality-assessment instruments are valid means of identifying the dimension of depression, which may or may not be present in the person suffering from psychosis. Personality inventories and rating scales are frequently used instruments for identifying aspects of depressive symptomatology. As specified in Chapter 7, depression is conceived in terms of three components:

- Cognitive
- Affective
- Physiological

Major personality inventories have multiple scales and subscales that address each aspect of depressive experience (Kleiger & Weiner, 2023).

Indications of cognitive correlates of depression on the Rorschach include a lower number of responses, a higher percentage of form-based responses, and, possibly, expressions of incompetence (e.g., "I just can't see anything – I'm not very good at this"). Test variables suggesting depressive affect include diminished use of color and attention to achromatic color (black and gray) in determining one's response. Thematically, responses reflecting damaged and broken contents (e.g., a butterfly with broken wings), along with attributions of sadness or dysphoria (e.g., a sad-looking face), may represent an outward manifestation of depressive experience. Finally, Rorschach responses given after a long delay and spoken in a slow, halting manner with frequent sighs may reflect fatigue and diminished energy and drive.

Mania

Mania can be deconstructed into several components (Kleiger & Weiner, 2023). The Reininghaus et al. study (2013) showed loading of excitement, hostility, uncooperativeness, and poor impulse control on the mania-symptoms dimension. Grandiosity is generally considered another aspect of mania; however, it also loaded on the positive-symptom dimension in the Reininghaus study. For our purposes, we consider test correlates of four overlapping subdomains of the mania dimension:

- Activation
- Irritability
- Expansiveness and grandiosity
- Disinhibition and dyscontrol

Activation

Numerous scales and subscales on personality inventories measure different aspects of mania and hypomania, including increased arousal, hyperactivity, lability, and pressure to act instead of think (Selbom & Whitman, 2023; McCredie et al., 2023). An increased number of responses on the Rorschach may occur in the context of hypomanic acceleration. Ideas come quickly, the subject speaks rapidly, and the examiner may have difficulty keeping up. Colored cards may elicit more responses as the patient's ideas and associations are activated by the evocativeness of the stimuli.

Irritability

Irritability and hostility are captured on myriad combinations of scales and subscales on the MMPI-2, MMPI-3, and PAI. Elevations on these scales suggest a propensity toward impatience, anger, hostility, and explosive behavior.

Rorschach indications of manic and hypomanic hostility may be reflected in the patient's behavior during the test. He may be impatient and ignore the examiner's repeated requests to slow down so that the examiner can record his responses. Other overt manifestations of hostility and uncooperativeness may permeate the testing session, punctuated with loud and angry comments about the test, the examiner, or the process of being examined. Representations of hostility may also emerge in response variables. Color may elicit immediate responses that are not well bounded by the form features of the blot. The content may reflect violent actions or images. For example, a hypomanic patient may look at Card II and quickly respond: "Looks like two guys fighting. There's blood all over the place. It's on the floor and all over them. Looks like they want to kill each other. No, I don't see anything else. Who made this stupid test?"

Expansiveness/Grandiosity

To the test indications of grandiosity mentioned previously, we add the concept of expansiveness to capture the behavioral aspect of over-striving and over-ambitiousness. Here, we wish to focus on Rorschach response variables that may reflect expansiveness. Not only does the patient produce a high number of responses, but he may attempt to over-synthesize and over-connect the details that he sees. The pattern of excessive combination of details without regard to whether or not they are appropriate and congruent with reality is a hallmark of a manic response style on the Rorschach. Using the TDI, researchers demonstrated that *combinative thinking* is emblematical of the manic record (Khadivi et al., 1997). The strained expansiveness of the manic patient is exemplified by the following response to Card III:

> They're clowns dancing with red balloons in the background, floating in the air, and they have a friendly butterfly that is coming from their chests, but they are trying not to step on the crab that is about to bite their feet.

This busy response leaves no detail unaccounted for. The combination of details into one response is not only strained but also attempts to integrate elements that are realistically incompatible.

Dyscontrol

We can find a range of scales on personality inventories indicating a lack of impulse control and behavioral restraint. Items include sensation seeking, impulsivity, immediate gratification, and sexual disinhibition.

Disinhibition on the Rorschach is typically indicated by combinations of response variables and specific contents. Using color on the inkblot without integrated form – combined with images of explosions, fires, or blood – may suggest a vulnerability to express affect and impulses in an unbridled manner. Hypomanic and manic patients may not inhibit comments made while responding to the cards. Research with the TDI demonstrated that flippant responses, like the following example, were characteristic of manic patients: "Well, that looks like another vagina . . . But, hey, between us, I guess you're the one with the dirty pictures, Doc!"

Assessment of Insight

In clinical assessment settings, insight has been conceptualized in terms of resistance to a psychological explanation of problems or component psychological processes, such as psychological mindedness, openness to experience (one's own and that of others), mentalizing capacity, and cognitive flexibility. We group those test variables associated with:

- Psychological mindedness/resistance to insight
- Openness to psychological experience

- Mentalizing capacity
- Cognitive flexibility

We believe that it is always important to assess the patient's capacity to observe himself. When he gives strange-sounding test responses on the Rorschach or endorses critical items on personality inventories suggestive of psychotic symptoms, we want to know if the patient can spontaneously step back, observe himself, and explain what he was thinking when he gave the response. At times, after testing has been completed, we may query the patient in a nonjudgmental manner about his thoughts or reactions to some of his more idiosyncratic responses to assess his awareness of how his response might have sounded to the examiner. If he does not spontaneously notice the bizarre nature of his response, is there any evidence of self-awareness when his attention is drawn to the response in question? Again, we find that the focus on "spontaneous" versus "assisted" insight, described in Chapter 7, is equally useful in psychological assessment.

Use of Psychological Tests in Assessment of Psychosis Proneness and Psychosis-Risk Syndromes

Psychological testing can be potentially useful in assessing psychosis proneness. Among personality inventories, the MMPI-3, PAI, and MCMI contain several scales and subscales that can be used to identify variables associated with psychosis proneness and attenuated psychosis. As discussed in Chapter 8, the Rorschach dominates the field of performance-based techniques for assessing psychotic phenomena. Several studies have used the Rorschach, and the TDI in particular, to assess a continuum of psychotic phenomena, including schizotypal personality and disordered thinking in nonpsychotic relatives of psychotic individuals (Coleman et al., 1996; Edell, 1987; Exner, 1986; Holzman et al., 1986; Johnston & Holzman, 1979; Shenton et al., 1989).

More recently, investigators have sought to identify Rorschach variables that might be useful in detecting individuals at high risk for conversion to psychosis (Illonen et al., 2010; Lacoua et al., 2014). In a seminal study by Kimhy and colleagues (2007), CHR individuals displayed substantial deficits in visual form perception (i.e., form quality of responses) that were comparable to the levels of poor form quality observed in patients with schizophrenia. Poor visual form perception was found to be a more significant factor than Rorschach indices of disordered thinking, which were generally more intact in those in the CHR group compared to their psychotic counterparts. The researchers concluded that poor form quality of Rorschach responses may represent a trait-like marker in CHR individuals, which could be identified before the occurrence of disturbances in thought organization. Adding weight to this hypothesis was their finding that individuals in the CHR group who had first-degree relatives with histories of psychosis had poorer form quality than CHR persons with no such family history. Inoue et al. (2014) also found more evidence of poor Rorschach form quality and less indication of disordered thought processes in a UHR sample. By contrast, other research has identified problems with visual form perception, along with indices of thought disorganization and impaired self-other representations to be present in the Rorschach responses of CHR individuals (Illonen et al., 2010; Lacoua et al., 2014; Brener, 2014). The studies led by Lacoua and Brener were extended beyond help-seeking patients and included non-clinical adolescents who might be at risk while not actively seeking support. (See Appendix A for a list of psychological testing variables that have conceptual and empirical relationships with proneness and psychosis-risk states.)

Clinical Assessment Points

1. Two central tenets of psychological assessment bear repeating. All assessment, especially diagnostic evaluations of psychotic functioning, requires multiple perspectives, multiple methods, and a search for converging patterns on which to base inferences. The second tenet is that psychological tests do not diagnose disorders but assess psychological functioning. As tempting as it might be to use a single method to establish a complex diagnosis, it never works this way. We select a range of empirically sound procedures to assess aspects of an individual's functioning, search for patterns in our data, and make representative inferences that closely follow the data. Linking together primary inferences enables us to make diagnostic inferences about different clinical syndromes.
2. Negative symptoms pose challenges for psychodiagnosticians. As we demonstrate in this chapter, we can form links between aspects of negative symptomatology and scores and scales from different psychological assessment instruments. The problem is that most, if not all, scales and scores we identify as suitable representations of negative symptoms also reflect signs and symptoms of depression and other conditions that affect psychic energy levels and increase cognitive and emotional constriction. Thus, most of the scores and scales we posit as representative measures of negative symptoms may be sensitive but not very specific measures.
3. Personality inventories can be useful adjuncts to test batteries in assessing psychosis. The multi-scale format of broadband inventories provides a great deal of information about the individual's personality functioning beyond addressing questions of whether

this individual might have some degree of psychotic functioning. Most provide measures of the patient's test-taking style, openness in answering questions, and bias in responding. However, the use of personality inventories without performance measures is insufficient. As self-report measures, personality inventories have clear limitations. Patients are limited in what they can or are willing to acknowledge about themselves. It is especially difficult for individuals to objectively respond to questions about aspects of their thought organization, such as reasoning, concept formation, and abstract thinking.

4. Many clinicians might ask how much testing is required to rule out the presence of a psychosis that is not immediately obvious from the patient's behavior. Is an interview sufficient? Is the Rorschach required? We believe that both are necessary. Some may feel that a Rorschach alone provides sufficient information about the nature of a patient's thought processes and that no other measures are needed. However, most of us have encountered cases of delusional patients with clean Rorschachs. Likewise, we are all familiar with patients who reveal no oddities of thought content or expression during the interview but produce a severely thought-disordered Rorschach. When evaluating patients for whom a central question has to do with ruling out psychosis, or a thought disorder in particular, and provided that there are no broader questions that must be answered, we recommend using a focal battery. Beginning with a clinical interview and using the kinds of questions presented in Chapter 7, we would administer a screening measure of intellectual functioning like the WASI-II (Wechsler & Hsiao-pin, 2011); either the MMPI-2, MMPI-3, or PAI; the Rorschach; and the Sorting and Proverb Tests from the D-KEFS (Delis et al., 2001). The WISC-V/WAIS-IV Comprehension subtest could even be added to elicit an extended sample of the subject's spontaneous verbalization. A battery such as this tells us about the individual's intellectual abilities, personality functioning, and aspects of her verbalization, thought organization, concept formation, and abstract thinking.
5. As we have seen, psychological tests can be blunt instruments that may not clearly distinguish between psychosis proneness, attenuated signs and symptoms of a psychosis-risk syndrome, or even a syndromal psychotic disorder. Although MMPI-3 and PAI scale elevations may signal the presence of psychotic phenomena, as studies have demonstrated, poor form quality of Rorschach responses may be a marker to assist in the early detection of high-risk individuals (Kimhy et al., 2007). While the Rorschach may help to distinguish psychotic phenomena, additional information is required to

make a differential diagnosis. Thus, we need to know about recent changes in the patient's level of functioning, genetic risk, and the patient's levels of emotional distress and stability. Furthermore, the psychotically prone individual may come to our attention for other reasons, whereas the risk-syndrome patient, by definition, may come to our attention because he or she is in great distress and search of help.

9

ASSESSING PSYCHOTIC PHENOMENA WITH RATING SCALES

As described in the last chapter, psychological assessment methods are used in clinical settings to identify unique aspects of an individual's experience and functioning for diagnostic clarification and treatment planning. In contrast, research-based methods are intended to assess symptom-related constructs in a broader population of patients and non-patients. Research-based scales can be grouped into categories that distinguish the instruments' purpose, intended use, nature, and scope. Some instruments were developed for research purposes and intended for scientific investigations. Others were designed to be used in a clinical setting.

Many research-based instruments consist of structured interviews and rating scales typically completed by the interviewer, while others are based on self-report. Additionally, instruments can be divided into multidimensional methods and single-symptom instruments. Finally, some instruments have been developed in single studies, with single samples and limited external validation, whereas others have been used in multiple studies and have well-documented psychometric properties. We restrict our focus to those instruments with broader empirical support.

Following a brief discussion of the characteristics of each category, we review the most popular and empirically valid instruments according to the dimensional framework we have used in the preceding chapters. In addition to the scales presented in this chapter and Appendix B, readers are directed to the edited volumes of Waters and Stephane (2015) and Weiner and Kleiger (2021) to review rating scales for assessing psychosis and psychotic symptoms in research and clinical settings.

Research-Specific versus Dual-Purpose Instruments

Research-Specific Methods

Regardless of type, research instruments, like their clinical assessment counterparts, must meet standard psychometric criteria to be used in empirical studies or be classified as evidence-based methods (Hunsley &

 DOI: 10.4324/9781003415206-13

Mash, 2008). To be more specific, the measurement of *reliability* (internal consistency, interrater, and test-retest) and *validity* (fact, content, construct, discriminative, and criterion-related) are central tenets of test construction and critical to determining the adequacy of a measure. Additionally, it is important to know how well the instrument predicts group membership and outcome. Knowledge about a measure's sensitivity and specificity helps determine the proportion of cases correctly identified by the positive scores on the measure and the proportion of non-cases correctly identified by negative scores, respectively.

Some procedures were developed primarily for use in research studies and not intended for use with clinical populations. Two such instruments include the Comprehensive Assessment of Symptoms and History (CASH; Andreasen, 1985; Andreasen et al., 1992) and the Signs and Symptoms of Psychotic Illness (SSPI; Liddle, Ngan, Duffield, et al., 2002).

The CASH focuses on past and current signs and symptoms of the illness, in addition to sociodemographic status, premorbid functioning, cognitive functioning, and course of illness. The instrument includes nearly 1,000 items which are divided into three primary sections: present state, past history, and lifetime history. Ratings are based on interviews with patients and relatives and include an assessment of global functioning and the severity of specific symptoms. The thoroughness of the CASH makes it a valued instrument for researchers interested in comprehensive assessment that goes beyond categorical diagnosis.

Liddle, Ngan, Duffield, et al. (2002) developed a 20-item scale to assess major signs and symptoms of psychotic illness as well as insight into illness severity. The factor structure of the SSPI is similar to that of the PANSS and includes five symptom factors:

- Poverty (psychomotor poverty)
- Disorganization
- Reality distortion
- Psychomotor excitation
- Anxiety/depression

Dual-Purpose Methods

In clinical settings, interview-based rating scales are used to establish diagnosis, determine immediate treatment, and gauge response to treatment interventions, which typically involve medication trials. Additionally, these measures can contribute to longer-term treatment planning by assessing and monitoring the level of impairment on social and self-care dimensions.

Two prominent instruments have been widely used for establishing diagnoses of psychotic disorders such as schizophrenia. The Structured

Clinical Interview (SCID) for DSM-IV and DSM-5 is a well-validated diagnostic measure that includes both research and clinical versions (First, 2014; First et al., 2007; First et al., 1996; Sbrana et al., 2005; Shankman et al., 2018; Ventura et al., 1998). The Present State Examination (PSE) is a similar, interview-based instrument used primarily in the UK (Luria & Berry, 1979; Wing, 1970). The SCID and PSE have high levels of reliability and validity for diagnosing schizophrenia; however, both require extensive training and clinical interviewing experience and take from one to two hours to complete.

Several semi-structured instruments with well-established reliability and validity are used for the assessment of individual symptoms. One of the most common instruments is the BPRS, which was originally developed to assess the efficacy of antipsychotic medications and evaluate changes in clinical symptoms (Hedlund & Vieweg, 1980; Overall & Gorham, 1962; Overall, 1974). The original version consisted of 16 items rated on a seven-point scale. It required anywhere from ten to 40 minutes to administer and could be used by anyone who knows the patient well. However, according to Johnson (2010), the original version of BPRS did not adequately assess specific psychological symptoms, lacked anchor points for determining symptom intensity, and did not provide an adequate assessment of negative symptoms. To address these limitations, the BPRS was revised and later expanded to 24 items (Hafkenscheid, 1993; Lukoff et al., 1986).

Whereas the BPRS was developed as a general psychiatric interview-rating scale for the assessment of a broad range of symptoms of severe psychopathology, the PANSS (Kay et al., 1987) was developed specifically for the assessment of positive and, to a lesser extent, negative symptoms of schizophrenia. The PANSS was designed to be an improvement over the BPRS, which was used as a source for more than half of its 30 items. The overlap in symptoms between the two scales yielded similar factor structures for both instruments, which have included dimensions of thought disorder, negative symptoms, anxiety/depression, disorganization, and activation (Long & Brekke, 1999; Mueser et al., 1997; van der Gaag et al., 2006).

Like the BPRS, the PANSS includes interview probes and clearly articulated descriptions of target symptoms. Each item on the PANSS is rated along a seven-point scale, and the items are organized into positive, negative, and general psychopathology scales. An additional composite score was included to capture the direction and magnitude of the difference between positive and negative symptoms. A combined SCID – PANSS interview-rating scale has also been used as a two-tier system for the diagnosis of psychotic disorders to supplement categorical diagnosis with functional-dimensional assessment (Kay et al., 1991). The hour-long interview results in a diagnostic classification and ratings of symptoms and dimensional scales, including positive and negative syndromes, depression, thought disturbance, and severity of illness.

Multidimensional versus Single-Dimension Instruments

Most dual-purpose methods have scales for measuring multiple dimensions of psychosis. These are the gold-standard instruments such as the PANSS and BPRS, which contain a large pool of items pertaining to different symptoms of psychosis. Large pools of heterogeneous items lend themselves to factor-analytic studies and the identification of relevant factors or dimensions that define psychosis.

In contrast, many research-based instruments were designed to measure single dimensions of psychosis. At first, the narrow, single-symptom focus might seem to reduce the multidimensional nature of the psychosis or the complexity of the individual to the presence of an isolated symptom. However, the most effective single-dimension scales go beyond the binary question of whether the symptom is present or absent and attempt to delineate the complex nature of the symptom. In other words, instead of simply measuring the presence or absence of a symptom, many of these scales were designed to examine the structural aspects of the symptom being measured. The purpose of this structural approach to assessment is to contribute to an understanding of the nature and severity of the symptom and to link structural elements with potential treatment interventions.

In their review of scales for assessing hallucinations, Ratcliff et al. (2010) noted the trend toward measurement of the individual's beliefs, attitudes, and interpretation of symptoms. Thus, instead of assessing only symptom severity, scales are increasingly sensitive to what the person thinks and how they feel about the symptom(s). Relatedly, and with particular relevance to planning treatment, scales also seek to identify the degree of insight the individual might have into the particular symptom.

Structured Interviews and Rating Scales versus Self-Report Questionnaires

Whereas the assessment methods reviewed in Chapters 7 and 8 include clinical interviews, multi-scale self-report inventories, and performance measures, research-based instruments are generally a combination of structured interviews and rating scales. The interviewer completes most rating scales based on the respondent's answers to structured questions, follow-up queries, and the interviewer's observations of the subject's behavior. However, some instruments, such as the PANSS, employ ratings from other treatment team members (such as nurses or other staff members involved in the patient's treatment). Although structured interviews can be exhaustively thorough, the comprehensive nature of these methods might make them too costly and time-consuming for single clinicians in a typical outpatient practice setting. For this reason, researchers and clinicians have sought simpler, more practical, and more economical tools for assessing symptom dimensions.

Researchers and clinicians tended to eschew the use of self-report measures with psychotic individuals. Traditionally, there were concerns that the presence of an active psychosis would interfere with an individual's ability to concentrate, synthesize, and make valid self-assessments of his symptoms (Christopher et al., 2007). However, despite conventional beliefs, Liraud et al. (2004) found that patients with acute psychosis were able to accurately assess their positive, negative, and depressive symptoms using the PANSS, Scale for the Assessment of Negative Symptoms (SANS), and Calgary Depression Scale.

Ratcliff et al. (2010) also noted an increased acceptance of self-report instruments. Such scales are frequently used for practical time-saving and cost-cutting reasons. However, Ratcliff's group pointed out that as interest has shifted from describing and quantifying symptoms to concern about the individual's beliefs and attitudes about his symptoms, self-report measures have been deemed more suitable for assessing a patient's subjective experiences. For example, a recent review of three self-report psychosis risk measures showed the strengths and limitations of measures intended to identify the experiences of at-risk individuals (Williams et al., 2022). Further, a recent review of self-report methods of paranoia showed some scales had acceptable psychometric properties (Statham et al., 2019) that make them worth using.

However, despite promising findings of some self-report measures, Ratcliff sounded a cautionary note that is equally important – namely, that psychotic individuals often require additional support from the interviewer to clarify the meaning of questions and monitor their approach to completing questionnaires and self-report scales. Although these researchers did not discourage the use of self-report measures, they indicated that cognitive functioning (focusing, concentration, frustration tolerance, motivation, and conceptual understanding) may be compromised by the acute nature of the psychotic symptoms and associated cognitive impairment. In particular, those symptoms reflecting impoverished thinking, disorganization, and reality distortion may be associated with impairments in focusing, comprehension, and insight, which prevent the individual from accurately endorsing symptoms on self-report scales and questionnaires.

Structured Interview and Rating Scale Assessment of Psychotic Dimensions

Assessment methods developed in empirical studies can be organized along most of the contemporary dimensions presented in Chapters 7 and 8. In addition to standard dimensions, we include instruments pertaining to insight and self-reflection. The instruments discussed, along with others, are presented in Table B1 in Appendix B (Johnson, 2010).

Hallucinations

Ratcliff et al. (2010) aptly note that hallucinations are an internal experience and, as such, cannot be directly observed. Although some individuals who hear voices may reveal observable behavior, such as addressing an unseen voice, hallucinations are private phenomena that rely on the subject's reports. Thus, as we pointed out in Chapter 7, direct inquiry is the most effective means of assessment.

The Ratcliff review of structured instruments for assessing hallucinations is one of several such reviews (Frederick & Killeen, 1998; Aleman & Larøi, 2008). Ratcliff selected only instruments developed in English and designed to measure auditory hallucinations, by far the most common type of hallucination in psychosis. Assessment of visual and olfactory hallucinations is typically part of a broader assessment of psychosis with instruments such as the PANSS or a more syndrome-specific assessment of visual or olfactory hallucinations in neurological disorders such as Parkinson's Disease or seizure disorders. The instruments chosen by Ratcliff include multidimensional methods that capture multiple characteristics of the hallucinations as well as more focal instruments seeking to identify the individual's beliefs, coping strategies, and degree of acceptance of the hallucinatory experiences.

Waters et al. (2003) evaluated the psychometric properties of the revised Launay Slade Hallucination scale (LSHS-R, Morrison et al., 2000). They found the LSHS-R demonstrated excellent convergent and discriminant validity as a measure of self-reported hallucinatory experiences.

Multidimensional Rating Scales

Two multidimensional instruments are highlighted. The Psychotic Symptom Rating Scales (PSYRATS; Haddock et al., 1999) is a structured interview that focuses on characteristics of auditory hallucinations (PSYRATS-AH) and delusions (PSYRATS-D). The PSYRATS-AH assesses eleven dimensions of the hallucinatory experience, including:

- Formal characteristics, such as frequency, duration, location, and loudness.

- Content features, such as the amount and degree of negative content.
- Beliefs regarding the origin of voices.
- Level of subjective distress and degree of disruption caused by voices.

The strength of the PSYRATS-AH lies in its dual-purpose utility. Ratcliff, Farhall, and Shawyer noted that the PSYRATS-AH has been the subject of extensive reliability and validity studies and can be used in clinical practice. It provides a brief and structured method of organizing the interviewer's questions regarding multiple aspects of a patient's hallucinatory experience. Ratcliff and colleagues encouraged further refinement of the scale to increase its value in clinical settings. In particular, they recommended changes to enhance the scale's sensitivity in assessing conviction of beliefs about the origin of voices.

The Auditory Hallucination Rating Scale (AHRS; Hoffman et al., 2003, 2005) is a brief structured interview that has been used in transcranial magnetic stimulation studies. Like the PSYRATS-AH, it measures formal characteristics of the hallucinatory experience (frequency, loudness, length of time, number of voices), as well as the degree to which the voices demand attention (attentional salience), seem real, and cause distress. The advantage of the AHRS is that it is brief and includes two dimensions absent in the PSYRATS-AH: attentional salience and perception of the reality of the voices. However, several factors make the AHRS less suitable for clinical use. First, it is the product of a narrow investigation that focused on the efficacy of repetitive transcranial magnetic stimulation in reducing refractory auditory hallucinations and has not been used outside this context. Additionally, the scale is limited in the information it provides regarding the voice hearer's subjective experience of his hallucinations. Thus, the limited scope may make this a less useful instrument in planning psychotherapy.

The Hamilton Program for Schizophrenia (HPSVO; Van Lieshout & Goldberg, 2007) and the Characteristics of Auditory Hallucinations Questionnaire (CAHQ; Trygstad et al., 2002) are brief self-report scales that take little time to administer. Both focus on formal characteristics of the hallucinatory experience, level of distress, and compliance with commands. However, neither scale has been widely studied, resulting in scanty information about psychometric properties.

Finally, in a study of the phenomenology of auditory hallucinations, McCarthy-Jones and colleagues (2014) conducted a cluster analysis on a lengthy semi-structured research interview, the Mental Health Research Institute Unusual Perception Scale (MUPS; Carter et al., 1995) to identify four subtypes of auditory hallucinations. They argued that each subtype might suggest a different approach to treatment. The most frequently occurring cluster – occurring in 86% of their predominantly male sample of individuals, most of whom were diagnosed with schizophrenia – included constant voices in the first or third person, which were repetitive, commanding, or issued running commentaries. Thus, the first cluster represented the prototypic auditory hallucination associated with schizophrenia. The remaining three clusters occurred less frequently. The second cluster consisted of first-person voices that did not address the individual and were similar to memories, perhaps more reflective of PTSD. The third cluster was made up of nonverbal or nonsensical words or sounds. The final cluster included voices identical to a memory of heard speech.

Beliefs, Interpretations, and Coping Scales

Structured approaches to assessing how individuals attempt to make sense of and cope with their hallucinations can deepen our clinical understanding of patients' subjective experiences of hearing voices. The Belief About Voices Questionnaire-Revised (BAVQ-R; Chadwick et al., 2000) is a self-rating scale that measures beliefs about and emotional and behavioral responses to auditory hallucinations. The developers changed the yes/no response format of the original BAVQ (Chadwick & Birchwood, 1995) to a four-point Likert scale and added items to increase the scale's sensitivity. The revised BAVQ yields three factors measuring belief in the voices' benevolence, malevolence, and omnipotence. Additionally, the BAVQ-R measures the degree of engagement with and resistance to the voices. Chadwick and colleagues found an association between perceived malevolence, omnipotence, and resistance efforts on the one hand and perceived benevolence of voices and engagement on the other. Other studies supported the validity of the BAVQ-R's omnipotence and malevolence scores, which showed both to be related to the perception of threat, use of safety-seeking strategies, and emotional distress (Hacker et al., 2008). Furthermore, omnipotence scores were found to be related to the degree of compliance with threatening command hallucinations (Shawyer et al., 2008). Finally, several studies found that cognitive therapy had different levels of effectiveness on post-treatment BAVQR scores of malevolence, omnipotence, and resistance (Pinkham et al., 2004; Trower et al., 2004).

Examining the factor structure of the BAVQ-R, researchers subsequently found that a two-factor solution was superior to one consisting of three (Strauss et al., 2018). In addition to a Benevolence factor, the study found that constructs of Malevolence and Omnipotence fit better within a Persecutory factor.

Two additional self-report scales provide information about the perceived relationship between the voice hearer and his voices. The Voice Power Differential (VPD; Birchwood et al., 2000) and the Voice and You Scale (VAY; Benjamin, 1989) examine different aspects of the perceived power differential and relative dominance, power, and intimacy vis-à-vis voice hearers and their voices. Ratcliff concluded that both measures provide brief and reliable measures of relationship qualities that exist between the subject and his voices.

Acceptance and Mindfulness Scales

In their comprehensive review, Ratcliff and colleagues (2010) described two self-report scales that measure the degree to which the subject has achieved acceptance of his voices on the one hand and seeks to be present with the hallucinatory experience on the other. Both the Southampton Mindfulness of Voices Questionnaire (SMVQ; Chadwick et al., 2007) and the Voices Acceptance and Action Scale (VAAS: Shawyer et al., 2007) provide new ways of thinking about the phenomenology of auditory hallucinations; however, both lack substantial research support at this time.

Delusions

Like the assessment of hallucinations, scales to measure delusions have evolved from simple categorical instruments designed to determine delusional presence/absence, content, and severity to more nuanced measures that examine the multidimensional structure of delusions. In particular, assessment has moved far beyond traditional classification in terms of content and is now concerned with understanding the formal features of the delusional experience. Researchers and clinicians have become more interested in the continuous and multidimensional nature of delusions.

As we saw in Chapter 5, all psychotic symptoms, in one form or another, occur across the general population and among a broad range of clinical groups. Delusional thinking is *not* an exception. Similarly, researchers have moved beyond classification on the basis of content (e.g., delusions of persecution, jealousy, grandiosity, etc.) and have sought to understand the different defining dimensions that distinguish one person's delusional experience from another's. Deconstructing delusions into separate dimensions has also allowed clinicians and researchers to assess responses to different treatment interventions.

Dimensional Structure of Delusions

Bell et al. (2006a) described six dimensions of delusions, including conviction, insight, systemization, disorganization, stability, and bizarreness. Garety and Hemsley (1987) developed a visual analogue scale, Characteristics of Delusional Experience, which contained 11 items to characterize formal features of delusions. A principal analysis component of their scale resulted in four factors:

- Distress
- Belief strength
- Obtrusiveness
- Concern

Perhaps one of the most interesting studies by Harrow et al. (2004) examined three characteristics of delusions and their relationship to outpatient versus inpatient status, length of hospitalization, rates of re-hospitalization, differential diagnosis, and effectiveness in work settings. The three dimensions were

- Belief certainty or strength of belief in delusions.
- Emotional commitment, which reflects the importance, urgency, and immediacy that the individual ascribes to his delusions.
- Self-monitoring, including self-editing, self-awareness, and, most importantly, a perspective that others regard one's delusions as strange.

The researchers found that the strength of these dimensions was greater during the acute phase of the psychosis when affective arousal and activation intensified positive symptoms such as delusions. They also concluded that, along with cognitive deficits and negative symptoms, higher levels of emotional commitment and poorer self-monitoring interfered with work functioning. Lower levels of self-monitoring were associated with poorer social functioning, as patients lacked sensitivity to the impact of their delusions on other people. They demonstrated an "impaired social perspective," which, as noted in Chapter 2, is associated with deficits in insight. Elevations in emotional commitment and lower self-monitoring measures also shed light on why certain patients are re-hospitalized more often than others. A heightened emotional commitment and lower self-monitoring demonstrated a sense of urgency and a lack of social perspective that affected their self-control and judgment, increasing their rates of hospitalization. Conversely, even though a broader range of patients may exhibit equally strong beliefs in their delusions (elevated belief certainty), those individuals with lower emotional commitment and higher self-monitoring may behave more adaptively and thus remain in the community.

Scales for Assessing Delusions

The list of self-report scales and clinician-guided interviews increases yearly. A variety of instruments have been developed and well-researched to measure the qualities of the delusional experience in a variety of populations. The instruments we review can be organized into two categories:

- Those developed to measure delusional thinking in the general population.
- Those that purport to distinguish qualities of delusional experience among different psychotic and nonpsychotic patient groups.

Scales for Delusional Thinking in the General Population

Consistent with the concept of a continuum of psychotic phenomena in the general population, researchers have studied delusional thinking in clinical and nonclinical populations. The PDI (Peters et al., 1999, 2004) is one such instrument. Consisting of 21 items, the PDI is a self-report questionnaire that was not designed to assess florid psychotic delusions among patients. Instead, like other psychosis-proneness instruments, it was constructed to measure delusional ideation in the general population. The PDI attempts to ascertain both the presence/absence of delusional thinking and to identify the level of distress, preoccupation, and strength of certainty for each delusional belief. The authors found that these structural dimensions were likely to be more important than the content of the belief for placing an individual on the continuum between normal and delusional thinking (Peters et al., 2004).

As indicated earlier, research (Statham et al., 2019) found that the Green Paranoid Thought Scales (Green et al., 2008), used in clinical and nonclinical populations, was a valid and reliable scale for assessing paranoid thoughts and dimensions of preoccupation, conviction, and distress. An eight-item version (GPTS-8), developed as a quick measure of paranoid ideation in schizophrenia, was shown to have adequate psychometric properties (Bianchi & Verkuilen, 2021; Raffard et al., 2023).

The Magical Ideation Scale (MagId; Eckblad & Chapman, 1983) was developed to study delusional thinking in psychotically prone individuals in the general population (see Chapter 11). However, the MagId contains items representing severe first-rank symptoms, which very few people in the general population endorse, as well as items reflecting superstitious beliefs that are so frequently endorsed that they are less sensitive to delusional thinking. Nonetheless, the MagId has been used extensively in research on psychosis proneness.

Scales for Delusional Thinking among Patient Groups

Several measures purport to assess multiple dimensions of delusions among different clinical groups. As described previously, the PSYRATS-D is an interview-based scale for assessing aspects of delusional experience. Six dimensions are rated, including:

- Preoccupation, or how often the subject thinks about the delusion
- Duration of preoccupation, from seconds to hours at a time
- Conviction or strength of belief
- Distress
- Intensity of distress
- Disruption in one's life

The PSYRATS-D is intended to be used in a clinical population and provides a simple screening tool for characterizing the qualities of a patient's delusions.

The Brown Assessment of Beliefs Scale (BABS; Eisen et al., 1998) was developed to assess delusionality across a range of psychiatric disorders, including OCD, body dysmorphic disorder, psychotic mood disorder, and hypochondriasis. A seven-item, clinician-administered, semi-structured scale, the BABS begins with identifying the patient's dominant belief, obsession, worry, or delusion, then includes specific probes and five anchors for each item. Convergent validity was demonstrated with the Characteristics of Delusions Rating Scale (CDRS; Garety & Hemsley, 1987) and the Dimensions of Delusional Experience Scale (DDE; Kendler et al., 1983), both of which assess multiple dimensions of delusions similar to those described previously. It is interesting to note that developers of the BABS advise caution in its use with patients who have current thought disorder or cognitive impairment associated with schizophrenia or dementia because these patients may be unable to respond meaningfully to the questions. Thus, these researchers draw attention to an inherent limitation of using self-report scales with some actively psychotic patients.

The Delusions Symptoms State Inventory (DSSI; Foulds et al., 1975) is an older instrument developed for use in diagnosing more florid delusional content in a clinical population. Unlike the other measures, the DSSI assesses content categories as opposed to dimensions of delusional thinking. As such, the sections of this 84-item self-report scale include content qualities such as delusions of grandeur, contrition, dis-integration, persecution, and associated symptoms that include anxiety, depression, elation, conversion, dissociation, rumination, and phobias. The DSSI has been used in numerous studies over the years to provide a reliable measure of categories of delusional thinking.

The Simple Delusional Syndrome Scale (SDSS; Forgácová, 2008) is a diagnostic-specific instrument developed to study the characteristics of patients diagnosed with delusional disorders. Delusions characteristic of delusional disorders are distinguished from delusions in patients with schizophrenia by their logical consistency, their stability, and their systemization. The scale is completed by the clinician-interviewer, who rates the patient based on clinical observations and the individual's verbalizations. The dimensions include:

- Logical organization
- Systemization
- Stability
- Conviction
- Influence of action or behavior
- Extension, or how broadly a person's life is affected
- Insertion, or whether the delusion has some grounding in reality

What is most interesting about this scale is its focus on distinguishing simple, systematized, and logically based delusions typically characteristic of patients with delusional disorders from more bizarre, scattered, and variable delusions found in schizophrenia.

Finally, the GPTS-8 was mentioned previously. It was developed as a unidimensional measure of paranoid ideation in schizophrenia. The GPTS-8 was shown to have respectable reliability and validity (Bianchi & Verkuilen, 2021; Raffard et al., 2023).

Cognitive Disorganization (Thought Disorder)

While it makes sense to assess dimensions of hallucinations and delusions with interviews and self-report measures, measuring disorganized speech and errors in reasoning typically requires the use of observational and performance-based instruments. As indicated in the previous chapters, ratings based on speech samples and quantifying speech abnormalities in response to Rorschach inkblots are generally more common methods of assessing formal thought disorder and errors in reasoning and conceptual thinking. However, the issue of whether self-report of symptoms such as formal thought disorder and errors in reasoning is a valid method of assessment is not settled.

Speech Samples and Clinician Rating Scales

In previous chapters, we have described the TLC (Andreasen, 1978, 1979) as an interview-based method for assessing formal thought disorder. The TLC consists of 20 subscales, which catalog a broad range of positive and negative types of speech and language disorders. The definitions are clearly defined and well worth learning. Subsets of the TLC are incorporated into the positive and negative thought disorder subscales of Andreasen's Scale for the Assessment of Positive Symptoms (SAPS;

Andreasen, 1984) and in the alogia subscale of the SANS (Andreasen, 1983b). Ratings are made by the clinician following an interview with the patient that includes an uninterrupted sample of the patient's speech. Andreasen summarized research on the TLC that demonstrated adequate interrater reliability of the subscales (Andreasen & Grove, 1986b). However, in their comprehensive review, Straube and Oades (1992) concluded that the TLC is less sensitive to subtle anomalies of disordered thinking and speech.

We recommend that clinicians become familiar with the TLC, if for no other reason than to understand the variety of forms of positive and negative formal thought disorders. However, for practical purposes, routine use of the TLC will require time and training. Furthermore, rating the presence of subtypes of formal thought disorder in live speech samples is challenging without the ability to make a tape recording to review before giving ratings. However, obtaining permission to tape record a clinical interview is complicated, and even if permission is granted, it is time-consuming for the clinician to listen to the recording again in order to rate the incidence of formal thought-disorder subtypes.

The Thought and Language Disorder Scale (TALD, Kircher et al., 2014) is an alternative to the TLC. Like the TLC, the TALD is another interview, clinician-based rating scale of spontaneous speech. Clinician ratings on the TALD correlated well with other clinician-rated scales and divergence from scales rating depression and mania (Boyette & Noordhof, 2021).

An interesting interview and performance-based measure combination is Liddle's TLI (Liddle, Ngan, Caissie, et al., 2002; Liddle, 2019), which was developed to detect subtler varieties of formal thought disorder. The TLI requires the patient to produce eight one-minute speech samples in response to cards from either the Rorschach or TAT. The speech samples must be recorded verbatim and then analyzed for the presence of eight carefully defined types of speech/thought abnormality. The researchers found three factors:

- Two items loaded on an impoverishment of thought and speech factors.
- Four items loaded on disorganization factors describing looseness, illogicality, and peculiarity of language.
- Two items described attentional variables, including perseveration (set-shifting difficulties) and distractibility.

The impoverishment factor correlated with the SANS, and the disorganization factor correlated with the SAPS. The scoring of the TLI was patterned after four levels of severity adopted by the TDI, which is described in Chapter 8 as a Rorschach method for assessing forms of thought disorder. Scores at the least severe level were found among nonpatients, thus reinforcing the notion of a continuum of disordered thinking in the population.

The TLI is an appealing instrument. It has the potential to provide a more structured and efficient measure of thought disorder, including both formal disorganization of speech and errors in reasoning. Using standard testing stimuli like Rorschach and TAT cards may appeal to psychologists who already use these instruments. However, this may be somewhat of a disadvantage to nonpsychologist assessors who do not use psychological testing instruments. The other potential disadvantage is that the TLI does not have a substantial body of research supporting its use with a broader range of patients in a variety of settings.

Shifting away from traditional concepts of thought disorder, Chen and colleagues (Chen et al., 1996) developed an alternative measure to classify speech symptoms according to levels of linguistic structure. The Clinical Language Scale (CLANG) provides a broader evaluation of speech beyond thinking and discourse and includes voice quality, fluency, and articulation disturbances. The CLANG is an interviewer-rated scale that assists in assessing speech's syntactic, semantic, and production aspects. Like the TLC, the interviewer must elicit a sample of the subject's speech. Although the CLANG might sound more appropriate at first for speech and language assessment, each of the factors it assesses is associated with familiar qualities of disordered speech and thinking. For example, syntactic dysfunction affects the structure of language expression (how things are said), while semantic dysfunction has to do with the ability to map thoughts onto language and communicate ideas in a logical manner. Production dysfunction has to do with poverty of speech, lack of intonation, and scarcity of details – all of which characterize negative forms of thought disorder.

Self-Report Scales

Waring et al. (2003) argue that thought disorder can be assessed directly. Citing evidence that many individuals with schizophrenia are aware of and can describe their disturbances in thinking, Waring and his group developed the Thought Disorder Questionnaire (TDQ) as a self-report measure to aid in the early detection of psychosis. A 304-item scale developed over the course of a decade, and it was eventually pared down to 60 items which were organized into six areas, including:

- Content of thought
- Control of thought
- Orientation
- Perception

- Fantasy
- Symptoms

The TDQ includes validity scales to assess infrequent responding and social desirability, making this a more sophisticated measure that guards against response styles that can invalidate self-report measures. Although Waring et al. believe that patients with schizophrenia can reliably complete the TDQ, they also indicate that the questionnaire may be too challenging for more disturbed patients. Furthermore, they found that while the TDQ distinguished healthy nonpatients from those with schizophrenia, the scale did not distinguish disordered thinking and speech, among other diagnoses. For example, it was found that individuals with personality disorders had the highest scores on the TDQ. For this reason, we do not think this is the most useful scale for assessing thought disorder.

Two additional scales, one completed by a caregiver/informant and one by the patient, were developed to examine formal thought disorder (FTD) from a pragmatic, linguistic perspective (Barrera et al., 2008; Barrera et al., 2015). The FTD-Patient and the FTD-Carer scales contain questions covering pragmatic, semantic, syntactic, memory, attentional, para-linguistic, and nonverbal aspects of communication. The factors derived from both scales have an experience-near quality more descriptive of actual speech behavior than traditional terms employed in other instruments such as the TLC. For example, factors from the self-report scale include self-descriptions such as:

- I lose track in conversation.
- I mutter for no reason.
- Too many words come into my head.
- I do not get to the point.
- I talk in ways that other people find strange.

Similarly, the caretaker version has four factors labeled descriptively as

- Goes around in circles in conversation.
- Draws the wrong conclusions when speaking.
- Speech is suddenly blocked.
- Hard to give instructions to find a place.

Barrera and colleagues thus argued that psychotic patients are able to reliably describe their symptoms, including cognitive difficulties and communication deficits. Additionally, they noted that almost half of patients had insight into their formal thought disorder (Amador et al., 1994).

The FTD scales are nontraditional measures employing both self-report and ratings from an informant caretaker. The latter version provides something unique among thought-disorder scales – namely, obtaining ratings from a family member or other caretaker who is familiar with how the patient thinks, reasons, and speaks on a daily basis. In their 2015 study, the FTD was used with nonclinical subjects and a parallel rating scale with their relatives or friends. A principal component analysis found three factors: odd speech, conversational ability, and working memory deficit. However, correlations with parallel forms completed by informants thought statistically significant were low.

Whether these scales are ready for clinical use is another matter. Although intriguing, there does not appear to be a broad research base to justify routinely employing these instruments in clinical assessments. Nonetheless, clinicians need to understand more about the linguistic dimensions of thought disorder when trying to make sense of a patient's speech and thought organization. The utility of self-report measures for assessing cognitive disorganization or formal thought disorder remains unsettled. The question of whether an intrinsic aspect of one's speech organization can be assessed in the same way as symptoms such as hallucinations and delusions is controversial.

Negative Symptoms

There are a number of scales that have been developed to assess negative symptoms of schizophrenia. Most are clinician-rated; however, some, like the SDSS (Jaeger et al., 1990), involve a subjective assessment of negative symptoms.

Perhaps the best known measure is Andreasen's SANS, which was developed to assess the subtler features of schizophrenia (Andreasen, 1983b). The SANS contains 30 items, which are rated on the basis of observation and interviews with the patient and key informants. One large factor-analytic study yielded a three-factor solution comprised of blunted affect, apathy–anhedonia, and alogia–inattention (Sayers et al., 1996). As noted in Chapter 2, negative symptoms are classified into two domains, one describing restricted emotional expression and the other avolition. Two more recent additions include the Brief Negative Symptom Scale (BNSS; Kirkpatrick et al., 2011) and the Clinical Assessment Interview for Negative Symptoms (CAINS; Horan et al., 2011). Of these scales, the BNSS has shown better discrimination between these factors (Kirkpatrick et al., 2011; Horan et al., 2011). The BNSS has recently been recommended as a focal measure of negative symptoms (Weigel et al., 2023).

Bizarre and Disorganized Behavior

As indicated previously, assessing abnormal behavior is best accomplished by listening to and observing the patient's verbal and nonverbal behavior. However, catatonia is a more discrete category of abnormal behavior that has been assessed with clinician rating scales. The Bush – Francis Catatonia Rating Scale (BFCRS; Bush et al., 1996; Zingela et al., 2021) is the best-studied measure for rating the presence and different signs of catatonia. Nonetheless, some have pointed to its limitations as a sufficiently sensitive and specific measure of catatonia.

Cognitive Impairment

In the previous chapters, we described screening instruments for assessing deficits in cognitive functioning. We mentioned the RBANS (Gold et al., 1999; Hobart et al., 1999) as a performance-based screening measure and the MOCA (Nasreddine et al., 2005) as an interview-based instrument for assessing cognitive impairment. The Mini-Mental Status Exam (MMSE; Folstein et al., 1975) is another well-known interview method for assessing orientation, word-recall language, attention, and visuospatial ability. Compared to the MOCA, the MMSE may be somewhat shorter, but overall, the MOCA is a more sensitive instrument for picking up subtle aspects of cognitive impairment.

As with the measurement of disordered thinking, objective assessment may be preferable to self-report measures when screening for cognitive deficits. Having a family member's ratings may provide a more valuable measure of a patient's level of cognitive impairment. The Schizophrenia Cognition Rating Scale (SCoRS; Keefe et al., 2006) contains 18 items describing the individual's day-to-day functioning that were rated during an interview with either the patient or a relative. The cognitive domains include attention, memory, reasoning, working memory, language production, motor skills, and problem-solving. However, there are questions about how well ratings from the patient, and to some extent the family members, correlate with measures of cognitive functioning and functionality.

Another self- and informant-rated scale is the GEOPTE Scale, developed as a method for rapidly assessing a psychotic patient's level of cognitive impairment. Sanjuán and colleagues (Sanjuán et al., 2006; Sanjuán et al., 2003) demonstrated significant correlations between patients and family members regarding the level of cognitive impairment. Although caregivers assigned higher ratings of impairment than did the patients themselves, the differences were not significant. The key implication of this study was that psychotic patients retained some insight regarding deficits in their cognitive functioning. However, patients may be less aware of their deficits in social functioning than their caregivers or relatives.

Depression

There are numerous rating scales for assessing depressive symptomatology across the diagnostic spectrum. However, depression is such a ubiquitous symptom in mental disorders that the rating scales most germane to our review include those that pertain to the presence of depression in patients suffering from psychosis. At the top of the list is the Calgary Depression Scale for Schizophrenia (CDSS; Addington et al., 1993), which has nine items rated on a four-point scale. The CDSS offers several advantages. First, it was developed to identify depression among patients with schizophrenia. Second, it does not contain psychomotor items, which might be associated with negative symptoms. Finally, it correlates with other gold-standard self-report measures of depression, such as the Beck Depression Inventory, Second Edition (BDI-II; Beck et al., 1996) and the Hamilton Psychiatric Rating Scale for Depression (HRSD; Hamilton, 1960).

An interesting-sounding scale named the Schizophrenia Suicide Risk Scale (SSRS; Taiminen et al., 2001) was developed to identify patients with schizophrenia who are at risk for suicide. The scale contains 25 items, nine from the CDSS and 13 having to do with personal history. Two groups of patients were contrasted – one was living, and the other had committed suicide. Consistent with commonly held risk factors, the best predictors of suicide were items involving communicated plans for suicide, suicide attempts, observed depression, and job loss. Johnson (2010) pointed out that the absence of information about the suicide group limits the generalizability of this scale.

Mania

Readers are directed to an updated review of screening instruments for assessing aspects of bipolar-manic symptoms (Kleiger, 2023). Two rating scales, one interview-based and the other a self-report measure, represent the state-of-the-art in brief screening methods for assessing mania. The Young Mania Rating Scale (YMRS; Young et al., 1978) provides a quick screening of mania. Consisting of 11 items, the YMRS is easily administered in 15 to 30 minutes. It includes subscales covering different aspects of mania, including elevated mood, increased motor activity, heightened sexual interest, speech/language/thought disorder, content, disruptive/aggressive behavior, and appearance and insight.

The Altman Self-Rating Mania scale (ASRM; Altman et al., 1997) is another widely used measure that provides an even briefer screening than the YMRS. The ASRM consists of a mere five items, rated on a Likert scale. The items have to do with happiness, sleep, talking, and activity level. The brevity and informal nature of the ASRM are appealing; however, it does not have the comprehensive scope of the YMRS. For example, there are no items pertaining to aggressive behavior or insight.

Insight

Although not a formal dimension of psychosis, we have pointed out the importance of assessing the degree of insight, self-awareness, and self-monitoring because of their relationship to treatment compliance, prolonged duration of illness, and severity of positive and negative symptoms. Johnson (2010) reviewed several scales that have been researched. Three of the most popular include the Insight Scale-Birchwood (IS-B; Birchwood et al., 1994), the Beck Cognitive Insight Scale (BCIS; Beck et al., 2004), and the Scale to Assess Unawareness of Mental Disorder (SUMD; Amador et al., 1994).

The IS-B has been used primarily as a research instrument in a range of studies investigating the severity of symptom dimensions and insight in patients with psychoses. As indicated in Chapter 2, insight is a multidimensional construct. The IS-B is a brief, self-report measure that addresses the three primary dimensions of insight:

- Awareness of illness
- Need for treatment
- Attribution of symptoms to psychosis

The BCIS purports to measure different aspects of self-reflective capacity, including the ability to correct mistaken judgments and certainty about mistaken conclusions. The BCIS is another self-report scale that can be completed relatively quickly. The researchers found two predictive factors: self-reflective capacity and self-certainty in beliefs.

Finally, the SUMD was developed to assess noncompliance with treatment when associated with a lack of awareness of one's illness. The scale has been used in research and clinical trials but less often in clinical settings because of its length (74 items). Recently, Michel and his team developed a reliable and valid abbreviated version of the SUMD for clinical use (Michel et al., 2013). Although the original version of the SUMD appears to provide a comprehensive assessment of insight, the shorter version is more likely to be used in routine clinical assessments.

The VAGUS Insight into Psychosis Scale (Gerretsen et al., 2014) is a self-report and clinician-rated measure of clinical insight into psychosis. The VAGUS has been shown to identify small changes in insight that may be of use in intervention studies.

Clinical Assessment Points

1. For clinicians interested in research, many of these scales offer a wealth of criterion measures for assessing specific symptoms or functions. Even for those of us not engaged in clinical research, learning about developments in psychosis research is an enlightening discipline

that surely enriches our understanding of psychopathology and enables us to serve our patients better. For this reason, we recommend that clinicians become familiar with scientific journals that publish cutting-edge studies and commentaries regarding the assessment of psychotic phenomena. Journals such as *Schizophrenia Bulletin, Clinical Schizophrenia and Related Psychoses,* and *Schizophrenia Research* not only publish studies relating to the biological underpinnings of severe mental illness (not just schizophrenia) but also the cognitive and subjective experiences and characteristics of individuals who have psychoses. When one is evaluating patients suspected of having psychotic illnesses, it is imperative to look beyond our own journals and the psychological assessment literature and connect with the impressive research being done in the field of psychosis.

2. If there is a downside to the research proliferation of scales that have been developed, beyond the fact that most were not developed and are not available for clinical use, it is the fantasy that we can learn complex things about a person whose thinking, reasoning, receptive language functioning, and level of trust might be compromised by directly questioning them. Therefore, as attractive and user-friendly as many of these scales appear, there is always the risk that they overestimate an individual's ability to know himself sufficiently and be able to report about himself accurately. In no way is this observation intended to dismiss the importance of first-hand, subjective points of view, which continue to contribute to the psychosis literature. Our point is that self-reports based on binary, closed-ended questions might be misleading, especially when these questions are asked of individuals struggling with issues of information-processing and interpersonal rapport.
3. Contrasting research scales with psychological assessment also reminds us of the essential difference between these traditions of assessment. Researchers develop interviews and rating scales as tools to measure a particular phenomenon. The approach is essentially nomothetic, and findings are valid if methodological procedures are sound and the results can be generalized with a certain level of confidence. In clinical assessment, we employ empirically validated assessment instruments, but our mission is more to understand the whole individual and less to classify individual functions or symptoms per se. Symptom identification is, of course, important for treatment planning purposes, but symptom classification is not the primary purpose of conducting a psychological evaluation. We need to be reminded of this when evaluating a patient suspected of having a thought disorder. Although, as clinicians, we should always be mindful of the referral questions, it is also important not to lose the forest by concentrating on the trees and reducing the person to a set of isolated symptoms when conducting our evaluations.

Part IV

ASSESSING SPECIAL ISSUES AND POPULATIONS

10

ASSESSING PSYCHOSIS IN A CULTURAL CONTEXT

While performing a religious ritual in a local church, Ms. B., a 40-year-old woman, reports hearing voices of spirits and goes through a trance-like experience. Shortly afterward, she passes out and is taken to a medical emergency room.

Mr. R., a 19-year-old male international student, becomes increasingly alienated from his peers at a local college. While at home on spring break, he begins to hear "voices of spirits" and believes that "evil spirits" possess him. In response to command hallucinations from these evil spirits, he attempts to mutilate his genitals in what amounts to a near-lethal suicide attempt. He is found by a neighbor and rushed to the hospital.

Finally, there is Didia, mentioned in Chapter 1, who hears the voice of a tribal elder telling her she is bad for having sex with her boyfriend. The resident on call worried she was psychotic and in need of hospitalization.

All three individuals are highly religious, first-generation immigrants from a non-Western culture. None had a prior history of psychiatric illness or substance abuse. As these two examples illustrate, differentiating cultural experiences or beliefs from psychotic symptoms is a common diagnostic challenge for clinicians, especially those practicing in metropolitan cities with large immigrant populations. Clinicians who encounter patients like Ms. B., Mr. R., and Didia have the daunting task of determining what aspect of the patient's clinical presentation is normative within a cultural context and what, if any, is reflective of psychotic phenomena.

Hallucinatory experiences will alert clinicians and most lay people to the possible presence of psychosis. Furthermore, astute clinicians realize that immigration and the urban environment can combine to produce a sense of "social defeat" that may increase the risk for psychosis (Selten et al., 2007). Additionally, in clinical encounters with patients such as those described previously, diagnostic decisions are further complicated by the fact that delusions frequently occur with religious themes (Siddle et al., 2002).

DOI: 10.4324/9781003415206-15

This chapter discusses the challenge of assessing psychosis within a cultural context. Consistent with the assessment focus of the book, we accept DSM-5 and 5-TR operational definitions to frame our approach. The DSM-5 defines culture, which refers to

> the values, orientation, and assumptions individuals derive from membership in diverse social groups (e.g., ethnic groups, military, and faith communities). Culture also refers to aspects of a person's background that may affect their perspective, such as ethnicity, race, language, or religion.
>
> (Black & Grant, 2014, p. 443)

With this definition in mind, we accept as a standard of practice the importance of considering cultural, ethnic, religious, and socioeconomic factors when assessing psychosis in individuals from diverse backgrounds.

Challenges in Assessing Psychosis in Culturally Diverse Individuals

Assessing psychosis is a challenging task on its own, but when the evaluation involves someone from a different cultural, religious, and spiritual background, the assessment task becomes even more complex. To begin with, there is considerable variability within individuals from the same culture (Black & Grant, 2014). Not everyone with the same cultural background expresses their cultural beliefs in the same manner. The concept of "cultural humility" holds that there is a difference within similarity or that individuals internalize their cultural, religious, and spiritual beliefs and experiences in a highly individualized manner. The culture may set broad norms, but individuals within that culture may differ in myriad ways. Moreover, this internalization process is filtered through one's personality functioning in the context of any unique psychological difficulties (Bushra et al., 2007). As a result, when evaluating individuals with mental disorders, the task of differentiating cultural experiences or beliefs from personality functioning and psychological symptoms is inherently complex.

The following case of Ms. M. illustrates the interplay of cultural factors with personality and psychological symptoms.

> Ms. M., a 32-year-old woman with a history of bipolar disorder, had previously made sexualized comments toward her male psychiatrist. During her outpatient treatment, she became increasingly hypomanic, and during the holiday season, she offered a set of men's underwear to her psychiatrist in a seductive manner.

> Ms. M. is from a culture in which gift-giving is a prevalent practice. As such, a gift would seem to fit within an acceptable cultural context for her. However, both the nature of the gift and how she presented it to her psychiatrist were consistent with features of her bipolar disorder and aspects of her personality functioning. Thus, her actions could be construed as an erotic transference that had become exacerbated by her hypomanic symptoms. What also made her gift-giving gesture appear more reflective of her illness and personality was the fact that there were other patients at the clinic from the same cultural background as Ms. M. who did not engage in gift-giving to members of their treatment team. As one can see from this case, disentangling the threads of culture, personality, psychopathology, or transference is unclear.

There is consensus in the field that accurate diagnosis and development of an effective treatment plan depend on understanding the cultural variations in the clinical presentation of mental illness (Geltman & Chang, 2004). A culturally competent evaluation seeks to capture the uniqueness of the individual and assess the impact of cultural experiences and beliefs without generalizing or stereotyping the individual (Tseng et al., 2004).

This is particularly important when attempting to understand how cultural factors impact the presentation of psychotic symptoms. In assessing psychotic disorders, our task is to capture how one person with a psychotic disorder is different from another with a similar disorder in terms of cultural identification, the meaning they attribute to their illness, and their perception of treatment. However, discerning issues of cultural identification or the culture-specific meaning of symptoms is further complicated by the fact that psychotic symptoms can impair a patient's reality testing and ability to communicate coherently or logically. According to Smith (2021), culture significantly impacts both the content of thought and the thought process. He emphasizes that it is incorrect to assume that all cultures utilize the same reasoning process, such as the "Aristotelian logic." Smith cites the work of Werner (1957) and other psychologists who have acknowledged that the variation in reasoning reflects the unique logic inherent in each culture. Similarly, Larøi et al. (2014), citing the literature review, argue that culture significantly influences various aspects of hallucinations, including identification, content, experience, meaning, and level of distress caused. Furthermore, the authors demonstrate that culture plays a role in both normal and pathological forms of hallucinations, and it can also shape the way people respond to this phenomenon.

Given these potential challenges in cross-cultural assessment of psychosis, we clinicians may err in two opposite directions. On the one hand, we may run a risk of prematurely attributing the patient's psychosis to cultural factors, thus overlooking the presence of treatable psychotic symptoms. Erring in the direction of extreme cultural correctness may lead to under-interpreting the significance of symptoms that might have distinctive meanings for this individual. On the other hand, we may err by over-pathologizing an individual, seeing only the psychotic-like nature of the symptoms while overlooking the cultural context for his experiences or beliefs. Either way, we end up stereotyping and missing what is most salient for an individual patient.

The cultural background, values, and lack of cultural understanding of the evaluating clinician may be another source of bias, skewing the results of an assessment (Banerjee, 2012). Banerjee cites a significant study by Barnes (2004) that illustrates the impact of clinicians' cultural background on assessing psychosis. This study found that in comparison to Caucasian patients, African American hospitalized patients were significantly more likely to be diagnosed as having schizophrenia and were five times more likely to receive a diagnosis of a primary psychotic disorder than a mood disorder. In addition, earlier studies demonstrated similar findings that Latino and African American patients were more likely to be diagnosed as having paranoid schizophrenia than affective psychosis (Mukherjee et al., 1983; Strakowski et al., 1996).

In addition to bias and cultural insensitivity among evaluating clinicians, official diagnostic systems have traditionally been slow to recognize the role of culture in mental illness and psychosis. For example, the DSM-III was criticized for not being sensitive to cultural factors in mental illness, which led to the development of an outline for a cultural formulation in the DSM-IV-TR (Lewis-Fernández & Díaz, 2002). The DSM-5 further expanded the framework for assessing cultural aspects of individuals with mental illnesses and developed a brief, semi-structured Cultural Formulation Interview (CFI) consisting of 16 questions. The CFI was designed to assess the cultural definition of the problem, the cultural perception of cause and context, and the cultural factors impacting treatment. The information is obtained from the patient. In addition, and more critically, the CFI has an informant version that can be used with family members. The CFI is a significant development that standardizes and systematically assesses cultural factors in any clinical context (Black & Grant, 2014). Aggarwal et al. (2020) reviewed the studies using CFI, showing the instrument has good content validity. In most studies, clinicians and patients reported that using the CFI improved the therapeutic alliance.

Nonpathological and Pathological Psychotic Experiences and Beliefs across Cultures

In the review of cross-cultural psychosis studies, we identify two significant findings that have implications for clinical assessment. First, many individuals with diverse religious or cultural backgrounds have nonpathological psychotic-like experiences that are normative. For example, Latino and Caribbean patients attending outpatient clinics have a significantly higher percentage of nonspecific hallucinations in the absence of any other psychotic symptoms. In addition, compared to other patients, they were more likely to experience hearing their name being called (Geltman & Chang, 2004). Similarly, Moreira-Almeida and Cardeña (2011) reviewed studies that differentiated mental disorders from spiritual experiences in Latin America. Their review found that nonpathological psychotic-like experiences, including hallucination and dissociation, were widespread in the general population.

Second, significant findings from cross-cultural studies of psychosis indicate that there is considerable variability in the expression of psychotic symptoms in patients from diverse cultural backgrounds. For example, transient psychotic breaks with full recovery are reportedly ten times more common in non-Western cultures (Castillo, 2006). Furthermore, Aleman and Larøi's (2008) review of the literature on hallucinations indicated that in comparison to Western cultures, visual hallucinations are more commonly experienced in developing countries, and the content of auditory hallucinations is more likely to be of a superstitious or religious nature as opposed to being experienced as abusive, commanding, or derogatory. In addition, patients from non-Western cultures experienced fewer Schneiderian-type hallucinations (e.g., voices giving a running commentary) or voices issuing commands.

Similar cross-cultural variability is seen in the expression of delusional symptoms (Bentall, 2003). Studies show that individuals from the Far East were more likely to have delusions that were sexual and involved fears of sexual assault, vampires, and poisoning compared to patients from India, the Middle East, and the Caribbean. Bentall also argues that cultural factors, including socioeconomic status and religion, impact the expression of psychotic symptoms within the same culture. He cites a study by Sendiony (1976) that showed middle- or upper-middle-class Egyptian patients had paranoid delusions that centered around nonreligious themes. In contrast, economically disadvantaged patients had paranoid delusions regarding religious institutions. Other studies (Dutta & Murray, 2010) conducted in the UK have shown that the prevalence of schizophrenia is greater in West Indian immigrants living in the UK than in those individuals who remain in their country of birth and do not immigrate. Furthermore, these studies also point out the impact that emigration and dislocation from family and culture can have on the psychological functioning of individuals. Overall, these findings indicate how culture, socioeconomic factors, and immigration can affect the nature, type, and content of psychotic symptoms.

Differentiating Psychosis from Cultural Experiences or Beliefs

The DSM-5-TR recognizes the importance of distinguishing cultural experiences and beliefs from actual psychotic symptoms by expanding the discussion of cultural issues for selected psychotic disorders and developing the CFI. However, the DSM does not provide specific guidelines on how to differentiate actual psychotic symptoms from normative cultural experiences or beliefs. However, scholars have proposed helpful guidelines to assist clinicians in determining the nonpathological nature of cultural experiences or beliefs from actual psychotic symptoms.

Moreira-Almeida and Cardeña (2011) proposed six features that may suggest the nonpathological nature of spiritual experiences. These include:

1. Absence of subjective distress.
2. Absences of social or functional impairment.
3. Compatibility with the patient's cultural background and peer group.
4. Lack of psychiatric comorbidities.
5. Degrees of personal control over the spiritual/religious experience.
6. Personal growth because of the spiritual experience.

In another review, Clark and Harrison (2012) summarized guidelines to help clinicians differentiate delusions with religious content from culturally normative religious or spiritual beliefs. Their recommendations to clinicians include:

- Never be too quick to assign a diagnosis of a psychiatric disorder and risk pathologizing normative religious beliefs.
- Go beyond the content of beliefs and focus instead on the degree of conviction, pervasiveness, bizarreness, and distress.
- Consider the religious or spiritual context of the belief and examine the extent to which the current belief deviates from accepted cultural, religious, or spiritual norms.
- Remain cognizant that some forms of delusions with religious content that involve grandiose antichrist ideation, persecution, and guilt may potentially be associated with harm to self and others.

- Perform a careful evaluation, including assessing suicide risk factors such as past self-harm, substance misuse, and severity of any mental illness.
- Establish a therapeutic alliance, rapport, and openness with the patient and family, and respect other cultural, religious, and spiritual professionals who may become involved with the patient.

A final complicating issue in assessing psychosis within a cultural context is the validity of our assessment instruments in our diagnostic practices. A core principle in conducting competent, culturally informed assessments is knowledge about the limits of these methods, for which patients they are designed, and the conditions they indicate. Those of us who use psychological tests, structured interviews, and rating scales need to know when these instruments are not appropriate for patients from cultural backgrounds that differ from the normative samples for which these instruments were developed. Relying on traditional testing methods to aid in diagnostic decision-making may have limited value with patients whose cultural and ethnic backgrounds diverge from Western cultural norms.

Clinical Assessment Points

1. Transient hallucinations in the context of spiritual or religious experiences and the absence of any other psychotic symptoms are more likely to be normative.
2. Similarly, cultural, religious, and spiritual beliefs, such as belief in voodoo, witchcraft, ghosts, and various conspiracy theories, without any accompanying psychiatric symptoms as part of the patient's presenting problems, are not uncommon and more likely to be culturally normative.
3. Given the difficulty of reliably assessing the bizarreness of the belief, it is more beneficial to evaluate the pervasiveness of the belief, the degree of preoccupation, the action taken in response to the belief, the degree to which the belief is related to the presenting problem, and the level of subjective distress and social/functional impairment.
4. Utilizing a cultural, religious, or spiritual consultant or professional familiar with the individual's culture is an effective way of assessing the degree of deviation from cultural and religious normative beliefs, experiences, and practices.
5. Cultural beliefs or experiences that move the individual toward harming self or others should be carefully evaluated for the presence of psychosis or other psychiatric disorders.

11

ATTENUATED PSYCHOSIS, PSYCHOSIS-PRONENESS, AND RISK FACTORS FOR PSYCHOTIC ILLNESS

Gary Brucato, Ph.D.

Several constructs have been proposed for conceptualizing individuals who might share similar features that render them vulnerable to developing psychotic disorders. These concepts include prodromal psychosis, clinical high-risk and ultra-high-risk categories, attenuated psychosis syndrome, psychosis proneness, schizotypy, and psychoticism. While there is some overlap in these designations, there are key theoretical and clinical distinctions between them, which we will address in detail in this chapter. We will discuss how subthreshold psychotic signs and symptoms generally present in clinical settings and summarize current views and controversies related to identifying and evaluating psychosis risk. The literature regarding psychosis proneness and schizotypy will be reviewed, and we will consider various demographic, environmental, and contextual risk factors for psychotic illness.

The Concept of Attenuated Psychosis

While schizophrenia, the most common psychotic disorder, is associated with a relatively low global prevalence of about 1%, it imposes significant, sometimes devastating personal disability and a disproportionately severe financial burden of approximately 23 billion dollars per year (Desai et al., 2013; Switaj et al., 2012). It has long been understood – for instance, by Bleuler (1911) and Sullivan (1927) – that this and other psychoses occur on a continuum, with the onset of one's first episode of *syndromal* or full-blown illness preceded by a period of subthreshold signs and symptoms, with the latter ranging from a brief interval to several years (Fenton & McGlashan, 1991, 1994; McGlashan & Fenton, 1993). Researchers hoped that this subthreshold phase might constitute a window for intervention, permitting curtailment of the onset of more severe illness and reducing the psychosocial difficulties associated with

 DOI: 10.4324/9781003415206-16

psychotic disorders (Beiser et al., 1993; Broome et al., 2005; Crow et al., 1986; Klosterkötter et al., 2001; Loebel et al., 1992; McGlashan et al., 2001; Morrison et al., 2004; Riecher-Rössler, 2006; Yung & McGorry, 1996a; Yung et al., 1998; Yung et al., 2003).

The term *attenuated psychosis* refers to positive signs and symptoms – specifically, delusions, hallucinations, or thought disorder – which occur at clinically significant levels but without the frequency, intensity, behavioral impact, and/or degree of conviction associated with syndromal illness. Notably, affected persons may or may not have initially been predisposed to psychosis. The term *prodrome* was introduced into the literature nearly a century ago (Mayer-Gross, 1932) to describe this period of subthreshold psychotic illness, which would later be more extensively defined by Häfner and colleagues (1992, 1995), followed by a worldwide initiative to understand better its phenomenological and clinical attributes and effects. This label, alongside the term *pre-psychosis*, has fallen out of favor, as a constellation of subthreshold psychotic signs and symptoms should only be labeled a *prodromal* phase retroactively, following conversion to full-blown psychosis (Yung & McGorry, 1996a, 1996b). Importantly, it is impossible to determine if those found to meet the criteria for supposed psychosis risk who never progress to syndromal illness within two to three years (Fusar-Poli, Bonoldi et al., 2012; De Pablo, Radua et al., 2021; Shrivastava et al., 2011) had, in fact, been false-positives, with signs and symptoms better accounted for by some other condition. More will be said about this point later in the chapter.

Further complicating the matter, psychotic disorders are heterogeneous in nature, with wide variation between individuals in terms of clinical presentation, course, degree of functional impact, and the efficacy of treatments. This heterogeneity can also render the distinctions between normal and especially subthreshold versus syndromal psychotic signs and symptoms daunting to disentangle. Moreover, those considered to be at risk for the development of psychotic conditions will often demonstrate cognitive, interpersonal, psychomotor, attentional, emotional, and language-related deficits, which might be comorbid with the risk syndrome, or else be better accounted for by an unrelated neurodevelopmental or psychiatric disorder.

Development of Specific Criteria for Psychosis Prediction

Working in Germany in the 1960s, Gross (1969, 1989) created an early scale for predicting psychosis from subthreshold features, which was further developed by other investigators in that nation (Klosterkötter et al., 1997; Schultze-Lutter et al., 2006). The Bonn Scale for the Assessment of Basic Symptoms (BSABS) evaluated cognitive, perceptual, and energy-related deficits, termed "basic symptoms," subjectively perceived by individuals as possible indicators of emergent psychosis. These included mild but troubling experiences involving drive, affect, sensory perception, thinking, and motor behavior. This work yielded a constellation of nine symptoms suggestive of a schizophrenia risk phase (Klosterkötter et al., 1997). In a subsequent prospective study with 160 high-risk patients over a ten-year period, titled the Cologne Early Recognition Study, nearly half were found to have developed the condition, and the presence of self-perceived basic symptoms predicted conversion to schizophrenia with a probability level of 70% (Klosterkötter et al., 2001).

The Cologne study and the BSABS served as springboards for the creation of another instrument designed to identify risk symptoms at an even earlier juncture in the course of psychotic illness, the Schizophrenia Proneness Instrument for Adults (SPI-A; Schultze-Lutter et al., 2007). A semi-structured interview containing guiding questions and inquiries, the SPI-A was subsequently streamlined into a 32-item instrument with six dimensions: (1) impaired tolerance to normal stress, (2) emotional deficits, (3) cognitive impediments, (4) cognitive disturbances, (5) body perception disturbance, (6) perception of motor disturbances and estrangement. It has been demonstrated to be both reliable and valid in terms of assessing early subjective alterations in functioning that characterize subthreshold psychosis.

The early 1990s saw additional promising work from European research groups. In England, Falloon (1992) demonstrated a reduction in progression to first-episode schizophrenia among young people with suspected attenuated symptoms but raised concern that false-positive cases might incur stigma and prompt unnecessary treatment. In 1994, Häfner and colleagues (1994) retroactively examined individuals who had experienced first-episode psychosis and observed that only 10–20% could not recall a preceding prodromal period.

These efforts prompted groundbreaking research by Yung, McGorry, and colleagues at the Personal Assessment and Crisis Evaluation (PACE) clinic based in Melbourne, Australia. They sought to maximize the identification of persons at risk for psychotic disorders based on their clinical presentations, with the hope of learning how to prospectively, rather than retrospectively, examine signs and symptoms and prevent conversion to syndromal illness. They developed an *ultra-high risk* (UHR) construct (Yung & Nelson, 2013), incorporating age, presumed genetic risk, and clinical risk factors, such as decline in functioning and subthreshold psychotic symptoms. Three UHR subgroups were established, which have influenced virtually all subsequent psychosis-risk research: (1) An attenuated psychotic symptoms (APS) group for young people with subthreshold positive symptoms in the past year, (2) a brief, limited intermittent psychotic symptom (BLIPS) group for those who have experienced frank psychosis lasting less than a week and abating without treatment, and (3) a trait and state risk factor group, containing persons with first-degree relatives with psychotic disorders and/or schizotypal personality disorder, in addition to a major functional decline or chronically low functioning in the past year (Yung et al., 2004). An initial validation study found that over 40% of UHR individuals developed syndromal psychosis within one year (Yung et al., 2003).

To facilitate identification of individuals potentially at risk of psychosis, the UHR subcategories were developed into the Comprehensive Assessment of At-Risk Mental States (CAARMS; Yung et al., 2000, 2004, 2005; Yung & McGorry, 1996a, 1996b), widely used in Australian, Asian and European research. The CAARMS manual operationalized definitions, questions, and anchor points for eliciting and rating 27 signs and symptoms, organized into seven dimensions (Yung et al., 2005): (1) positive symptoms, (2) cognitive changes in attention and concentration, (3) emotional disturbance/decreased stress tolerance, (4) negative symptoms, (5) behavioral changes/impairment in role functioning, (6) motor/physical changes, including sleep disturbance, and (7) general psychopathology.

In early studies, the measure demonstrated good reliability and validity (Yung et al., 2003, 1996). A revised version, the CAARMS-II, has shown comparable to superior validity and reliability (Yung et al., 2005). With participants followed for one to two years, the CAARMS increased prediction levels of conversion to psychosis in high-risk groups up to 30–50% over the 10% level, based on family genetic factors alone (Yung et al., 1998).

In 1999, Yale University's Prevention through Risk Identification, Management and Education (PRIME) Clinic in New Haven, Connecticut, developed the Structured Interview for Prodromal Symptoms (SIPS; Miller & McGlashan, 2000; Miller et al., 2002; Miller et al., 2003; McGlashan et al., 2010), later titled the Structured Interview for Psychosis-Risk Symptoms. Generally favored in North America, the SIPS divides the constellation of psychosis-risk features delineated in previous research into positive, negative, disorganized, and general categories, ascertained by way of a semi-structured interview. Across these domains, it utilizes 29 questions to elicit ratings on the Scale of Prodromal Symptoms (SOPS) regarding the presence and severity of 19 signs and symptoms. The Yale group also established a distinct set of criteria to identify the three psychosis-risk syndromes originally identified by the Melbourne group, called the Criteria of Prodromal Symptoms (COPS).

The clinical high-risk (CHR) categories utilized in the SIPS were found to be reliable and valid (McGlashan et al., 2010). A large multisite study using SIPS demonstrated excellent reliability and acceptable levels of predictive validity (Addington et al., 2007; Woods et al., 2009). Within one year, 25% of individuals who met psychosis-risk criteria developed psychotic illness, and within two years, 35% converted to psychosis (Cannon et al., 2008).

Of note, the present version of the SIPS contains separate categories for whether the Attenuated Positive Symptom Syndrome (APSS) is of the "progression" type (a new or worsening attenuated positive sign or symptom with the required frequency in the past year) or "persistence" type (one or more active attenuated positive signs or symptoms, occurring at the required frequency, but with none of these being new or worsening in the past year). Criteria for partial and full remission are also indicated.

Attenuated Psychosis Syndrome in the DSM-5 and DSM-5-TR

Of note, the progression type of the SIPS APSS would serve as the basis for an Attenuated Psychosis Syndrome (APS), included as a condition for further study in the Appendix (section 3) of the fifth edition of the *Diagnostic and Statistical Manual of Mental Disorders* (APA, 2013). In its original form, this category required, on Criterion A, at least one positive symptom (delusions, hallucinations, disorganized speech) "in attenuated form, with relatively intact reality testing," which is "of sufficient severity or frequency to warrant clinical attention." To satisfy Criteria B and C, the symptom(s) must have "been present at least once per week for the past month" and "begun or worsened in the past year." For Criterion D, the symptom(s) are "sufficiently distressing and disabling to the individual to warrant clinical attention." Finally, Criterion E required that the symptom(s) are "not better accounted for by another mental disorder, including a depressive or bipolar disorder with psychotic features, and is not attributable to the physiological effects of a substance or another medical condition." In a subsequent text revision (DSM-5-TR; APA, 2022), Criterion A was modified to enhance its clarity. The phrase "with relatively intact reality testing" was removed and the three symptoms (i.e., attenuated forms of delusion, hallucination, and disorganized speech) were defined more accurately, using a "gatekeeper" to distinguish the attenuated from the non-attenuated form.

Comparison of the UHR, CHR, and DSM-5-TR Constructs

When the UHR and CHR constructs are compared, it is noted that they assess similar signs and symptoms using rating scales, with a predominant focus on positive signs and symptoms, while also evaluating negative symptoms, behavioral disorganization, general symptoms, such as concentration difficulties and dysphoric mood states; and functional impairment. Both instruments delineate the APSS, BLIPS, and GRD psychosis-risk categories. A 2015 meta-analysis by Fusar-Poli and colleagues determined that both the CAARMS and SIPS successfully identify individuals who go on to convert to syndromal psychosis at comparable rates.

These categories differ, however, in some key respects. Persons meeting the criteria for the SIPS and CAARMS psychosis-risk categories, most of whom fall into the APSS designation (Fusar-Poli, Bonoldi et al., 2012), are help-seeking and symptomatic at the time of baseline assessment and, as previously noted, have no histories of syndromal psychosis. Similarly, in the DSM-5-TR APS diagnosis, signs and symptoms "are sufficiently distressing and disabling to the patient and/or parent/guardian to lead them to seek help" (APA, 2022, p. 903). The CAARMS category requires at least one attenuated positive symptom present in the past year, and at least one attenuated positive symptom occurs outside of peak intoxication from a substance known to be associated with psychotic experiences (e.g., hallucinogens, amphetamines, cocaine). At least one attenuated positive sign or symptom also occurs one or more days per month, for more than one hour a day or three or more days weekly. One is only deemed to be at risk for psychosis by the CAARMS if there has been a significant decline in psychosocial functioning. In this measure, a diagnosis of syndromal psychosis requires at least one positive sign or symptom occurring at a fully psychotic level for three or more days per week for one hour or more a day, or at least daily, for a period of one month, unless antipsychotic medication is newly being taken or there has been an increase in dosage (Yung et al., 2005; Woods et al., 2023).

The SIPS APSS and DSM-5-TR categories, by contrast, require at least one attenuated positive symptom present in the past month, occurring at an average frequency of at least once weekly in that period, and at least one attenuated positive sign or symptom must have begun or significantly worsened in the past year (McGlashan et al., 2010; Woods et al., 2010; APA, 2022). The SIPS defines threshold psychosis as at least one positive sign or symptom occurring at a fully psychotic level for one hour or more at an average frequency of four days a week for at least one month or, if the sign or symptom is seriously disorganizing or dangerous, as little as a single day (Powers et al., 2021). Alternatively, the DSM-5-TR APS does not diagnose syndromal psychosis, where a sign or symptom is disorganizing or dangerous.

Recently, the U.S. National Institute of Mental Health (NIMH) launched an effort to harmonize the SIPS and CAARMS instruments into an additional measure that would permit an individual to meet for the syndromes defined in both (Woods et al., 2023). The result has been the development of the Positive Symptoms and Diagnostic Criteria for the CAARMS Harmonized with the SIPS (PSYCHS), offering unified criteria for how attenuated positive signs and symptoms are rated and how syndromal psychosis is defined. The CAARMS frequency ratings were edited and harmonized with those from the SIPS. The "better accounted for" convention was also adapted. The CAARMS definition of threshold psychosis was used, but incorporating a SIPS criterion, the frequency and duration requirements were waived if a positive sign or symptom is "imminently dangerous." Further specification has been given that this danger is physical in nature or "to personal dignity or to social/family networks."

The PSYCHS contains partially consistent criteria for how the progression of attenuated positive signs and symptoms is defined. For instance, individuals who would not have met CHR progressive criteria on the SIPS do meet this category on the PSYCHS because of the CAARMS UHR groupings. This can yield a complicated diagnosis summary, for example, "CAARMS APS subthreshold intensity, UHR grouping and vulnerability group and SIPS APSS persistent."

It is important to note that the PSYCHS was not intended to render the SIPS and CAARMS obsolete. Rather, its purpose has been to facilitate the comparison of findings from worldwide research centers and to allow for more comprehensive meta-analyses.

While the various instruments we have been reviewing have been shown to possess acceptable psychometric characteristics, there are subtle differences. In a 2012 review, Addington and Heinssen noted that BSABS and SPI-A appear to pick up high-risk features earlier than the CAARMS or SIPS. In advocating the use of the SIPS/SOPS, McGlashan noted that these instruments provided a broader scope of diagnostic information than the CAARMS. Specifically, they pointed out that while the CAARMS was designed to be a diagnostic instrument, the SIPS was intended not only to diagnose psychosis-risk symptoms but also to assess the severity of risk symptoms over time and determine the likelihood of conversion to syndromal psychosis (McGlashan et al., 2010). The most widely used and best-validated instruments for assessing the CHR state are listed in Appendix B.

Clinical Presentation of Attenuated Signs and Symptoms

Attenuated Delusions

As noted earlier in this volume, a delusion is a false belief about external reality, which an individual unshakably maintains despite incontrovertible contrary evidence. The phrase *attenuated delusion* might be considered contradictory, as it connotes a false belief about external reality which is held with some, but not a full conviction, with skepticism that can be elicited by persistent questioning or confrontation. A more appropriate term might be *overvalued ideas*. Any of the numerous subtypes of delusion can occur at an attenuated level. For instance, a patient in a clinical setting demonstrating attenuated grandiosity might state that several times weekly over the past few months while taking her first-ever writing class, she has wondered whether she is a "literary genius" who "might win the Nobel Prize," despite never having been told by her instructor, classmates, or anyone that she possesses any particular ability in this area. She notes, however, that this is "maybe not true," adding, "Maybe what constitutes good writing is more a matter of opinion." Such individuals might demonstrate *expansiveness*, characterized by an inflated sense of self-importance, heightened enthusiasm, and excessive friendliness.

Another patient might describe several months of sensing, daily, that a specific individual is following him, explaining, upon further inquiry, that he generally dismisses this notion "after thinking about it" because "it probably doesn't make sense for anybody to be doing that." This would constitute attenuated paranoia, termed *suspiciousness* in the psychosis-risk field. Here, the aforementioned "disorganized or dangerous" criterion utilized in the SIPS APSS and the PSYCHS but not included in the DSM-5 APS might be well-illustrated: If the patient just described had additionally stated that, despite his statement that he can, with contemplation, dismiss suspicious ideas, he has decided to attain a firearm and confront the person possibly following him "to get to the bottom of it once and for all," this dangerousness would require a designation of syndromal psychosis on the SIPS and the PSYCHS measures. The DSM-5 category, by contrast, would not rule out attenuation in this instance, although, in practice, a clinician might wish to take this into consideration when making a judgment regarding an overvalued idea versus frank paranoia.

A wide array of unusual ideas might be reported by individuals in the psychosis-risk state. Some such persons will describe dissociative symptoms, including derealization, depersonalization, perplexing déjà vu or jamais vu, or a sense of losing track of time. These might be distinguished from similar experiences associated with trauma or severe anxiety by probing the individual's sense of whether these began following a specific negative event or are triggered by a particular worry or stimulus. For instance, someone experiencing derealization might state that this symptom began within the weeks following a physical assault, or a patient might notice depersonalization during panic states or when exposed to a stimulus associated with a phobic disorder. In the psychosis-risk state, individuals might provide peculiar explanations for dissociative phenomena with delusion-like premises, such as, "I feel like I might be living in a simulation," "I've been wondering if I'm a ghost of somebody on an operating table somewhere," or "I feel like I'm having déjà vu a lot because my dreams are somehow coming true." Some CHR persons will describe feeling as if they are on "The Truman Show," a reference to the 1998 film in which a man's seemingly ordinary life has been, without his knowledge, aired to the public as a reality show, with the people he knows all secretly being actors.

Attenuated ideas, which, in fully psychotic form, would constitute Schneiderian first-rank symptoms, can occur in the CHR state. These might include subthreshold thought insertion or withdrawal, thought broadcasting, or feeling that one's thoughts, emotions, or actions are being influenced or caused by some external agent. Some individuals will report altering their thoughts, affect, or behavior due to a vague sense that others can somehow read (i.e., attenuated mindreading) or hear (i.e., attenuated thought broadcasting) their thoughts. Others might conversely describe feeling that they can read or hear other people's thoughts. This idea sometimes arises in individuals who are adept at intuiting or empathizing with the feelings of those around them, who subsequently misinterpret themselves as utilizing a telekinetic ability. Some might discuss a sense of somehow being able to anticipate future events by way of premonitions, dreams, or revelations from God, angels, deceased persons, or some other metaphysical being. Note that the latter might overlap with attenuated grandiose ideas. It is also important to be sensitive to cultural and religious beliefs when evaluating the potential delusionality of ideas about communications from spiritual entities.

Attenuated ideas of reference can occur, often described as being associated with finding irrelevant stimuli salient and then feeling compelled to make some meaning out of them. Some research suggests that, in schizophrenia, the formation of delusions may be associated with dysregulation of the mesolimbic dopamine system, leading to over-attending to irrelevant stimuli (Heinz & Schlagenhauf, 2010; Kapur, 2003). Of note, a study by Crump and colleagues (2018) examined whether attenuated first-rank symptoms might be especially predictive of conversion to psychosis and, in particular, a subsequent diagnosis of schizophrenia. No significant relationship emerged between these factors.

Some individuals in the CHR state might describe or demonstrate preoccupations with scientific, political, philosophical, and/or religious constructs beyond what would be considered average in one's cultural paradigm or idiosyncratic notions that are not typically held by proponents of these schools of thought. For example, a patient might report confusing friends and family with an intense focus on concepts from theoretical physics, such as multiverses, wormholes, or the possibility of time travel. Another might describe existential concerns, such as whether he "actually" exists, or display epistemological concerns, fixating on whether it is possible for a given statement to be entirely truthful or for any piece of information to be fully "knowable." Moving beyond the commonly shared beliefs of a certain religious faith, a patient might describe a bizarre idea not held by the wider group, such as worry that God will punish her if she touches a religious text with a particular finger. An attenuated delusion of guilt can also occur.

Individuals in the CHR state might describe unusual somatic preoccupations, such as thoughts about having a medical condition despite reassurance by professionals that this is not the case or excessive concern about the appearance or symmetry of one's body. Notably, these ideas might overlap with perceptual disturbances. For instance, a patient might describe concern that his nose is "the same size as a cell phone" when this is demonstrably not so, possibly influenced by a disturbance of visual perception when viewing himself in a mirror. Another might describe concern about a parasite moving in her abdomen, arising from tactile perceptual experiences that feel like "tickling" across her stomach.

Some unusual ideas and associated behaviors in the CHR state might be challenging to distinguish from Obsessive-Compulsive Disorder (OCD). In general terms, it should be noted that, in peculiar or magical ideas associated with OCD, there should be no co-occurring negative symptoms, nor any suspiciousness or other attenuated delusions, thought disorder, or perceptual aberrations. Moreover, OCD is associated with a bimodal age distribution. In child-onset OCD, the condition typically emerges in childhood, at a mean age of 11, while in adult-onset OCD, it generally arises between ages 19–23 (Roessner et al., 2022). The attenuated positive signs and symptoms of the CHR state, by contrast, have been shown in several studies to generally first appear or to be at least first ascertained in mid-adolescence through young adulthood (Brucato et al., 2017; Mensi et al., 2021; De Pablo, Radua et al., 2021). Kennedy and colleagues (2021) explored whether a transition to psychosis was more likely in persons whose obsessive-compulsive ideas were implausible and magical in nature, such as blinking one's eyes in a particular pattern to prevent the death of a loved one, rather than simply preoccupations with plausible matters, such as germ contamination. No significant relationship was observed. Given the difficulty of distinguishing between qualitative differences in attenuated psychosis and obsessive-compulsive signs and symptoms, the authors proposed that clinicians encountering adolescent or young adult patients with new-onset OCD or obsessions or compulsions not meeting full DSM-5 criteria for the condition in the past year should monitor these for a minimum of two years to assess for the possible emergence of psychotic illness.

Attenuated Perceptual Disturbances

Perceptual disturbances in attenuated psychosis occur along a wide spectrum of intensity and loss of contact with reality. Some may perceive an actual stimulus in an inaccurate or exaggerated way, while others may perceive stimuli that do not exist in the external world while retaining insight that these likely arise from one's own mind. The maintenance of this insight regarding the origin of such experiences in the self is key to whether a perceptual disturbance remains at an attenuated level. The alternative notion that such experiences are arising from an external source, such as God, the devil, some electronic device, other people, animals, or extraterrestrials, might be associated with some delusional belief, which should be evaluated as a potential additional positive symptom. As noted for other psychotic-like phenomena, one should remain sensitive regarding the role of one's cultural and spiritual beliefs in how perceptual aberrations are interpreted.

While perceptual disturbances can occur in any sensory modality in the CHR state, they are predominantly auditory and visual in nature. These are encountered to similar degrees in attenuated psychosis, but some evidence suggests that auditory aberrations are predictive of progression to psychosis, while abnormal visual experiences are somehow protective against conversion (Lehembre-Shiah et al., 2017).

Visual and auditory perceptual disturbances in the CHR state sometimes take the form of illusions, in which stimuli that actually exist in the external world are misapprehended. For instance, an individual might overhear a stranger on the street shouting out a random word and misperceive that his name is being called. There can also be an intensification of the intensity, brightness, or color of visual stimuli; light sensitivity, called *photophobia*; or, in a phenomenon known as *hyperacusis*, exaggerated sensitivity to sound. Interestingly, the latter is a commonly stated reason among individuals in the CHR state for isolative behavior, akin to how persons on the autism spectrum might evade experiences that overwhelm the sensorium.

Where an auditory or visual experience occurs in the absence of an actual external stimulus, the visual type generally consists of briefly glimpsed flashes, shadows, trails, or amorphous patches of color, sometimes perceived out of the corner of one's eye. Less frequently, these are more fully formed and intense. Where the latter occurs, the potential effects of illicit drugs or alcohol or an underlying medical condition are generally considered. Improbable visual phenomena are also sometimes described by persons malingering psychosis due to some external motivation, such as evasion of military duty or work, attainment of financial compensation, avoiding criminal prosecution, or obtaining medications to abuse or sell.

With auditory aberrations occurring in the absence of an actual external stimulus, sounds or verbiage can occur very briefly or for longer patches of time. These can be perceived as arising from inside or outside of one's head. One or more voices may make commands of the individual. While the latter does not necessarily imply full loss of contact with the reality that these experiences originate in the self, the reader should bear in mind the aforementioned "disorganized or dangerous" rule associated with the APSS categories in the SIPS and PSYCHS measures.

The author of this chapter (GB), who has over 15 years of experience evaluating and treating CHR individuals, has observed that some such persons come to be more convinced that voices and other auditory aberrations are arising from a source other than themselves because these sounds gradually feel farther away in space or more external to the self, which may reflect some presently unclear gradual change to the brain associated with an insidious psychotic disorder. He also notes that some CHR individuals perceive that auditory aberrations are transitioning from feeling inside their heads to sounding outside. Such individuals sometimes describe these sounds or hallucinations as generally feeling close to the head or body, "flowing" from their eyes, nostrils, mouth, or ears. Hence, some individuals in the CHR state will attempt to block or cover these orifices with dark glasses, bandanas, headphones, a medical mask, their hands, or some other means. For this reason, it is best to inquire about the rationale for such behavior before deeming it disorganized in nature. In one instance, a patient whom a previous evaluator had described as displaying "flat affect" reported that he intentionally limited the rage of his facial expression, especially his smiling, because of a sense, without full conviction but with considerable behavioral impact, that auditory perceptual experiences were escaping his mind through his canine teeth. Note that, in this way, an apparent negative symptom revealed itself to be a purposeful behavior stemming from a positive symptom.

Tactile perceptual disturbances can include pins and needles sensations, called *paresthesias,* a sensation of what feels like insects crawling on or moving beneath one's skin, known as *formication*, vibrations, or cold or hot spots on the body. Where these are reported, the need for a neurological work-up is sometimes considered. Unusual olfactory and gustatory perceptual experiences are rare, although possible, in the CHR state and might be more consistent with some organic etiology, also potentially warranting further evaluation.

Disorganized Communication in the CHR state

Attenuation versus syndromal-level thought disorder can be distinguished by way of observing or eliciting insight from an individual that other people might struggle to understand his or her attempts at communication, or that comprehension of the self might be impaired. The disorganization in communication might be oral or written. Commonly reported or seen are vagueness, stereotyped language, difficulties with derailment in which there is eventually a return to one's original point (i.e., *circumstantiality*)

Table 11.1 Syndromal psychotic versus attenuated positive psychotic signs and symptoms

Psychotic-Level Signs and Symptoms	*Attenuated-Level Signs and Symptoms*
Delusions	Overvalued ideas, ideas of reference
Paranoia	Suspiciousness
Grandiosity	Expansiveness
Hallucinations	Perceptual abnormalities • Hearing odd noises • Hearing one's name being called • Hearing muffled or distant voices • Illusions • Seeing flashes of light or geometric shapes • Shadows seen out of the corner of one's eye • Less commonly, olfactory, gustatory, or tactile sensations • Recognized to be arising from one's own mind
Disorganized speech	Discursive speech • Use of peculiar words or phrases • Speech that is tangential or circumstantial, vague, or stereotyped
Impaired insight and reality testing	Maintenance of some insight • Doubt and lack of conviction are reported or can be elicited regarding the nature of one's experienced symptoms

or else the point is lost entirely (i.e., *tangentiality*), pressured or excessive speech, a sudden inability to think or speak clearly, followed by a change in topic (i.e., *thought blocking*), connecting of irrelevant or loosely-associated topics, or idiosyncratic use of language, such as neologisms, rhyming or clanging. Entirely unintelligible *word salad*, when not associated with an aphasic or other general medical condition or use of an illicit substance or alcohol, is generally more associated with syndromal psychosis.

- Signs and symptoms are distressing and disabling.
- Signs and symptoms are not better explained by another nonpsychotic mental disorder.
- Criteria for a full-blown psychosis have never been met.
- In addition to being less severe and frequent, insight and reality-testing are relatively intact.

Experience of Multiple Signs and Symptoms in Attenuated versus Syndromal Psychosis

The previously-referenced author of this chapter (GB) has observed in conducting research and clinical practice with CHR individuals that, in the attenuated phase, they generally experience more than one positive sign or symptom simultaneously. For instance, a patient might describe, over the past six months, a period of collectively hearing vague "footstep-like sounds," seeing "shadows" in the corner of his eye, feeling vaguely suspicious, and sensing that random things heard on television "might mean something." When asked about how these might relate to one another, the individual will typically describe the phenomena as disparate and not coalescing into a meaningful theme or narrative.

As the attenuated phase progresses and the patient converts to syndromal psychosis – into what an observer might call a *break-down* – he or she sometimes experiences a coming together of previously disconnected signs and symptoms into a meaningful narrative that feels to him or her more like a *break-through*. Losing contact with reality and a willingness to question these ideas and experiences as improbable or false, the patient might now state,

> Now it all makes sense! The footsteps are those of the people I'm seeing in the corner of my eye . . . the ones I sensed wanted to hurt me . . . and God was trying to warn me through messages on the television to stay away from them.

Here, the patient's newfound certainty may prevent willingness to trust caretakers who are not "in the know" about these conclusions or meanings or to enter now especially needed treatment. The author has thus utilized the method in evaluations of persons with psychotic illness to probe for the connectedness of positive symptoms and the meaning patients make of their experiences as an indicator of severity and capacity for reality testing. Moreover, there is some evidence that this point of conversion to syndromal psychosis might constitute a period of heightened risk for violent acts, which may occur within an average of seven days of the transition to full-blown illness (Brucato et al., 2018, 2019).

The newness and intensification of positive signs and symptoms may also be key to predicting conversion to syndromal psychosis. Brucato and colleagues (2021) reported that the likelihood of progression increases with the number of positive signs or symptoms determined by the SIPS to be present, and new or worsening in the past year. The authors suggested that the severity and number of attenuated positive symptoms, per se, are less predictive of progression to syndromal psychotic illness than the timing of their emergence and intensification. They also suggested that the earliest phase of psychotic illness may involve a rapid, dynamic process, beginning before an individual's first episode of syndromal psychosis.

Other Signs and Symptoms

While positive signs and symptoms are central to determining psychosis risk, negative symptoms may be present in the psychosis-risk state. These might include social anhedonia, avolition, reduced affective range, diminished verbal spontaneity, a decreased sense of oneself or difficulty experiencing one's own emotions, a lessening of ideational richness, or impaired psychosocial functioning. Disorganization signs and symptoms, including odd behavior or appearance, bizarreness in ideas, trouble with focus and attention, and hygiene difficulties, are sometimes observed. More general signs and symptoms that can be associated with the CHR state or which may reflect other comorbid conditions include impaired sleep, dysphoric mood states, motor abnormalities, and impaired tolerance to normal stress.

Outcomes for Persons in the CHR State

Rates for conversion to syndromal psychosis within two to three years among CHR persons range from 20% to 50% in several long-term prospective studies (Fusar-Poli, Bonoldi et al., 2012; De Pablo, Radua et al., 2021; Shrivastava et al., 2011). Those who progress show a mean time to conversion following baseline assessment of 21.6 months or 1.8 years (Powers et al., 2020). Notably, Brucato and colleagues (2017) explored whether the average conversion time might vary between those who transition to schizophrenia versus other psychotic disorders. They found that conversion time averaged 7.97 months for 60% of 200 prospectively examined CHR individuals who developed schizophrenia and 15.68 months for those who developed psychotic mood disorders or other psychoses. The mean conversion age was 20.3 for males and 23.5 for females, consistent with previously-referenced research.

Importantly, long-term functional impairments are common among non-converters. A systematic review of the pertinent literature by Beck and colleagues (2019) yielded approximately half of the non-converters present with poor psychosocial outcomes at two- and six-year follow-up time points. Lin and colleagues (2015) found that individuals determined to be at risk for psychosis two to 14 years previously who did not transition to syndromal illness were at significant risk of chronic attenuated positive signs and symptoms. In terms of outcome diagnoses, the authors noted that 68% experienced nonpsychotic disorders (mood disorder in

49%, anxiety disorder in 35%, and substance use disorder in 29%). For 90% of the sample, the nonpsychotic disorder was present at baseline and persisted for 52% of them. During follow-up, 26% of the cohort had remission of a disorder, but 38% developed a new condition.

One question that has remained unanswered in the CHR literature is whether individuals with attenuated positive signs and symptoms that remain chronic but never develop into syndromal psychotic illness constitute a portion of those who are diagnosed with Cluster A personality disorders. These would include the paranoid, schizoid, and schizotypal personality disorders presently defined in the DSM-5-TR (APA, 2022). Indeed, in the year in which such individuals first experienced their characteristic, unusual ideas, thought disturbances, perceptual aberrations, and psychosocial impairments, these might have occurred with the frequency and impact associated with one of the aforementioned CHR categories. At present, the demarcation point is presently unclear between someone with a Cluster A personality disorder and an individual who was at high risk for psychosis and did not convert to syndromal illness but developed chronic subthreshold positive signs and symptoms.

Psychosis Proneness

Unlike attenuated psychosis, *psychosis proneness* is a non-clinical concept and does not constitute a diagnostic category. It encompasses a far larger group of individuals across the psychosis spectrum, including some who meet DSM-5-TR (APA, 2022) criteria for schizotypal personality disorder and those who do not and may well never come to the attention of mental health clinicians. Unlike the smaller CHR group, these individuals are not necessarily in acute distress, may not demonstrate any degree of disability or deterioration in functioning, and may not be help-seeking. The relationship between psychosis proneness and syndromal psychotic illness is a complex one that is far from settled.

Those falling into the proneness category may be relatively stable schizotypal individuals or people experiencing isolated, ego-syntonic, psychotic-like phenomena (e.g., perceptual aberrations, magical thinking, suspiciousness, expansiveness, or discursive speech) that do not create major functional disruptions or satisfy DSM-5-TR (APA, 2022) diagnostic criteria. The proneness concept is compatible with contemporary models proposing a continuum or spectrum of psychotic experiences varying in degree of sign and symptom severity. As in the CHR construct, some persons on this continuum may develop florid psychotic disorders over time, but many may never, hampering prediction and yielding a high false-positive rate.

As described in Chapter 5, the concepts of psychosis proneness, schizotypy and psychoticism (which we will refer to as "psychosis proneness") have drawn a great deal of interest from researchers who hypothesize a continuum of psychotic phenomena across the general population (Bentall et al., 1989; Chapman et al., 1978; Claridge et al., 1996; Eysenck, 1960; Eysenck & Eysenck, 1976; Meehl, 1962). Reviewing available studies, van Os and colleagues (2009) found the mean prevalence rate of psychosis proneness in the general population to be roughly 5%, with a median incidence rate of nearly 3%.

Assessment of Psychosis Proneness and Schizotypy

The majority of the instruments for assessing psychosis proneness were developed for research purposes. While some involve self-report, most utilize structured interviews and guided follow-up questions. See Appendix B for a list of these assessments.

One of the most comprehensive measures for evaluating psychosis proneness is the Wisconsin Manual for Assessing Psychotic-Like Experiences (WMAPLE). This interview-based assessment system rates psychotic proneness on a continuum, ranging from deviancy from normal to extremely psychotic. The original manual included six scales for assessing psychotic-like symptomatology: thought transmission, thought withdrawal, aberrant beliefs, passivity experiences, auditory experiences, and visual experiences. Later, a seventh was added to assess deviant olfactory experiences.

The WMAPLE was based on the Chapman Scales (Kwapil et al., 1999), which had been developed over a number of years to assess a broad range of experiential and behavioral features of *schizotypy*, a personality organization posited to reflect vulnerability to schizophrenia or more generally, psychosis-proneness (Chapman et al., 1995). Chapman and colleagues developed five self-report scales, presented in a true-false format: (1) The Perception Aberration Scale (PerAb), which assesses unusual bodily and sensory phenomena (Chapman et al., 1978), (2) the Magical Ideation Scale (MagId), which measures magical thinking and erroneous inferences about causality (Eckblad & Chapman, 1983), (3) the Revised Physical Anhedonia Scale (PhyAnh), measures deficits in the ability to experience physical pleasures (Chapman & Chapman, 1978), (4) the Revised Social Anhedonia Scale (SocAnh; Eckblad et al., 1982), developed to assess deficits in the ability to experience pleasure from social, nonphysical sources, and (5) the Impulsive Non-Conformity Scale (ImpNon) evaluates impulsivity and failure to conform to social expectations regarding the rights of other people (Chapman et al., 1995). The scales have been beneficial in studies attempting to distinguish between positive and negative forms of schizotypy. *Positive schizotypy* includes psychotic-like symptoms such as odd beliefs, unusual perceptual experiences, and mood dysregulation, while *negative schizotypy* is associated with asociality, avolition, diminished positive affect, and anergia (Vollema & van den Bosch, 1995). Kwapil et al. (2008) found that both the PerAb and MagId scales load on the positive schizotypy dimension and are related to psychotic-like experiences, substance abuse, and mood disorders. Negative schizotypy is associated more with blunted affect, diminished sensation-seeking, and schizoid phenomena. The scales have been studied extensively and shown to have good psychometric properties (Kwapil et al., 1999), including sensitivity and specificity ratios of .64 and .82, respectively. Notably, a ten-year follow-up study predicted the development of psychotic disorders (not exclusively schizophrenia-spectrum disorders) and poorer adjustment in a subgroup of high-risk participants. Chapman and colleagues (1994) demonstrated that young adults identified by elevations on the PerAb and MagId scales demonstrated significantly higher rates of mania and hypomania at ten-year follow-up.

Despite these favorable qualities, the WMAPLE poses two challenges for clinicians wishing to employ them in clinical assessments. The authors caution that the scales have limitations for use among non-white individuals. Moreover, the scales are essentially research tools that were developed in a college setting. Nonetheless, while their clinical use may be contraindicated, the scales help reinforce the construct validity of dimensions of psychosis-proneness that interest diagnosticians seeking to understand subthreshold presentations of psychotic-like phenomena.

The Schizotypal Personality Questionnaire (SPQ; Raine, 1991) has been extensively studied and repeatedly revised in the forms of the SPQ-B (Raine & Benishay, 1995) and the SPQ-BR (Cohen et al., 2010). Raine developed the original 74-item self-report scale to measure psychosis-proneness and, in particular, schizotypal personality patterns. Modeled on DSM-III-R (APA, 1987) criteria for schizotypal personality disorder, which have remained grossly unchanged in the DSM-5-TR (APA, 2022), it includes individual subscales to assess each of the condition's nine features: ideas of reference, social anxiety, odd/magical beliefs, unusual perceptions, odd/eccentric behavior, no close friends, odd speech, constricted affect, and suspiciousness. Three-factor solutions were identified in multiple adult and adolescent samples (Chen et al., 1997; Raine et al., 1994), including cognitive-perceptual deficits, disorganization, and interpersonal deficits. While the SPQ's psychometric properties were shown to be adequate, some problems were noted with the 22-item SPQ-B revision (Axelrod et al., 2001). In an effort to address these concerns, Cohen and colleagues (2010) revised the format of the SPQ and SPQ-B and designed a three-factor, 34-item scale, which they felt improved upon the SPQ-B while still providing a briefer version of the full SPQ. In a comprehensive review of psychosocial measures, Johnson (2010) determined that the SPQ, although originally developed within a college population, was a psychometrically sound questionnaire that could be beneficial in clinical groups.

The Structured Interview for Schizotypy (SIS; Kendler et al., 1989) was developed to measure a broad range of schizotypal characteristics, such as magical ideation, referential thinking, and social anxiety in family members of patients with schizophrenia and non-clinical subjects. This comprehensive measure assesses mild features and distinguishes between signs and symptoms. In order to address inadequacies in the original SIS, Vollema and Ormel (2000) developed the SIS-R, which contained clearer definitions and scoring criteria for assessing the previous version's three dimensions. Although Johnson (2010) commented that the original SIS has proved to be an excellent predictor of schizophrenia-proneness and possibly schizophrenic illness, there are no indications that it has been utilized as a clinical diagnostic tool.

Finally, the Structured Clinical Interview for the Psychotic Spectrum (SCI-PSY; Sbrana et al., 2005) is based on a spectrum model encompassing soft signs and subthreshold conditions, including temperamental and personality traits and disorders that reflect psychotic-like phenomena. Employing an interview-based scale, the instrument consists of 164 items, coded *yes* or *no*, organized into the five domains of paranoia, schizotypy–schizoidism, interpersonal sensitivity, misperceptions, and typical psychotic symptoms. The authors' preliminary investigation yielded acceptable validity and reliability for the measure in patients with psychotic and nonpsychotic disorders. The SCI-PSY identifies a continuum of delusions, hallucinations, interpersonal sensitivity, misperceptions, grandiosity, and anger over-reactivity that was able to detect psychosis-spectrum features in patients without diagnosable psychotic disorders.

Clinical Assessment of Psychosis Proneness and Psychosis-Risk Syndromes

As the previous sections have indicated, it has been researchers in the areas of psychotic illness and personality, rather than mental health professionals exclusively in clinical practice, who have developed various assessment methods for identifying psychosis proneness or psychosis-risk syndromes. The instruments these teams of researchers have developed, though comprehensive in scope, are often unsuitable, impractical, or unavailable to clinical practitioners faced with diagnostic decisions regarding psychosis potential in the patients they evaluate and/or treat. Even the DSM-5-TR's (APA, 2022) APS syndrome, which can be clinically utilized as a subtype of the diagnosis of psychotic disorder not otherwise specified, is often not understood by mental health professionals. For instance, in the absence of specialized training, they might struggle with the question of whether a sign or symptom is attenuated or fully psychotic in intensity or how to define whether it is "new or worsening in the past year" without referring to a scale like the one given in the SIPS instrument, upon which the APS category was based.

Clinicians typically rely on unstructured clinical interviews and standard psychological testing instruments to determine whether a patient might be at risk for developing psychosis. The following clinical vignette demonstrates how difficult it can be to determine whether an individual has a critical mass of clinical features to be considered at imminent risk for developing a psychotic disorder.

"Eddie:" Attenuated Psychosis or Unstable Schizotypy?

Eddie was initially evaluated when he was ten years old after the school he attended had raised concerns about his behavior and some organizational difficulties. Testing showed significant elevations in Rorschach indices of disordered thinking. Additionally, stories he told regarding the Children's Apperception Test (CAT), a projective measure used to examine personality, family, and other interpersonal dynamics and aspects of emotional disturbance, were particularly odd, both in thematic content and test organization. As a result of the assessment, the psychologist referred Eddie for psychotherapy and a medication consultation. He was treated with psychotherapy for a period of two years. Although he demonstrated some improvement in his behavior, he continued to demonstrate a certain level of oddness in his speech and behavior. Eddie was taking medications to address poor attention and anxiety. He had not, however, been prescribed any neuroleptic medication.

Eddie was referred for a second consultation two years later when his therapist became concerned about his thinking, judgment, and poor hygiene. This time, the test responses showed fewer signs of florid disorganization and idiosyncratic thinking, although he continued to give confusing explanations when the examiner asked about some of his behaviors.

Finally, at the age of 16, Eddie was referred for testing a third time because his new therapist and psychiatrist had become concerned about his disorganization, odd preoccupations, and confused thinking. Although his hygiene was still poor, and he seemed to harbor some odd concerns, there continued to be no indication of positive signs. Eddie denied hallucinations or even reported perceptual anomalies, and he gave no indications of delusional-like thinking, which might suggest his insight and reality testing were psychotically impaired. His Rorschach, however, now revealed severely disorganized and illogical thinking, which again raised concerns about the level of acute risk for psychosis. It was concluded that, while Eddie was not obviously psychotic, he demonstrated a pattern of schizotypal personality features that had persisted over the past six years. The key question was whether, in the context of these attributes, Eddie had or had not demonstrated marked deterioration in his functioning from the previous year. The challenge for the treatment team was to determine how much, if any, his functioning had declined during that period.

Of particular importance from a clinical perspective, Eddie does not meet the criteria for the proposed attenuated psychosis syndrome delineated in the DSM-5-TR (APA, 2022). Functional decline across the past year would satisfy Criteria D if "sufficiently distressing and disabling" to the patient "to warrant clinical attention." However, he presented with no entirely new positive signs or symptoms over the year preceding his most recent evaluation. Delusions and perceptual disturbances, attenuated or otherwise, were not present in his case. While some odd speech and thinking are present, there is no indication in the case history that these significantly increased in the past year.

Notably, were the current version of the SIPS clinically applicable, it is possible that Eddie would meet the criteria for the Persistence subtype of the APSS category, but we do not have adequate information in the vignette provided here regarding frequency, degree of insight, or behavioral impact to determine SIPS scores at the various timepoints of evaluation.

Psychological Testing

Compared to structured interviews and rating scales developed by researchers to study narrow groups of symptoms or syndromes, psychological tests are generally fewer specific measures. Furthermore, tests do not establish diagnoses. Using psychological testing variables to identify specific dimensions of psychosis or, more specifically, to distinguish psychosis proneness from attenuated psychosis, on the one hand, and full-blown psychotic illness, on the other, may not yield the precise set of differential testing scores and indices that we might desire. While psychological testing variables may yield useful information, especially regarding questions about psychosis-risk syndromes, they are not sufficient grounds for making diagnostic decisions. Like all diagnoses, psychosis-risk syndromes require information about the history and duration of signs and symptoms. It is important to remember that testing instruments measure psychological functions, not diagnostic entities. Since the psychotic phenomena found in psychosis-risk syndromes overlap with the phenomena associated with psychosis proneness, many of the same psychological testing variables will apply to both groups. The distinctions between these groups may not be found in measures of psychotic symptoms per se but in measures of psychological stability, coping, and emotional distress.

Controversies Regarding the DSM-5-TR Attenuated Psychosis Syndrome

Paris (2013) notes that one of the most controversial proposals for the DSM-5-TR (APA, 2022) was the aforementioned inclusion of the APS category as a condition in need of further study. Although the working group on schizophrenia recommended including a psychosis-risk syndrome in the manual, there were disagreements among prominent researchers in the field about whether it should have been included as a diagnosis (Yung et al., 2012). The crux of the controversy contrasts the value of correct early detection and intervention efforts with the risks associated with false-positive identifications. Those in favor of official recognition of the diagnosis point to the growing body of research identifying psychosis-risk syndromes and the fact that irrespective of whether many such individuals never convert to syndromal psychosis, they are symptomatic, distressed, and may need some type of treatment (Shrivastava et al., 2011).

Those opposed to including the APS as a diagnostic category point out the high number of false positives in research that sought to identify these patients. As previously noted in this chapter, several long-term prospective studies have yielded rates for conversion to psychosis within two to three years among CHR persons ranging from 20% to 50% (Fusar-Poli, Bonoldi et al., 2012; De Pablo, Radua, et al., 2021; Shrivastava et al., 2011). It is unclear if the remaining 20–50% of individuals might experience longer periods of attenuation before developing syndromal psychosis at later time points, if they have had conversion prevented by treatment or some unclear resiliency, if they might develop more chronic signs and symptoms, or if they might never have been on the psychosis spectrum, with signs and symptoms that are better accounted for by some other condition.

The potential negative consequences of high false-positive identifications include stigma and unnecessary treatment. Paris (2013) also notes that research has not convincingly demonstrated that early intervention with CHR individuals is always effective. Thus, while the APS was maintained in the Appendix of the APA's 2022 text revision of the DSM-5, its ultimate fate awaits further empirical support.

Other Psychosis Risk Factors

In addition to assessing biogenetic variables and psychopathological dimensions that predict risk for developing or converting to a psychotic disorder, other risk factors include developmental, demographic, social, environmental, and stress-related variables. For example, delays in development may predispose some children to later learning and social difficulties in adolescence. Children with learning difficulties may develop behavioral problems, which may possibly lead to being bullied at school or elsewhere. Social stress may further affect brain development and exacerbate behavioral, learning, and social difficulties. Furthermore, environmental factors such as poverty, drug abuse, immigrant status, social adversity, and isolation and urbanization were found to be risk factors associated with schizophrenia (Kelly & Murray, 2000).

A range of relational factors have been associated with risk for psychotic illness. In particular, an increasing number of studies have focused on the possible impact of traumatic events. These might include, but are not limited to, the following (Beck & van der Kolk, 1987; Grivel et al., 2018; Kelly & Murray, 2000; Larkin & Morrison, 2006; Moskowitz et al., 2009; Read et al., 2005):

- Insecure attachment
- Early loss of parents
- Exposure to parental or community violence
- Childhood sexual, physical, and emotional abuse
- Emotional or physical neglect
- Socioeconomic stress or poverty
- Social isolation
- Bullying
- Immigration status
- War trauma
- Early heavy use of marijuana in adolescence

As noted in Chapter 3, psychosis itself can be a traumatic experience. Thus, it appears as if the causal pathway may work both ways with trauma and psychosis, with traumatic experiences playing a possible etiological role in psychosis and a psychotic episode serving as a traumatic precipitant for the subsequent development of post-traumatic stress disorder (PTSD; APA, 2022).

Recent studies have found a relationship between childhood sexual abuse, but not trauma, generally, and subsequent conversion to psychosis in groups of CHR individuals (Thompson et al., 2009; Bechdolf et al., 2010). Methodological shortcomings, however, limited the generalizability of these findings. Employing a larger sample size, a longer follow-up period, and a comprehensive diagnostic interview using the CAARMS, Thompson and colleagues (2014) confirmed a positive relationship between sexual abuse in childhood and adolescence and medium- to long-term conversion to psychosis.

Clinical Assessment Points

1. Mental health professionals should be aware of a growing number of clinics throughout the United States and elsewhere around the globe specializing in the early detection of psychosis. The website Schizophrenia.com offers a directory of specialized clinics that provide early detection and treatment for emergent psychoses.
2. Even with well-researched instruments, detecting patients who will convert to psychosis is a difficult diagnostic task, leaving us with the problem of how to best address the issue of false positives. Nonetheless, early detection and intervention should be the primary concerns for consulting clinicians. Criteria for the APS category presently proposed in the DSM-5-TR (APA, 2022) should be examined. Unfortunately, research instruments developed for the early detection of psychosis risk are not easily accessible to clinicians or approved for clinical use. Although the SIPS, CAARMS, and PSYCHS may not be suitable for clinical practice, we recommend that mental health professionals become aware of these instruments and the criteria for psychosis-risk syndromes for the evaluation of patients who might be vulnerable. The concepts underlying these research instruments and risk syndromes can offer clues to clinicians regarding what to look for – in particular, which psychological tests to select and what interview questions to ask when evaluating patients.
3. To become alert to a possible psychosis-risk syndrome, clinicians need to pay particular attention to functional changes in their patients. In other words, well before the onset of positive signs and symptoms of psychosis, the first indications of an emergent disorder are new or worsening signs of deterioration in social, intellectual, and organizational domains. If possible, clinicians want to obtain estimates of GAF levels at the time of the evaluation and compare these to levels from a year ago. Although this might be somewhat subjective, it is important to have some measure of functional decline and be able to describe what specific changes have occurred.
4. When evaluating patients who are at risk for psychosis, trauma is a key concept. Not only is evidence of childhood trauma a significant risk factor in the psychotically vulnerable person, but converting to psychosis can become a traumatic event for the individual. Thus, trauma may predispose the individual to psychosis, and conversely, psychosis can be a traumatogenic event in a person's life. The traumatizing consequences of having a psychotic break underscore the importance of early detection and prevention efforts.
5. It is further recommended that assessors add a previous history of sexual trauma during childhood or adolescence to the set of criteria used to identify CHR patients.

12

ASSESSING PSYCHOSIS IN A FORENSIC CONTEXT

In many forensic psychological evaluations, it is vital to assess accurately whether a person has a psychotic disorder. In some cases, such as insanity evaluation, establishing the presence of a psychotic disorder is essential and directly related to psycho-legal questions (Goldstein et al., 2013). In other forensic examinations, like sentencing mitigation, establishing the presence, degree, or severity of psychosis can be an indirect but critical mitigating factor (Khadivi, 2017).

Assessing psychosis is a crucial aspect of forensic criminal psychology, which will be the focus of this chapter. Although forensic psychological evaluations may also involve the assessment of psychosis in civil, immigration, or custody cases, it is more commonly required in criminal cases.

Criminal Responsibility Evaluation

The assessment of criminal responsibility, which includes insanity evaluations, is aimed at determining the defendant's state of mind during the alleged crime (Goldstein et al., 2013). Although different jurisdictions have varying definitions of insanity, the purpose of these types of evaluation is to determine whether the defendant, due to mental illness, lacked the substantial capacity to understand the nature, consequences, or wrongfulness of their actions (cognitive capacity) or whether they were unable to refrain (volitional capacity) from committing the alleged crime.

As such, it is crucial to determine whether a primary psychotic disorder exists and how severe it is in a criminal responsibility evaluation. Studies indicate that individuals who are acquitted by reason of insanity (NGRI) by the court are more likely to have a diagnosis of a significant psychotic disorder (Packer, 2009).

When assessing criminal responsibility, it is crucial to understand the link between psychosis and the instant offense. Based on the literature (Rogers & Shuman, 2000; Packer, 2009; Resnick & Knoll, 2018) and

DOI: 10.4324/9781003415206-17

our experience, there are six possibilities to consider when evaluating this relationship. They are as follows:

1. There is a direct connection between psychosis and the instant offense, and the severity of symptoms significantly impairs the defendant's ability to comprehend the nature, consequences, or wrongfulness of their actions.
2. There is a nexus between psychosis and instant offense, but it does not significantly impair the defendant's ability to comprehend the nature, consequences, or wrongfulness of their actions.
3. Psychosis is present at the time of the instant offense but is unrelated to the crime.
4. Psychosis is not present during the instant crime.
5. Psychosis may or may not be present, but the defendant is malingering symptoms of psychosis regarding the alleged offense at the time of evaluation.
6. Psychosis is present at the time of the instant offense, but it is secondary to substance use (substance-induced psychosis).

Competency to Stand Trial Evaluation

In contrast to determining criminal responsibility, which looks back in time, a competency to stand trial evaluation focuses on the defendant's mental state. As such, assessing the presence of any active, positive psychotic signs and symptoms and their impact on the defendant's ability to participate in his defense in a rational and meaningful manner is essential. Defendants who are deemed incompetent to stand trial are most likely to exhibit active psychotic symptoms and have a diagnosis of psychotic disorder (Pirelli et al., 2011; Warren et al., 2006).

Various models have been proposed to operationalize domains needed to assess competency to stand trial (Bonnie, 1992; Kruh & Grisso, 2009). A Four-Capacity model (see Krun & Grisso, 2009) is instrumental in assessing the impact of psychosis on competency to stand trial (CST). In this model, CST abilities are constructed along four domains, "Understanding" (factual understanding of the proceeding), "Appreciation" (rational understanding of the proceedings), "Assisting" (ability to consult and assist with an attorney), and "Decisional Capacity" (ability to consider alternative decisions regarding the legal case, to consider plea agreement offer, or considering going to trial). Using this model, one can see that disorganized speech, specific types of delusion, and paranoia could potentially impair all four domains.

In some cases, the acute and grossly psychotic clinical presentation of a person can cause marked impairment in all four domains of CST. In other cases, a specific delusional belief can potentially impact one domain of CST. Take the following example:

> Mr. J., a young man with a history of schizophrenia who had a delusional belief that the governor of New York was in love with him, and he was convinced that she would grant him clemency after conviction. As a result, he did not see any need to work with his counsel.

On the other hand, the presence of a delusion may have no impact on CST.

> Ms. S., a 45-year-old cisgender female with a delusional disorder, was convinced that she had a foul odor emanating from her and she would wear heavy perfume to offset her perceived smell; however, her delusions did not impair any domains of CST.

As discussed in Chapter 2, some individuals with a psychotic disorder may incorporate the examiner into their delusional system. Similarly, the person can include his counsel, judge, or prosecution in his delusional beliefs. For example, Mr. X., a 36-year-old male with a long history of schizoaffective disorder, believed that his counsel was a clone and was being manipulated by some outside alien force.

Sentencing Mitigation Evaluation

The purpose of a sentencing evaluation is to assess any mitigating factors that could affect the length of a sentence. The assessment usually happens after a defendant has pled guilty and is waiting for the court to determine their sentence. The sentencing evaluation is a comprehensive assessment that looks at different aspects of functioning, including developmental deficits, mental illness, interpersonal functioning, reality testing, emotional regulation, impulse control, and moral development (Cunningham, 2010). Therefore, identifying the presence of a psychotic disorder is a crucial mitigating factor in determining the sentence. Since it can be challenging to establish a psychotic disorder accurately (see Chapter 6), a multi-method assessment that includes reviewing records, gathering information from other sources, and conducting psychological testing is often recommended.

Additionally, the issue of malingering psychosis becomes more significant in any forensic evaluation (Glancy et al., 2015), including the sentencing examination. A review of federal court cases has shown that malingering defendants receive sentencing enhancements (Resnick & Knoll, 2018).

Malingering Psychosis

Research on the effectiveness of the diagnostic interview method in detecting malingered hallucinations or delusions is scarce. Most studies on malingering psychosis have focused on specialized interview-based measures such as the Structured Interview of Reported Symptoms, Second Edition (SIRS-2: Roger et al., 2010), the Miller Forensic Assessment of Symptoms Test (M-FAST; Miller, 2001) and the use of multi-scale personality inventories (see Chapter 8 on psychological testing). In terms of the multi-method psychological assessment of malingered disturbances in thinking and perception, readers are directed to chapters in Weiner and Kleiger (2021) and, in particular, the chapter by Acklin (2021) in that volume. Additionally, Kleiger (2017) reviewed the literature on Rorschach indications of malingered psychosis.

According to Resnick and Knoll (2018), detecting malingered disorders of thinking and perception with a clinical interview is a challenging and time-consuming task that requires a systematic approach involving multiple sources of information. They argue that no published study has examined the effectiveness of clinical interviews in assessing feigning psychosis. They urge that relying solely on the clinical interview is not enough. To recognize signs suggestive of malingered psychosis, clinicians must focus on the atypical clinical presentation of hallucinations and delusions while having a detailed understanding of how these symptoms present in genuine psychiatric patients. To help clinicians develop hypotheses regarding malingered psychosis, Resnick and Knoll (2018) compiled a comprehensive list of atypical clinical presentations of hallucinations and delusions that can be observed or probed during the interview. What follows is a selected summary of the atypical clinical presentation of hallucinations and delusions described by Resnick and Knoll (2018).

Atypical Auditory Hallucination (AH)

Voices that sound like animals; report of voice as always very distressing; voices that only yell; voices that ask questions; voices that are always vague or inaudible; hearing only voice of children or females; report of having no coping strategies to deal with distressing voices; voices addressing the individual as Mr. or. Mrs.; claiming that all command hallucinations are obeyed; AH without delusions.

Atypical Visual Hallucination (VH)

Visual hallucination that is in black and white; VH in the absence of AH (excluding substance-induced and neuropsychiatry conditions); seeing giant or miniature.

Atypical Delusions

Delusions that abruptly start and stop; behavior or conduct inconsistent with the delusional belief; bizarre delusions without disorganization; eagerness to discuss the delusion.

Clinical Assessment Points

1. When conducting a criminal forensic evaluation, it is important to assess for malingering using all available information and specialized psychological measures.
2. In cases of criminal responsibility, it is crucial to determine the connection between the offender's psychosis and the instant offense. This involves assessing the severity of signs and symptoms and their impact at the time of the crime.
3. To examine the impact of psychosis carefully, it is recommended to use a conceptual model for competency to stand trial (CST) examination.
4. In sentencing evaluation, it is important to conduct a comprehensive and multi-method assessment of psychosis

13

DIFFERENTIATING DELUSIONAL DISORDER FROM THE RADICALIZATION OF EXTREME BELIEFS

Mark D. Cunningham

Differentiating delusional disorder from extreme religious or political beliefs is a diagnostic challenge for mental health professionals. When the radicalization of these extreme beliefs leads to violent expression, this differential becomes important to courts as well (e.g., questions of insanity or competence to stand trial). These challenges are paradoxical, considering the long history of the syndrome in the scholarly literature and the straightforward definitions and associated diagnostic criteria. More specifically, delusions are fixed beliefs that are not amenable to change in light of conflicting evidence; delusional disorder involves the presence of delusions in the absence of other significant psychopathology (see DSM-5-TR). When the fixed false beliefs are thoroughly idiosyncratic (e.g., a spouse is conspiring with various Fed-Ex workers to deliver toxic packages to the home), there is little need for additional diagnostic guidance. More problematic is the presentation of fixed beliefs having some overlap in content or theme with extreme religious or political beliefs held by others in a culture.

Challenges In Differentiating Delusional Disorder

The diagnostic challenge for clinicians and courts is exacerbated by the *encapsulated* nature of delusional disorder. Generalized psychopathology is typically absent and, outside of the delusional system, these patients are quite functional. This presentation was described as early as 1838, with Esquirol observing that patients with "monomania" were distinct from broad "insanity" (later termed schizophrenia) in having odd or eccentric beliefs but otherwise retaining good reality-testing in most arenas, as well as logical thought processes, accurate memory, and lively curiosity (Hoff, 2006). Kraeplin, writing in the late 1800s and early 1900s, described a "partial insanity" characterized by an encapsulated delusional system.

DOI: 10.4324/9781003415206-18

He described a distinct illness (i.e., "dementia paranoids") characterized by a chronic, unshakable system of non-bizarre delusions, but without thought disorganization or a major disturbance in affect or volition seen in "dementia praecox" (i.e., schizophrenia) (Tamburello et al., 2015). The encapsulated nature of delusional disorder has been emphasized by more recent scholars, as well:

> Perhaps the most unique feature of delusional disorder is the way in which a patient can move between delusional and normal "modes." In the former, the individual is overalerted, preoccupied with the delusional theme and often driven remorselessly by it. In sharp contrast, the normal has relatively calm mood, neutral conversation, and some ability to pursue everyday activities. The contrast is striking and often difficult for the lay person to understand.
>
> (Munro, 1995, p. 203)

Iterations of *The Diagnostic and Statistical Manual* of the American Psychiatric Association, beginning with DSM-III-R, have embraced that delusions with an encapsulated presentation, in the *absence* of other significant psychopathology, are the essential diagnostic feature of delusional disorder.

ICD-11 (World Health Organization, 2019) has classified encapsulated delusions that are the most conspicuous and the only clinical characteristic as "delusional disorder" (PDD). Illustrating the encapsulated nature of delusional disorder, ICD-11 noted the associated delusion or set of related delusions occur in the absence of a depressive, manic, or mixed mood episode, *without* characteristic symptoms of schizophrenia, such as clear and persistent hallucinations (unless directly related to the delusion), negative symptoms, disorganized thinking, or experiences of influence, passivity, or control. As compared to schizophrenia, personality functioning is relatively preserved in delusional disorder, with less deterioration or impairment in social and occupational functioning. ICD-11 further specified that, apart from actions and attitudes directly related to the delusional system, affect, speech, and behavior are typically unaffected.

In both delusional disorder and extreme beliefs, the content involves *reality-based content or culturally-anchored themes*. Scholars have long recognized that delusions may be both organized and reality-based. Kraeplin described that "dementia paranoids" had disturbed beliefs involving diseased interpretations of real events that often extended to events of recent date. In a differential with extreme beliefs, delusions are more likely to be paranoid and/or grandiose, unaccompanied by thought broadcasting, thought insertion, or other grossly disturbed reality testing. For this reason, most clinical rating scales for delusions have limited utility in a differential with extreme beliefs, as they are directed toward the delusions accompanying schizophrenia. Admittedly, the diagnostic criteria for delusional disorder expanded from DSM-IV-TR to DSM-5-TR to include bizarre as well as non-bizarre fixed false beliefs. This seems a nod toward the difficulty in parsing whether a false belief is sufficiently improbable to be bizarre. In any case, bizarre delusions are less common in delusional disorder, and frankly, bizarre or fantastic content is more diagnostically obvious (see the later discussion on improbability of belief content). A differential of delusions from extreme beliefs is thus unlikely to be based on general topical belief content alone.

Differentiating delusional disorder from extreme beliefs is also challenging because both are typically supported by *logic and "evidence."* Esquirol observed that "monomania" patients supported their disturbed beliefs with appeals to evidence (Hoff, 2006). Kraeplin similarly described that "dementia paranoid" patients held coherent delusions, recognizing and explaining contradictions and objections to their beliefs (Tamburello et al., 2015).

The presence of premorbid personality disorder is similarly of little benefit in the differential, as these are a common precursor to extreme beliefs or overvalued ideas (Rahman et al., 2021), as well as delusional disorder (ICD-11). Similarly, Rahman et al. vaguely proposed "the use of [life] narrative to formulate forensic cases" [of overvalued ideas], describing a chronology of an extremely overvalued belief as one that is shared by others in a person's cultural, religious, or subcultural group. The belief is often relished, amplified, and defended by the possessor and should be differentiated from an obsession or a delusion. The belief grows more dominant over time, more refined, and more resistant to challenge. The individual has an intense emotional commitment to the belief and may carry out violent behavior in its service.

However, Rahman et al. neglect that some degree of shared cultural component (e.g., political or religious) is ubiquitous in delusional disorders where a differential is at issue. More broadly, Cummings and Mega (2003) noted: "the content of delusional disorders varies across cultures and reflects the social and cultural setting of the delusional individual" (p. 62). Regarding the use of life narrative as a differential, Ernst Kretschmer (1988–1964) observed that biography and personality could grow into delusional states (Hoff, 2006). "Amplification" in delusional disorder is observed as patients seek confirmatory data and ignore contradictory data, experience grandiosity, and may experience compulsions to act. Further clouding the differential, ICD-11 noted: "Individuals may present with a combination of delusions and overvalued ideas, both drawing on similar cultural idioms and beliefs."

In subsequent scholarship, Meloy and Rahman (2021) have collapsed the differential between overvalued ideas and culturally anchored delusions by disputing delusional disorder as a diagnostic categorization: "We think that delusional disorder represents a potential misclassification of phenomenology, recognized internationally as overvalued ideas which are shared and held with an intense emotional commitment" (p. 183). To the extent that clinical and forensic mental health professionals orient their assessments to DSM-5-TR or ICD-11 diagnostic systems, disputing the validity of a diagnostic category embraced by both fails to advance that assessment and renders any associated differential irrelevant.

Also contributing to diagnostic uncertainty, many clinicians have *limited experience* in recognizing culturally anchored delusions as distinct from extreme religious or political beliefs. This is a function of infrequent self-presentation and low community prevalence. Because individuals with delusional disorder remain broadly functional and are typically without insight that their beliefs represent delusions, they infrequently present themselves for mental health treatment (Tamburello et al., 2015). With that caution, the prevalence of delusional disorder in the community is quite low: 0.03 point prevalence and 0.2% lifetime prevalence (Tamburello et al., citing DSM-IV-TR, DSM-5). Forensic mental health practitioners may have greater exposure, as an eight-fold greater prevalence, 0.24%, has been reported for delusional disorder in a corrections context (Tamburello et al., 2015).

Factors Illuminating the Differential of Delusional Disorder and Extreme Beliefs

In the face of the previously mentioned challenges with a diagnostic differential between delusional disorder and extreme beliefs, DSM-5-TR provides limited guidance at best, prescribing that whether a belief constitutes a delusion depends in part on the degree of conviction with which the belief is held despite clear or reasonable contradictory evidence regarding its veracity (p. 101). This broad metric is markedly subjective and fails to discriminate extreme beliefs, which may also be held with unwavering conviction despite ample disconfirmation. It also provides no mechanism for systematic assessment and resultant transparency in delineating the features of the analysis. Similarly, ICD-11 described "a continuum of delusional beliefs, attenuated delusional beliefs, overvalued ideas, and unusual or eccentric beliefs in the general population." However, no guidance is provided by ICD-11 on how to segment that continuum clinically.

Addressing this vacuum in operationalizing the assessment, Cunningham (2018) has proposed a structured professional judgment tool involving seven criteria of analysis in differentiating delusional disorder from extreme beliefs, further disaggregated into 17 factors (*Model of Analysis for Differentiating Delusional Disorder from the Radicalization of Extreme Beliefs*, *MADDD-or-Rad-17*). These seven criteria, 17 factors, and various sub-factors are drawn from scholarship regarding the presentation of delusions and forensic case studies involving delusions versus extreme beliefs. The *MADDD-or-Rad-17* specifies:

A. *Cognitive content of the belief* (What is believed?)

1. Idiosyncrasy: Idiosyncrasy is conceptualized as a continuum on which:
   a. Some elements of the belief are not commonly held by others, and/or
   b. The integrated totality of the belief is unique.
   Caveat: Idiosyncrasy is not considered to be a dichotomous determination of whether anyone else shares any element (theme) of the belief.

2. Improbability: Improbability is operationalized to mean the extent to which the beliefs reflect:
   a. Historical inaccuracy or erroneous linkage to historical events;
   b. Faulty interpretation of current events; and/or
   c. Inflated confidence in associated actions having the desired impact.
   Caveat: Improbability does not require that the belief be impossible.

3. Grandiosity: In its more subtle forms, grandiosity may be implicated by beliefs and actions reflecting:
   a. Special insight into the problem;
   b. Special recognition of the action needed;
   c. Perceived right to take that action;
   d. Expectations of profound influence; and/or
   e. Heroic identification.
   f. Publicly claiming responsibility for the act.
   Caveat: Grandiosity as a subtext does not require that the person overtly claim to be someone of special importance.

B. *Cognitive style of the belief* (How is it believed?)

4. Rigid adherence to a belief despite disconfirming evidence (i.e., the strength of the belief), as reflected by:
   a. Difficulty articulating disconfirming evidence;
   b. Difficulty specifying alternative hypotheses;
   c. Difficulty mentally manipulating alternative hypotheses;
   d. Unsubstantiated claims of broad social agreement;

e. Irritability/agitation when challenged; and/or
f. Failure to incorporate disconfirming evidence following challenge.

Caveat: Standing alone, claims of being open to disconfirming evidence do not controvert rigid adherence to belief.

5. Suspension of critical judgment, i.e., the extent to which the beliefs reflect:

a. Deficits in Theory of Mind, i.e., difficulty accurately recognizing and interpreting the emotions and cognitions of others;
b. Confirmation bias, i.e., selectively attending to information that is consistent with the belief, with failure to incorporate readily available disconfirming information regarding the accuracy, prevalence, scope, severity, and/or social primacy of the belief;
c. Personalizing bias, i.e., the tendency to view others rather than circumstances as responsible for negative events;
d. Externalizing bias, i.e., the tendency to avoid viewing self as responsible for negative events, with readiness to blame others or circumstances;
e. Jumping to conclusions, i.e., substantial generalization or elaboration from limited or erroneous historical or current anecdotal data;
f. Social reality testing deficits, i.e., not utilizing the absence of shared belief and/or the lower intensity of belief by others for reality testing purposes (e.g., If the belief is true, why are others not equally concerned?)

6. Preoccupation with the belief, as may be demonstrated by:

a. Relative predominance of the belief;
b. Spontaneous digressions to the belief;
c. Recurrent "scripts" in discussing the belief;
d. Emotional energy accompanying discussion of the belief;
e. The primacy and affect surrounding the belief coming to the attention of others.

Caveat: The ability to discuss other topics does not negate preoccupation.

C. *Distress and social dysfunction associated with beliefs* (What are the repercussions of the belief?)

7. Distress and functional impairment associated with the belief.
8. Extent the beliefs have constituted a social difficulty.

D. *Social influences* (How are the beliefs inspired, maintained, and/or operationalized into action by a social context?) *As these are operative, delusional disorder is less likely.*

9. Interaction with a community of like believers:

    a. Virtual community; and/or
    b. Actual community.

10. Social motivators, i.e., the extent to which the beliefs arise and/or continue in a social context of like believers, where the person with the belief gains:

    a. Structure;
    b. Identity;
    c. Role/purpose/meaning;
    d. Affiliation; and/or
    e. Status.

11. Social facilitation/tangible support, i.e., the extent to which the group has provided:

    a. Selection/recruitment;
    b. Training;
    c. Planning;
    d. Targeting;
    e. Resources; and/or
    f. Sanctuary.
    E. *Social inclusion* (To what extent is the adherent socially integrated and productive in the community?) *As social inclusion of the adherent increases, delusional disorder is less likely.*

12. Social acceptance of adherent and his beliefs:

    a. Social integration;
    b. Productivity.
    F. *Prodromal factors* (What indications are there of a developing psychosis?)

13. Prodromal symptomatology.

    Caveat: This is thus a unidirectional metric: prodromal symptoms of psychosis support the presence of delusional disorder, but the absence of these is not contraindicative.
    G. *Behavioral/Action factors* (Is the belief acted on? How is the belief acted on or exhibited? What disturbance accompanies that action?)

14. Willingness to act.
15. Compulsion to act on the belief, as reflected by:

    a. An increasing subjective press or tension to act on the belief.
    b. An idiosyncratic sense of personal responsibility to take action.

c. A sense of special obligation to act.
d. Perception of an acute necessity or imminent harm.
e. Framing action as defining representations of self (e.g., If I fail to act, I am no better than the oppressors; I am not an authentic citizen if I remain passive).
f. Grandiose identification with historic or heroic figures who took action.
g. Ill-conceived planning, particularly for follow-on actions (e.g., the first action is well-planned, but subsequent actions are hasty and improvised).

16. Rigid moral distinctions in acting on the belief.
17. Psychological disorganization associated with the belief, e.g.:

a. Inconsistency in planning and execution in acting on the belief;
b. Pressured and/or socially inappropriate verbalizing about the belief;
c. Act-related factors symbolizing the belief that draws attention to the individual and/or increases the likelihood of apprehension.

Caveat: Psychological disorganization as conceptualized herein is not typically manifested by grossly disorganized speech/thought, nor is planning or organized activity in the execution of the attack a contraindication of delusion.

Several observations regarding the previous model are important. First, consistent with the observation of ICD-11, many of the factors of analysis reflect continuums rather than dichotomous categories. Second, the model is intended to structure the analysis and is not a scale supporting counting or cut-scores. Third, distinguishing features of *delusional pathology* are emphasized, as the heterogeneous nature of "normal" persons holding extreme beliefs renders it impractical to specify their features. That said, "normal" persons holding or acting on extreme beliefs are hypothesized to be heavily motivated by factors in the social influence arena (Horgan, 2008). Third, the model conforms itself to the diagnostic stance of DSM-5-TR that psychopathology, including delusional disorder, arises *within* the disturbed individual. This convention reflects only a segment of false and potentially delusional beliefs having more overt social contagion, with correspondingly broader prevalence.

A more comprehensive literature review and explanation associated with each of the 17 factors accompanied the introduction of the *MADDD-or-Rad-17* (see Cunningham, 2018). The reader is encouraged to review that paper for the associated rationales and scholarly support. Rather than reproduce that discussion herein, the practical application of this SPJ tool may be better facilitated by illustrating its use in a forensic case. Accordingly, each factor will be briefly described, followed by how this factor was analyzed in the Christopher Monfort case.

Case Application of MADDD-or-Rad-17: Chris Monfort

In October 2009, Christopher Monfort firebombed Seattle police vehicles parked in a city maintenance yard. His plan was to draw law enforcement to the scene, then relocate to a sniper perch on a nearby hillside and open fire. His exit from the maintenance yard was observed, so the sniping phase was aborted. Nine days later, he assassinated a Seattle police officer and wounded another. When confronted by police a week later, Mr. Monfort was shot in the face and back and paralyzed from the waist down. His capital trial in 2015 turned on his mental state at the time of the offense (insanity), i.e., whether he suffered from a delusional disorder or, alternatively, held extreme beliefs.

A. Content of Beliefs

Content of beliefs: Delusions are first identifiable by their content. It is, therefore, essential to distill the beliefs in question so that they may be assessed for idiosyncrasy, improbability, and grandiosity.

Monfort beliefs

During extended interviews with mental health experts retained by the prosecution and defense, Mr. Monfort espoused the beliefs that follow. Though these have been distilled and organized, the terminology is his, repeated in recurrent digressions.

1. The police in the United States, and more specifically in Seattle and King County, had departed from the legitimate exercise of their lawful authority and were acting in a tyrannical, brutal, raping, and murderous fashion against the citizenry.
2. The police, in their current role, function as an officially sanctioned but criminal gang.
3. There are inescapable parallels between the Seattle and King County police (as well as the police in many other jurisdictions) and the British Redcoats leading up to the American Revolution, who [he believes] engaged in widespread pillage, assault, rape, and murder on the American colonial citizenry.
4. Even those police officers who do not themselves engage in criminal assaults against the citizenry (50–55% of the Seattle and King County Police Departments) are complicit because of their solidarity with the "gang" and their failure to police their own.

5. The criminal and murderous conduct of police officers represents the gravest threat to liberty and the most serious social problem confronting the United States.
6. It is an essential obligation of the citizenry to resist such tyranny with deadly force, as was demonstrated by the Founding Fathers and other American colonial citizens.
7. By his own singular action, he would fulfill this obligation and function as a modern Minute Man in rousing the rest of the populace to similar action in throwing off the yoke of police tyranny.
8. Only when a sufficient number of police officers had been killed would police departments and district attorney offices act to restore the police to behaving lawfully and resuming their legitimate role of serving the citizens.
9. Though recognizing that his offense-related conduct subjected him to arrest and prosecution under Washington law, he believed his plans, preparations, and actions in the charged conduct were not only morally right but also consistent with the higher law of the Constitution of the United States.
10. His offense-related conduct was required of him as an American citizen under the Constitution.
11. Thus, his offense-related conduct was both morally right and lawful.

Factor 1. Idiosyncrasy

Though delusions are culturally informed, they arise as individual pathology. Unique features are not just expected but are a core characteristic (see Taylor et al., 1994; Taylor, 2006). That said, idiosyncrasy will be relative in beliefs with political or religious content, i.e., unique interpretations of more culturally prevalent themes. From this rationale, some scholars have found that political ideologies such as the Sovereign Citizen Movement are sufficiently shared so they do not represent delusions (e.g., Parker, 2014; Pytyck & Chaimowitz, 2013).

CASE ANALYSIS

Though Mr. Monfort's offenses preceded the Black Lives Matter movement, many persons were also concerned or even alarmed by instances of police brutality in the United States, and distrust of the police was widespread at the time in some American subcultures. Similarly, many Americans held views of Constitutional rights that superseded particular state or federal laws, with appeals to the Founding Fathers. These contours of belief were not idiosyncratic. Mr. Monfort's elaboration on these more commonly held beliefs was idiosyncratic. His idiosyncratic elaborations include the purported social primacy of this problem, its strong linkage to events precipitating the American Revolution [historically inaccurate], the exaggerated prevalence of murderous misconduct by law enforcement, a "tipping point" strategy of sufficient police deaths to produce reform, his grandiosity that his actions would achieve this end, his identification with the Founding Fathers and Minutemen, and his belief that the killing of police officers was both legal under the Constitution and a duty of citizenship. Further, the combined/integrated totality of these beliefs was idiosyncratic.

Factor 2. Improbability

Improbability is a fundamental characteristic of a non-bizarre delusion, i.e., the "content of the delusion is objectively wrong or impossible" (p. 244, Jaspers, 1913; as cited by Hoff, 2006).

CASE ANALYSIS

It is self-evident that Mr. Monfort's beliefs were improbable. He was historically inaccurate in his view of the purported policing role and excesses (pillaging, raping, murdering) of the Redcoats that modern law enforcement was allegedly reenacting. There is no linkage of armed resistance to law enforcement in the present day with the Minutemen of the American Revolution. Mr. Monfort arguably grossly overestimated the prevalence of officers engaging in serious brutality.

Mr. Monfort exhibited inflated confidence that his campaign of officer assassination would result in broad social support and police reforms. Rather than the killing of police officers achieving a tipping point of community support and police reform, it seems more probable that a campaign of police officer assassination would result in both an escalation in the use of force, as officers were more fearful/stressed/angry, and an increase in public acceptance of escalated force as the police were viewed as under siege, with the police being further licensed to act with brutality by an outpouring of public support.

Factor 3. Grandiosity

When grandiosity is sufficiently pronounced, its delusional nature is obvious. A more subtle analysis occurs when differentiating an adherent's narcissism from psychotic grandiosity. This analysis often relies on examining how beliefs and actions may rise beyond narcissism to implicate grandiosity.

CASE ANALYSIS

By framing contemporary police brutality as synonymous with the behavior of Redcoats in colonial America, Mr. Monfort identified with and elevated his status to that of important figures in American history, i.e., the Minutemen and the Founding Fathers. His perspective that he had a *singularly* clear view of police brutality, the threat it represents, and the action required to address it was grandiose as well. Grandiosity was also reflected in his belief that his individual action could resolve what he viewed as a systemic and widespread problem in local and national policing. This grandiose confidence in personal appraisal neglected a fundamental reality-testing mechanism. More specifically, individuals typically utilize the views and attitudes of their fellows as a modifying or braking factor regarding the soundness of personal perspectives. Mr. Monfort, by contrast, viewed the absence of fellow adherents as evidence of his clarity of vision, courage, and patriotism.

B. Cognitive Style of Beliefs

Assessment of delusions involves not only their content but also *how* they are believed, or what Appelbaum and colleagues (1999) termed their non-content dimensions. Peters (2010) opined that these non-content characteristics were more pathognomonic of delusion than content: "Form may be more important diagnostically than content; it is not what you believe, but how you believe it" (p. 134). Features such as conviction, preoccupation, and distress may better differentiate delusion than content (Peters et al., 1999). Similarly, Pierre (2001) observed that whether a belief was delusional was not only a function of "the content of the belief per se, but to the manner in which the belief is held (i.e., excessive preoccupation, conviction, emotional valence [distress], and resulting functional impairment)" (p. 170) were important in identifying a belief as delusional.

Factor 4. Rigid Adherence Despite Disconfirming Evidence

The strength of conviction and associated imperviousness to disconfirmation is an important non-content dimension of a delusion. Jaspers (1963) specified two associated pragmatic criteria of *how* delusions are believed: "1. Unparalleled degree of subjective feeling of certainty; and 2. Cannot be influenced by experience or arguments ('incorrigibility')" (p. 244, Hoff, 2006). Clinical rating scales have also specified the strength of the belief as a non-content feature of delusions (e.g., Maudley Assessment of Delusions Schedule [MADS; Wessely et al., 1993], subsequently adapted as the MacArthur-Maudsley Assessment of Delusions Schedule [MMADS; Taylor et al., 1994]).

CASE ANALYSIS

In assessing the strength of Mr. Monfort's beliefs (i.e., conviction), it is notable that substantial disconfirming evidence was abundant but entirely neglected by Mr. Monfort. Hundreds of thousands of law enforcement officers go about their duties daily with professionalism and respect for the citizens of their communities. That reports and videos of police brutality receive media attention and notoriety arguably speaks to the infrequency of these incidents. Historical literature, including in college courses attended by Mr. Monfort, was widely available that would have provided a more informed understanding of the causes of the American Revolution and the *rarity* of murder, rape, and pillage by British soldiers during the pre-War era. Historical support was not found in the scholarship he specified for the proposition that abuses of the colonists were routine. In his belief that the American Revolution and resistance of the "Founding Fathers" were primarily driven by the abusive behavior of British soldiers toward American colonists, Mr. Monfort neglected many more compelling precipitating contributions to the American Revolution.

The historical record is also replete with evidence that nonviolent protest and democratic mechanisms can be quite successful in changing even well-entrenched social and political issues (e.g., women's suffrage, the civil rights movement, and LGBTQ+ rights). In his belief that the police would only be motivated to reestablish a proper role of protecting and serving citizens, as opposed to brutalizing them, and begin to police their own when a sufficient number of police officers, both brutal and complicit, had been killed, Mr. Monfort neglected consideration of other mechanisms of change: training, leadership, legislation, etc. The neglect of these considerations appears to have been driven by his exaggeration of the scope and severity of the problem, thereby requiring immediate and violent intervention, as well as by his own grandiosity.

Even Mr. Monfort's modest level of employment and relationship development was evidence that he was an unlikely candidate to single-handedly produce radical reform in a social institution – as his limited achievement was inconsistent with his grandiose self-appraisal.

During his interview, Mr. Monfort *claimed* to be open to alternative views but failed to *demonstrate* this when engaged in discussion. He did not retain the alternative perspectives presented to him from one interview to the next and was unable to mentally manipulate opposing views – despite good intellect and a bachelor's degree in political science. He was completely unable to acknowledge or discuss the merits of alternative perspectives. Mr. Monfort responded to alternative perspectives with irritation, insisting that his views were supported by particular scholarly sources (which did not stand for those propositions), assertion of additional historical or contemporaneous inaccuracies, and digression to verbal scripts.

Factor 5. Suspension of Critical Judgment

Persons holding delusions exhibit impairments in the way they think about their beliefs. Such belief development and belief maintenance factors in delusions include the *Theory of Mind deficit* (see Bentall et al., 2001; Bentall & Taylor, 2006; Garety & Freeman, 2011). Other scholars (e.g., Frith, 1992; Frith & Frith, 1999; Hoff, 2006) describe additional reasoning errors such as *confirmation bias* (Borum, 2014; citing Freeman, 2007), *personalizing bias* (see Bentall & Taylor, 2006; Hoff, 2006; Penn et al., 2008), *externalizing bias* (see Kaney & Bentall, 1989; Kaney et al., 1997; Garety & Freeman, 1999; Bentall et al., 2001; Carlin et al., 2005; Bell et al., 2006c; Bentall & Taylor, 2006; Hoff, 2006; but see Fear & Healy, 1997), and *jumping to conclusions* (see Bentall & Taylor, 2006; Taylor & Felthous, 2006; van Dael et al., 2006; Borum, 2014). For concise operational definitions of various thinking errors that, while not restricted to delusions, are often involved in the development and maintenance of delusions, see Borum (2014). An additional thinking error, a *social reality testing deficit*, was hypothesized by Cunningham (2018).

CASE ANALYSIS

Mr. Monfort formed and defended his beliefs with little critical judgment. He readily accepted accounts of police brutality from youths in juvenile custody without verification of these events (implicating confirmation bias). He similarly accepted accounts of widespread police "murder" of civilians by police in particular Seattle neighborhoods, as well as nationally, without examining the necessity of deadly force in particular lethal encounters or the number of officers involved in relation to the total police department (implicating confirmatory bias, jumping to conclusions, social reality testing deficits). In his belief that approximately 45% of police officers are brutal and unrestrained in carrying out their official duties, Mr. Monfort had no basis except his subjective reaction to videos and media reports of police brutality in Seattle, King County, and elsewhere in the United States that he repeatedly viewed on the internet (implicating jumping to conclusions). Mr. Monfort's attention to lurid accounts and/or videos of police brutality served to make these events seem pervasive and constant without consideration that these were distributed across two decades and drawn from a national context (implicating confirmatory bias). In characterizing the conduct of the police as broadly "murderous," Mr. Monfort neglected the obvious continuum of misconduct as more often reflecting excessive force and only rarely resulting in death. Mr. Monfort asserted that his beliefs were widely shared and endorsed, that his tipping point solution would be adopted by others, and that a jury might acquit him by a nullification verdict (implicating Theory of Mind deficits). He rationalized the absence of fellow adherents as evidence of his clarity of vision, courage, and patriotism.

Factor 6. Preoccupation With the Belief

Delusional thinking is often characterized by preoccupation with the belief, as delusions may be pervasive, intrusive, persistent, and recurrent (see Wessely et al., 1993; Junginger, 2006; Taylor & Felthous, 2006). The MADDD-or-Rad-17 model identifies five features that may be useful in qualitatively assessing preoccupation.

CASE ANALYSIS

Mr. Monfort exhibited steadily growing preoccupation with police brutality and the associated beliefs specified previously – particularly in the months preceding the offense conduct. Even when visiting a friend, Mr. Monfort watched YouTube accounts of police brutality and surfed the web on this subject. He referenced the Constitution and the Founding Fathers in casual interactions. Mr. Monfort routinely made animated comments about police brutality and about specific local incidents in social conversation. When walking a friend's daughter to the park, he would initiate conversations with strangers sitting on their porches regarding their observations of police brutality. Others were oriented to his energy and preoccupation with this topic. Mr. Monfort carried a pocket copy of the U.S. Constitution with him at all times and also kept a collection of these arrayed on his kitchen counter. He had a large American flag spread over his bed. Mr. Monfort's alcoholic beverage of choice was Apple Jack Brandy, a spirit favored by General George Washington (Laird and Company website). During post-arrest mental health interviews, he repeatedly digressed to discuss his views of police brutality, using the same repetitive phrasing (i.e., scripts).

C. Distress and Social Dysfunction Associated with Beliefs

Factor 7. Distress and Functional Impairment Associated with the Beliefs

As beliefs are associated with greater distress, they are more likely to be delusional (Peters et al., 1999). Similarly, Pierre (2001) observed that distress and functional impairment were more likely to be observed in religious delusions than in strong faith.

CASE ANALYSIS

Mr. Monfort was increasingly disillusioned with his family, acquaintances, community, and institutions as they failed to exhibit the degree of alarm and activism regarding the police that he experienced. He became more irritable and reactive in his interactions.

Factor 8. Extent the Beliefs Have Constituted a Social Difficulty

Social problems tend to arise from both the content and dimensional features of delusional disorders. This is contrasted with adherents of extreme beliefs, who are more likely to be strategic in disclosing these beliefs, e.g., to a like-minded subculture where affirmation is anticipated.

CASE ANALYSIS

Mr. Monfort did not express his beliefs regarding a tipping point of police officer deaths after he received negative reactions in preliminary discussions with two friends. Instead, he became more withdrawn. As will be addressed subsequently, as he began to take violent action on his beliefs, he had episodes of unsolicited monologues regarding his concerns to strangers. Following his arrest, Mr. Monfort had repeated outbursts in the courtroom and loudly expressed his disagreement or approval of testimony.

D. Social Influences

Social influences Factors 9, 10, and 11 are distilled from Horgan (2008), reflecting three primary social influences related to belief structuring and a motivational role in the evolution of non-mentally ill persons from radicalization to acts of terrorism. These emphasize the central role of social context in this pathway. Conversely, persons espousing delusions are unlikely to be viewed as operationally reliable for recruitment by terrorist networks (see Horgan, 2005; Spaaij, 2010). Unsurprising, rates of mental illness have been reported as five times higher in far-right lone offenders (40.4%) than group offenders (7.6%) (Gruenewald et al., 2013). It is thus hypothesized that the more extensive and organized the social support for the beliefs and for acting on them, the less likely these reflect a delusional disorder (see Pytyck & Chaimowitz, 2013).

Factor 9. Interaction With a Community of Like Believers

CASE ANALYSIS

Mr. Monfort accessed videos and reports online where it is quite probable that others expressed outrage. However, he did not participate in any virtual forums or actual community organizations. He vaguely broached his ideas for an assassination campaign against police officers with two male peers but discontinued these feelers when they did not respond favorably. There was no evidence of direct social motivation, facilitation, or tangible support from others.

Factor 10. Social Motivators

CASE ANALYSIS

Some of Mr. Monfort's beliefs regarding the magnitude of police brutality were facilitated by internet sites posting descriptions and videos of these events. There was, however, no social contact with like believers where he would gain structure, identity, role/purpose/meaning, affiliation, and/or status.

Factor 11. Social Facilitation/Support

CASE ANALYSIS

In developing Mr. Monfort's ideology or its operationalization, there was no evidence that a group provided selection/recruitment, training, planning, targeting, resources, and/or sanctuary.

E. Social Inclusion

Killaspy et al. (2014) observed that social inclusion (i.e., social integration and productivity) is reduced in many psychological disorders. Both features of social inclusion decline in psychosis. As social ostracism exacerbates delusions, a vicious cycle occurs. While greater life functionality is typically maintained in delusional disorder as compared to other primary psychoses, it is hypothesized that delusional disorder is likely to be inconsistent with ongoing high levels of occupation or broad-life productivity.

Factor 12. Social Acceptance of Adherent and His Beliefs

CASE ANALYSIS.

Mr. Monfort's social integration was marred by several characteristics. He lived alone and had only one or two friends. He was uncomfortable in larger social contexts. His romantic relationships were few and short-term. He rarely proceeded beyond superficial conversation to personal disclosure. He had difficulty viewing situations from the perspective of another on most topics and particularly had difficulty understanding the emotional reactions of others. He was inflexible and tended to overreact to minor events, absent himself from interacting for days or weeks, and then behave as if nothing had happened. This sequence was particularly likely to occur if an activity deviated from what he had anticipated. He had little patience with people and became easily irritated with them. Mr. Monfort's friends and dating partners were aware of his views regarding police brutality but did not share his investment in these views. Mr. Monfort's employment as a truck driver was well below his intelligence and bachelor's degree education. He was unemployed for several months preceding the offenses.

F. Prodromal Factors

No developmental or family history characteristic is pathognomonic for delusional disorder. Though tending to occur at a later age than other primary psychoses (see IDC-11), delusional disorder does not have a clear etiology or typical prodromal course. Arguably, to the extent that broader evidence of psychological deterioration or decremented functioning is present, delusional disorder, as opposed to radicalization, is implicated (see Golding, 2007; Pytyck & Chaimowitz, 2013). Thus, a unidirectional metric is suggested, where prodromal symptoms of psychosis implicate delusional disorder, while the absence of such history is not contraindicative.

Factor 13. Prodromal Symptomatology

CASE ANALYSIS

In his college interactions in the years before the offenses, Mr. Monfort was memorable for his unusual degree of dogmatism. In this academic context, he was unable to grapple with information he did not agree with or was not prepared to hear. Rather, he had already made up his mind and would use the course and course materials to reinforce his beliefs instead of developing a more nuanced view or challenging his beliefs. Nothing anyone said could influence anything that he thought. In his political courses, he was quite outspoken – sometimes to the point of annoying other students with dogmatic statements. He did not seem attuned to other students and their reactions to him. Other students were not in his consciousness; rather, he was preoccupied with ideas.

Mr. Monfort was generous and good-hearted in his romantic relationships but was observed to be rigid, impatient, intolerant, and prone to overreaction. He had broad difficulty establishing/maintaining interpersonal intimacy. Illustrative of this, he was briefly married to a woman who spoke no English. He exhibited obsessive concerns with germs and contamination, becoming quite anxious when confronted with shared finger dishes in an Ethiopian restaurant.

Mr. Monfort held other over-valued ideas regarding jury nullification, the corporate exploitation of labor, the hazards of the Patriot Act, the false bases for the Iraq and Afghanistan Wars, and the 2nd Amendment right to bear arms. As early as 2002, in a speech for a college class, he had expressed concerns that the system was ineffective in controlling police misconduct. In the months before the offenses, he became unemployed and more withdrawn in his interaction pattern. However, his general behavior and interactions in the community (pre-arrest) or King County Jail (post-arrest) were not grossly impaired or frankly bizarre.

G. Behavioral/Action Factors

Factor 14. Willingness to Act on the Belief

In a forensic evaluation context for differentiating delusional disorder from extreme beliefs, a violent act has been committed. Such action alone is thus not a conclusive differential. That said, a delusional disorder creates a strong catalyst to act, thus raising the index of suspicion. A strong linkage between belief and behavior has been postulated (see Taylor & Felthous, 2006), with Wessely et al. (1993) specifying "assertive action" as a recurrent feature of delusions. Bental and Taylor (2006) reported that 60% of delusional patients acted on their beliefs, with those having paranoid delusions being at increased risk of committing violent acts toward others. Junginger (2006) reported that the presence of delusions increased violence risk 2.6-fold, with the delusional content forming a blueprint for the parameters of violence.

CASE ANALYSIS

Mr. Monfort engaged in a series of purposeful, organized, and planned actions in response to his beliefs. These actions began with assembling weapons and pipe bombs, proceeded with an aborted trip to attack police in California, continued with planning and scouting the bombing of a police vehicle storage lot and shooting responding officers, continued with the bombing but aborted shootings, and culminated in the targeted killing of a police officer nine days later.

Factor 15. Compulsion to Act on the Belief

The linkage between delusion and action may result in the patient/defendant with delusional disorder feeling internally compelled to act, as opposed to an adherent of extreme beliefs who acts more strategically.

CASE ANALYSIS

Mr. Monfort described a personal obligation, rising to "a duty," to respond to what he repeatedly characterized as brutal and murderous police conduct. His sense of personal responsibility to take action appeared to stem from his grandiose identification with the Founding Fathers. Thus, if the Founding Fathers took action and he did not, he would be faced with abandoning this grandiose connection. He described: "I thought about the British and the Founding Fathers as I loaded the backpack and prepared my weapons [in preparation for the Charles Street bombing]. I had a sense of solidarity and connection to the Founding Fathers." He similarly described that a "real citizen" does not respond passively to the brutalizing of his fellows: "If I see somebody doing something bad, then I have a responsibility to stop them. . . . Knowing about it makes me culpable." Other statements also reflected an idiosyncratic sense of personal responsibility to take action:

> I was getting ready to move into the next section of my life – to go to Denver and be a juvenile probation officer. I had connections and family there. But I kept seeing all these people get hurt by those who are supposed to protect us – it hurts you personally. I thought something has to be done about this. I can't go help one kid at a time and let this stand. No one else seems to know about this or at least feel this way about the problem. I never see the kind of angst I felt. I just felt I had to do something. I had to try and make a difference.
>
> (Interview, 04-04-2015)

As will be discussed subsequently, in sharp contrast to the careful planning of his first action, Mr. Monfort described increasing internal pressure to act again in targeting police officers. He responded by improvising, inadvertently planting the seeds of his apprehension.

Factor 16. Rigid Moral Distinctions in Acting on the Belief

Terrorists often deliberately target "noncombatants" or at least regard property damage or civilian casualties as collateral damage. By contrast, persons acting in the service of a delusional disorder may parse moral distinctions of who is a legitimate target and be intolerant of collateral damage.

CASE ANALYSIS

In placing his pipe bombs in the city lot, Mr. Monfort only targeted police vehicles. He explained that other city vehicles were involved in services and repairs that benefited the citizenry. Mr. Monfort did not fire on a city worker who observed him in the maintenance lot and represented an apprehension hazard by notifying law enforcement. He explained that shooting a maintenance worker would make him like those he was fighting. He described: "I'm not there to shoot civilians. That's not my mission. My mission is to stop police brutality."

Mr. Monfort explained that he considered stealing a car to carry out the police shooting, rather than using his own vehicle, but did not as this would have victimized another citizen who needed the vehicle to go to work, pick up children from school, etc. His regret regarding the fatal shooting was that he had used a weapon (i.e., an assault rifle) with significant potential to strike innocent citizens downrange inadvertently.

Factor 17. Psychological Disorganization in Acting on the Belief

Mentally ill offenders often demonstrate organized motives, sophisticated planning, and effective execution of their violent attacks (see Fein & Vossekuil, 1999; Borum, 2014; Gill et al., 2014; Gill, 2015). That said, when the psychotic capsule is breached in delusional disorder, some degree of psychological disorganization may be observed in thinking about, discussing, and acting on the delusions. Several contexts of psychological disorganization are specified by this model. Again, a unidirectional analysis is implicated.

CASE ANALYSIS

Mr. Monfort repeatedly exhibited psychological disorganization around his police brutality beliefs. When a video of a local police brutality incident came on television when Mr. Monfort was at work several months before the offense, he was observed to become "transfixed – like there was a war going on."

Mr. Monfort spent an hour planting leaflets in and on police vehicles at the scene of the Charles Street bombing before igniting the bombs. This activity ultimately resulted in his being observed by a maintenance worker who notified the police, forcing Mr. Monfort to abort the shooting portion of his plan. He appears not to have considered that dissemination to the public and police of the purpose of the bombing and associated shootings (as originally planned) could have been achieved with much less risk through post-bombing mailings to media outlets – with offense-specific details to demonstrate authenticity. In other words, with great jeopardy to his "mission," he limited himself in the dissemination of purpose to the resources possessed by the Founding Fathers, i.e., physically placing fliers. A lack of critical judgment in acting on the delusion was also demonstrated by his self-reported failure to wear gloves to avoid leaving fingerprints or DNA on the fliers he prepared.

Similarly, Mr. Monfort described familiarity with Sun Tzu's principal, from *The Art of War*, of bringing the enemy to you and thus engaging the enemy on the field of your choice. He applied this principle in his planning for the Charles Street bombing. However, he had no follow-up plan beyond the bombing for bringing officers to him. Instead, he engaged in improvised "hunting" for opportunities to shoot police officers. His self-imposed pressure to act quickly following the October 22, 2009 bombing and apparent inability to develop more than one strategic plan demonstrated startling suspensions of critical judgment. Mr. Monfort used his own vehicle in the fatal shooting of Officer Brenton and left a witnessing officer alive to return fire and provide a report.

Importantly, it is not that Mr. Monfort lacked the capacity to develop a strategic plan of some complexity. In fact, it is the marked *inconsistency* rather than *incapacity* in Mr. Monfort's planning that points to the belief system as a zone of significant psychological disturbance. To illustrate, he systematically and effectively planned many aspects of the Charles Street bombing (e.g., researching pipe bombs and fuse delays, gathering supplies to build these bombs, purchasing higher quality magazines and ammunition, sighting in his rifles, cutting a hole in the fence days before, disguising his appearance, etc.). At the same time, he failed to consider far easier and less risky mechanisms to announce the purpose of his attack. He did not pause to develop a second strategic plan (e.g., set a fire with a pipe/gasoline bomb in a dumpster, call in a crime in progress, snipe from a distance, etc.).

Similarly, Mr. Monfort made extensive preparations to fortify his apartment for a "last stand" but continued to leave this "bunker" on a daily basis to go about his usual activities – where he could be confronted by law enforcement without the aid of these resources. His failure to establish a "safe house," externally placed resources, or procedures for leaving the Seattle area also reflect stunning lapses for an individual who had meticulously planned other aspects of his campaign.

An obvious approach to avoid apprehension and further future "operations" in the service of an extreme belief is to keep a low profile. Mr. Monfort did the opposite. His behavior called attention to himself in the midst of an intense police investigation. In the days between the maintenance lot bombing and the fatal shooting of a police officer, Mr. Monfort spoke in a pressured fashion to "anyone who would listen" on a city bus about how the police and government want "all black men in prison." An observer recalled there was "something odd about the way the man was so angry with the police and the government" and that he was "too forceful" and "wasn't talking on an even keel." Similarly, several days following the police officer's assassination, Mr. Monfort initiated a long monologue about the unfairness of the judicial system and the behavior of the police toward Black people with a physician who joined him on a hospital elevator.

Chris Monfort: Epilogue

At the conclusion of the guilt phase trial in 2015, the jury rejected the insanity defense, finding that Mr. Monfort did know that his conduct was wrong (i.e., in violation of Washington law). They deliberated only briefly, however, in returning a unanimous sentencing verdict of life in prison rather than the death penalty, potentially reflecting a view that he did suffer from delusional disorder. Mr. Monfort committed suicide in prison in January 2017 by an overdose of prescribed amitriptyline (antidepressant) medication he had secreted.

Assessment Professionalism, Objectivity, And Neutrality

In a forensic context, differentiating delusional disorder from extreme beliefs sometimes occurs in the aftermath of an incident of extreme violence. When such acts have socio-political overtones, they are particularly shocking to social consciousness. These disturb our sense of order, safety, and reciprocal community. Intense media coverage brings these events and their aftermath psychologically close and holds them in psychological proximity for days or weeks. As these cases are adjudicated, they are subject to particularly vigorous adversarial advocacy. These social-emotional-interpersonal factors impact mental health experts, as well as courts, attorneys, jurors, and the public at large. Such influences challenge the professionalism, objectivity, and neutrality of evaluating mental health experts. Evaluators finding themselves in such contexts are encouraged to self-assess periodically and actively consider alternative hypotheses. As the assessment methodology is structured, these goals may be facilitated.

Clinical Assessment Points

1. Recognize the continuum from extreme beliefs to delusional disorder and the associated shared features.
2. Use, adapt, or conceptualize a structured set of literature-derived factors that will guide the assessment and the interpretation of the associated data in making the differential between delusional disorder and extreme beliefs. If using the *MADDD-or-Rad-17*, access the associated article (Cunningham, 2018) and employ it as an aid to comprehensive inquiry rather than a scoreable scale. To facilitate the

use of this SPJ tool, a fillable template in Word is available from the author by request.

3. In interviewing the patient/defendant, encourage the patient/defendant to fully elaborate on the content of the beliefs, their evolution, and their social context. Be attuned to how the beliefs are held/described, as well as their content. Broadly seek information regarding life history and contemporaneous functioning and relationships. Anticipate multiple interviews. Delay challenging the beliefs until a fully elaborated description and history has been obtained. Gently probe the beliefs to test the capacity for alternative perspectives, as opposed to confronting aggressively.
4. Interview third parties and scrutinize records for broad history and for expressions of the beliefs and behaviors that would provide inferences regarding these beliefs. These alternative sources are particularly important when the patient/defendant is circumspect about the beliefs.
5. From the interviews and review of records, formally distill and memorialize the beliefs in question. This is an invaluable foundation for the subsequent analysis of the beliefs.
6. In the assessment of patients/defendants who have violently acted on the beliefs, be aware of social impacts that may cloud objectivity.
7. In reports (and testimony), be transparent regarding the factors considered and the application of these in variously confirming and disconfirming the differential.

14

ASSESSING SUICIDE RISK IN PSYCHOSIS

There is a consensus in the literature that the presence of psychotic symptoms increases the risk of suicide (APA, 2003; Jacobs & Brewer, 2006). The literature on suicide and psychosis has focused chiefly on schizophrenia, schizoaffective disorder, and first-episode psychosis, with less information on suicide risk in other psychotic disorders (Hor & Taylor, 2010).

Huang et al. (2018) conducted a comprehensive review of all published studies on psychosis and suicidal behavior until 2016. The findings showed that psychosis is a risk factor for suicide death, attempted suicide, and suicidal ideation.

Regarding the prevalence of suicidal behavior and psychosis, earlier studies showed that nearly 5–10% of individuals with psychotic spectrum disorders die by suicide, with 20–30% attempting suicide and 30–40% having suicidal thoughts (Radomsky et al., 1995; Palmer et al., 2005; Fialko et al., 2006).

In a recent study, Álvarez et al. (2022) conducted a systematic meta-analysis to examine the prevalence of suicide deaths and attempts among individuals diagnosed with various psychotic disorders between 1990 and 2020. The results of the study revealed that the incidence of death by suicide was 2.4% for schizoaffective disorder, 2% for schizophrenia, 2.2% for delusional disorder, and 1.9% for first-episode psychosis.

The study also showed that the prevalence of suicide attempts was 46.8% for schizoaffective disorder, 20.3% for schizophrenia, and 12.5% for first-episode psychosis, 11.1 % for delusional disorders. Practice guidelines consider the assessment of suicide risk as an essential aspect in evaluating patients with psychosis (APA, 2003). Research has also consistently demonstrated positive psychotic symptoms, including command hallucination and specific types of delusions, are more associated with increased suicide risk than negative symptoms (Huang et al., 2018).

A review of suicide risk factors in psychotic disorders reveals two distinct patterns of suicide. In the first pattern, the patient's suicide occurs in response to active symptoms of psychosis (Breier & Astrachan, 1984; Fenton et al., 1997; Hawton et al., 2005). Such individuals

DOI: 10.4324/9781003415206-19

may feel intensely negative emotions in response to active, positive symptoms of psychosis, as the following example illustrates: Mr. P. presented with a first-episode psychosis that included a persecutory delusion that he was being followed and monitored by "certain individuals" and that he would be "captured and tortured." Mr. P. felt "tormented" by his delusional belief and eventually tried to jump from his apartment window to end his anguish before being stopped by family members.

Other patients who experience psychotic symptoms may try to kill themselves not as a response to a tormenting emotional state but because they believe that suicide is the proper response to specific psychotic symptoms. Consider: Ms. J. suffered from a chronic schizoaffective disorder with a long-standing delusion that she was "a messenger of God."

While off her medication, she attempted to drink cleaning fluid as an "act of purification" to join God and set an example for others. Both Mr. P. and Ms. J. attempted suicide while in a psychotic state. While Mr. P. felt that killing himself would spare him from delusional persecution, Ms. J. viewed suicide as a grandiose form of purification, allowing her to join God and become an example for others. In some cases, individuals experiencing positive symptoms of psychosis may engage in actions that could result in their death without intending to harm themselves. For instance, a person with a delusion that they have the power to fly may jump from a cliff (Maris, 2019).

In the second type of pattern, a suicide attempt may follow a period of symptom stabilization and become a response to feelings of hopelessness and despair. This pattern often occurs in what is referred to as a post-psychotic depression state (McGlashan & Carpenter, 1979), in which the patients have sufficient insight into their illness. As a result, they are aware of their diminished functioning and other losses associated with a chronic psychiatric illness that can result in mental deterioration (Dingman & McGlashan, 1986; Fenton et al., 1997). In Chapter 3, we discussed how being hospitalized for a psychotic episode can be a distressing and life-changing experience that can lead to feelings of hopelessness and shame. We talked about Chadwick's (2014) personal experience with post-psychosis, where he described it as "particularly sickening, embarrassing, and humiliating" (p. 484). The journey to recover from the trauma of psychosis can leave behind a "deep scar" that affects one's sense of self and potentially increases the risk of suicide.

The risk of suicide further increases in individuals who are intelligent and have had good premorbid functioning before the onset of their illness (Westermeyer et al., 1991). Dr. L. was one such individual. A knowledgeable, doctoral-level patient with a history of several past episodes of psychosis, Dr. L. was admitted following a near-lethal suicide attempt. However, he did not demonstrate any active psychotic symptoms while in the hospital. He remained suicidal. Dr. L. was painfully aware of the impact that his psychosis had had on his life, and he remained pessimistic about his future. He told the hospital staff, "Look at me. I went from a private practice to a private insane asylum." Dr. L. would look out the window, point to a car, and say, "I will never be able to drive a car with a girl next to me like all my normal friends. Who would want to go out with a man who has schizophrenia?"

Assessing Suicide Risk and Protective Factors in Psychotic Patients

Risk factors:

Suicide risk assessment aims to identify individualized risk and protective factors and implement treatment strategies to decrease suicide risk rather than predict it. (APA, 2003; Simon, 2004). Many suicide-risk factors that are present in nonpsychotic individuals are also current and relevant for psychotic patients. A comprehensive review study of risk factors (see Hawton et al., 2005) indicated that being male, having a history of suicide attempts and a family history of suicide, dealing with a recent loss, misusing drugs and alcohol, being depressed, and being non-adherence with treatment recommendations have been strongly associated with increased suicide risk in patients with schizophrenia. In addition, agitation and restlessness in psychotic patients have also been associated with increased risk (Freeman, 2012).

The suicide-risk factors that are unique to psychotic disorders include:

- Insight into illness
- Higher level of education
- Higher premorbid level of functioning
- Anxiety about mental breakdown
- Active delusions
- Some type of command hallucinations in which the voices are experienced as familiar.
- A loss of insight regarding the experience of hearing voices.

(Erkwoh et al., 2002; Scott & Resnick, 2009)

Protective factors:

Certain non-symptom-related factors have been identified as protective factors. These include family support and shorter duration of psychosis (Ventriglio et al., 2016; Hor & Taylor, 2010), as well as adherence to medication treatment and appropriate follow-up care. These factors are essential in mitigating the risk of suicide.

Challenges in Assessing Suicide Risk in Psychotic Patients

Assessment of suicide risk in patients with psychosis is challenging because some patients do not give any recognizable clues about their potential for suicide (Resnick, 2002).

Furthermore, some patients are actively experiencing paranoia or are guarded to the point that they do not reveal their suicidal ideations, intent, or other risk factors.

Mrs. B, a 35-year-old mother who was diagnosed with postpartum psychotic depression, did not reveal to her medical team that she was experiencing command auditory hallucinations to kill herself. Instead, she showed this to a close friend, who promptly informed her family and the medical team. Mrs. B. later explained that she was fearful and convinced that revealing her symptoms would result in the loss of custody of her infant.

Suicidal thoughts may evolve and reflect an individual's changing reactions to her psychotic symptoms. Ms. Z. was such a person. Although this 46-year-old woman had no history of suicide attempts, she had a long history of auditory hallucinations in which she heard the voice of God. More recently, she had begun to listen to the voices of her dead parents, which replaced the voice of God. She started thinking about killing herself to join them. Sadly, she had interpreted that God no longer considered her a "special person" and that hearing her dead parents' voices was an indication that her "mission from God was over." Thus, the time had come for her to die. People with psychosis may also experience certain life events, such as uniquely stressful. This subjective sense of heightened stress may, in turn, exacerbate their symptoms and potentially increase their risk for suicide. Anthony, who has chronic schizophrenia, was stabilized on his medication and began having interviews at different residential facilities before his discharge from the hospital. Anthony became increasingly paranoid when rejected after the first interview, despite having other interviews set up. He began to believe that there was a conspiracy to keep him homeless and that he would never be able to have stable housing. Feelings of hopelessness and suicidal ideation followed this. Anthony tried to hang himself at the hospital before staff intervened.

Although there is limited research identifying protective factors against suicide in patients with psychotic disorders (Hor & Taylor, 2010), it is imperative to assess case-specific factors that may protect these patients by exploring their reason for living (Freeman, 2012; Simon, 2004). Empirically validated protective factors such as children living at home and cultural or religious beliefs against suicide (APA, 2003) may interact in complex ways with psychotic symptoms (Huguelet et al., 2007). In some cases, psychotic symptoms may mitigate the impact of protective factors.

Ms. G., who suffered from a schizoaffective illness, indicated that she would "never" kill herself because she loved her two children, who lived at home with her. When the interviewer pointed out that she had tried to kill herself while off her medication and in response to command hallucinations, she replied that, at the time, the voices had been telling her to jump in front of traffic. She had no other history of suicide attempts. However, having young children living at home was only a protective factor when she was not experiencing symptoms of psychosis.

Clinical Assessment Points

1. Obtain a detailed history of suicide attempts and severity of suicidal ideation.

   We strongly recommend that the clinician use a structured, multimethod approach to gather the history of suicide attempts – both actual attempts and aborted or interrupted attempts, which also increase the risk of suicide. In constructing the patient's history of suicide risk, it is essential to understand what case-specific risk factors drive the patient to suicide.
2. Assess positive symptoms of psychosis, paying particular attention to the degree of distress that the patient may experience in response to psychotic symptoms. For example, some patients are highly distressed when they experience auditory hallucinations. For others, the nature and content of their delusional thinking may cause them to become desperate in response to tormenting emotions.
3. Similarly, the clinician should explore the impact of delusions from the patient's perspective. In other words, what might happen if the delusional belief continues for the patient? For example, a patient with the somatic delusion that he has a mysterious disease should be asked what he would do if no one could diagnose or identify his disease.
4. The clinician should explore if there is a threshold beyond which the patient may consider suicide as a solution to their hallucination or delusions.
5. Assess for depression. While the presence of depression may be associated with improved insight, it may also substantially increase suicide risk. Patients with a diagnosis of schizoaffective disorder often have higher rates of suicide and suicide attempts (Radomsky et al., 1999). Assessment of depression should go beyond asking questions about depressed mood, anhedonia, thoughts of hopelessness, and negative cognition. Instead, carefully explore the presence of

insomnia, increased agitation, and anxiety. These symptoms have been associated with suicide attempts in both inpatient and outpatient settings.

6. Assess for substance abuse. Given the strong association of alcohol and drugs with suicide and the fact that certain drugs may exacerbate psychotic symptoms, substance abuse requires careful assessment. Particular attention should be paid to recent relapses, increases in drug and alcohol use, and types of substances used.
7. Assess the level of insight and the impact of the patient's awareness about his illness. For some patients, increased awareness of their psychotic illness may increase their suicide risk. Thus, it is vital to explore the level and impact of a patient's insight and assess: What are the individual's emotional reactions to having a psychotic disorder? What is the degree to which psychosis has impacted their functioning? How do they perceive their recovery and their future life?
8. Psychological assessments can be very helpful with patients who are at high risk for suicide. Testing can assess the severity of psychotic and depressive symptoms. It can also help evaluate the patient's degree of reality-testing and insight and can aid in developing case-specific interventions.
9. Assess adherence to treatment and medication. In assessing treatment adherence, clinicians should explore the extent of the patient's alliance and connection with the treatment team and outpatient providers, past and present. For former inpatients, this may require their permission to obtain collateral information. Refusal of patients to grant that permission is informative and should be explored.
10. Patients may feel connected and understood by their therapists or psychiatrists, but this does not necessarily translate into taking the recommended medication. Thus, medication adherence should be carefully assessed regardless of how positively patients may describe their relationships with the healthcare professionals who oversee their treatment.

15

ASSESSING VIOLENCE RISK IN PSYCHOSIS

The connection between psychoses and violence has produced conflicting findings. Earlier studies of civil psychiatric patients discharged from emergency room or inpatient services indicated that the link between psychosis and violence was negligible (Appelbaum et al., 2000; Monahan et al., 2001; Steadman et al., 1998). Also, Bonta (Bonta et al., 1998), using a meta-analysis, reported either a negative or small association between psychosis and violence in mentally disordered offenders.

However, subsequent meta-analyses and meta-regression studies of violence and psychosis present a different picture regarding the role of psychosis in violence. One such meta-analysis (Douglas et al., 2009) focusing on the association between psychosis and violence from 204 studies indicated that although there was considerable variability in effect sizes, the results showed that "psychosis was significantly associated with a 49–68% increase in the odds of violence" (p. 679). Similarly, another meta-analysis by Fazel et al. (2009) reported 20 studies showing a positive association between violence and schizophrenia. Another major study (Witt et al., 2013), using a meta-regression analysis of 110 studies, examined the risk factors associated with violence in 45,553 individuals with a diagnosis of psychosis. The results demonstrated that multiple dynamic factors were significantly associated with violence. Among these factors, positive psychotic symptoms, as measured by PANSS and lack of insight, were significantly associated with violence. Finally, Large and Nielssen (2011) conducted a meta-analysis of studies examining the prevalence of violence in individuals with first-episode psychosis before their initial treatment. They found that although severe violence leading to significant injury was very low (one in 100), a substantial number of first-episode patients engaged in violent behavior (one in three patients), and one in six patients assaulted another person before the start of their first psychiatric treatment.

The findings from their study showed that violence of any severity was associated with the following risk factors: male sex, younger age, lower level of education, duration of untreated psychosis, illicit drug

DOI: 10.4324/9781003415206-20

use, a forensic history, involuntary treatment, symptoms of mania, and hostile affect. Serious violence, defined as an aggressive act causing injury, was associated with the duration of untreated psychosis, total symptom scores, and having a forensic history (Large & Nielssen, 2011).

Despite the earlier findings, there is now a consensus among researchers that the presence of psychotic symptoms increases the risk of violence (Scott & Resnick, 2013; Douglas et al., 2009). However, this conclusion must be put in perspective. Most individuals with psychotic disorders *do not* engage in violence, and most violent individuals *do not* have psychosis (Douglas et al., 2009). Furthermore, only a tiny fraction of all murders are committed by patients with psychotic disorders (Large et al., 2009).

Pattern of Violence in Psychotic Disorders

Douglas et al. (2009) have identified three different ways in which psychosis can contribute to violence. We have found their typology to be a clinically useful way of understanding the role that psychosis may play in violence and an indispensable model in conducting violence risk assessment with individuals who have psychotic disorders.

Type One

Positive psychotic symptoms, including hallucinations and delusions, may compel the person to engage in a planned, organized act of violence in which a specific person, group of people, or institution can be the target. Mr. B. was such an individual. Mr. B., a 25-year-old separated male with a history of paranoid schizophrenia, was admitted to a psychiatric inpatient unit after he was found at home by his father, dressed in a suit and packing a large knife in a briefcase.

At the time of admission, it became clear that Mr. B. had a delusion that prominent law firms in a major city were responsible for his wife separating from him. His delusional belief was based on the fact that after his wife left him, he once saw her downtown with a man who "looked like a lawyer." He was convinced that the man was connected to various major law firms and was responsible for influencing his wife to leave him. Mr. B. planned to go to one of the largest law firms in the city and take matters into his own hands. From his perspective, he felt justified. The patient's father also revealed to the treatment team that Mr. B. had been sending threatening emails to various law firms for months. The father brought copies of the emails, along with printouts of Google Maps of these law firms.

Mr. B. was psychotic. He concluded that the man he saw *must* be an attorney because of how he dressed. From this, he developed the compelling delusional conviction that major law firms were conspiring against him.

Type Two

Positive symptoms may lead to disinhibition and dysregulation. As a result, an individual may become angry and engage in a disorganized and impulsive act of violence. The police brought Mr. S. to the psychiatric emergency room after he was found walking on the street carrying a pipe, which he was swinging at strangers while screaming at them, "You cannot touch me anymore!" On examination, the patient showed marked psychotic symptoms, including a delusional belief that strangers, such as those he encountered on the street, would somehow enter his apartment every day and night, touch his butt from behind, and then leave the apartment. He indicated that he saw only "flashes of their faces in the mirror."

This more bizarre-sounding delusion, accompanied by possible fleeting visual hallucinations, had a disinhibiting effect and compelled Mr. S. to engage in this self-protective violent behavior.

Type Three

Although there is consistent evidence that negative symptoms are not associated with violence, Douglas et al. (2009) indicated that under certain conditions, negative symptoms might contribute to violence. They argue that negative symptoms can lead to the development of depression, which in turn can have a disinhibitory role that results in anger directed at self or others.

Ms. A., a 20-year-old female student, dropped out of college following her first psychotic break because of prominent negative symptoms, including severe anhedonia and marked problems with initiation. While living at home with her family and despite receiving treatment, Ms. A. became progressively depressed and suicidal. On the day of admission to the hospital, she made a noose with a rope that she had bought earlier to hang herself. Fortunately, her older sister entered the room as she put the noose on the door handle. When the sister tried to intervene, the patient ran into the kitchen, grabbed a knife, and attacked her sister, who ran out of the apartment and called the police.

Ms. A. was not experiencing hallucinations or delusions compelling her to become violent. Her prominent negative symptoms were associated with depression and lowered her threshold to control her aggressive impulses.

Psychotic Symptoms and Risk of Violence

There are consistent findings that positive symptoms, including hallucinations and certain types of delusions, are more likely to increase the risk of violence than negative symptoms (Douglas et al., 2009; Keers et al., 2014; Witt et al., 2013). We summarize the association of specific positive symptoms with risk for violence.

Hallucinations

Nearly half of psychiatric patients with auditory hallucinations experience commanding voices (Shawyer et al., 2013). However, this figure may be even higher. In their study of subtypes of auditory hallucinations, McCarthy-Jones and colleagues (2014) found that 86% of patients hearing voices reported constant commanding and commenting hallucinations. Although close to 60% of patients endorse negative adjectives relating to the content of the voice(s) they hear (McCarthy-Jones et al., 2014), most patients hear nonviolent command hallucinations rather than violent ones (Chadwick & Birchwood, 1994). However, there is evidence that certain types of command hallucinations that direct the person to engage in acts of violence are associated with an increased risk of violence (Monahan et al., 2001).

Several factors increase the likelihood of acting on hallucinations. These include;

- A sense of superiority in response to the voices.
- The perception of hallucinations as powerful.
- A delusional belief that command hallucinations have a positive benefit for the person.
- Delusional beliefs with themes consistent with the command of the hallucinations (Fox et al., 2004; Shawyer et al., 2008).
- Experience of negative emotions in response to hallucinations (Cheung et al., 1997).

Delusions

Case histories and empirical studies indicate that persecutory delusions are most likely to be associated with violence (Wessely et al., 1993). Others (Buchanan et al., 1993) have argued that seeking evidence to support or refute the delusions moves the person toward action. Although the action is not always violent, several factors – including the nature of delusions and the degree of emotional distress, especially anger – may turn the action in a violent direction. Research by Link and Stueve (1994) focused on certain kinds of persecutory delusions that are called threat/control override (TCO), in which the person has two distinct forms of delusional beliefs, both of which are likely to increase the risk of violence. The first form includes delusional beliefs that center around a perceived threat, including beliefs of being harmed, spied on, experimented on, poisoned, or followed. The second form consists of delusional beliefs that involve losing internal control to an external source, such as beliefs that one's thoughts are being controlled, that others' thoughts are being inserted into one's mind, or that others are exerting control over one's actions.

Swanson et al. (1996) assessed the relationship between psychotic symptoms and violence using the Epidemiologic Catchment (ECT) area survey. The results indicated that individuals who reported TCO symptoms were more likely to engage in violent behavior than those who had other types of psychotic symptoms. Furthermore, the risk of violence increased significantly in individuals with comorbid substance use and TCO symptoms. In addition, Link et al. (1998) conducted a study demonstrating that both symptom domains of TCO were independently associated with violence.

A study by Appelbaum et al. (2000) used the data from the MacArthur research project, a multisite study of civilly committed psychiatric patients discharged into the community (Monahan et al., 2001). In contrast to earlier findings, the results of their study demonstrated that TCO symptoms and delusions, in general, were not associated with an increased risk of violence in psychiatric patients living in the community post-discharge. Similar findings were reported in a study that compared patients with schizophrenia who were found not guilty because of insanity to a matched control group of nonoffending patients with a diagnosis of schizophrenia. The prevalence of TCO symptoms was not significantly different between the two groups. However, a study by Ullrich et al. (2013) reanalyzed the MacArthur study data. It showed that when there is temporal proximity between persecutory delusions and anger associated with delusions, the risk for violence increases significantly.

Using a longitudinal study design, Keers et al. (2014) followed UK prisoners diagnosed with psychotic disorders after they were released into the community. The results indicated that prisoners with schizophrenia who were untreated during the study period were more likely to become violent compared to those who received treatment. Furthermore, persecutory delusions in the untreated group were associated with post-release violence.

All the above studies show that despite some negative findings, persecutory delusions – particularly TCO symptoms – continue to play an active role in triggering violence, especially when the symptoms go untreated and are associated with anger. These delusions need careful assessment (Scott & Resnick, 2013; Keers et al., 2014).

Other Psychotic Symptoms and Risk for Violence

Non-delusional paranoia and suspiciousness with hostile intent have been associated with violence (Monahan et al., 2001). The results of another recent meta-analysis (Douglas et al., 2009) indicated that symptoms of disorganization were also significantly associated with violence. The authors suggested that disorganization potentially disrupts executive functions and impairs the patient's ability to solve problems effectively.

Nonpsychotic Violence Risk Factors in Individuals with Psychosis

There is considerable evidence that a history of violence and a criminal history that includes arrest for nonviolent crimes significantly increase the risk of violence (Monahan et al., 2001; Witt et al., 2013). A consistent finding across many studies has been the presence of comorbid substance abuse as a strong predictor of violent behavior in psychotic disorders (Monahan et al., 2001; Swanson et al., 2006; Fazel et al., 2009). Additional dynamic factors that have been associated strongly with increased violence are impulsivity, a high level of hostility, lack of insight, and nonadherence to treatment, including medication (Witt et al., 2013).

Mass Murder, Use of Firearms, and Psychosis

A comprehensive study conducted by Steadman et al. (2015) showed that only 2% of individuals with mental illness, including those with psychotic disorders, were involved in firearm violence. Another study by Swanson et al. in 2016 examined the arrest rate among 81,704 adults in Florida and found that only 13% of all violent crimes involving firearms were perpetrated by individuals with mental illness, compared to 24% of the general population in the same counties.

Regarding mass shootings, defined as killing three or more people, Brucato et al. (2021) conducted a comprehensive review of 14,785 mass murders from 1900 to 2019 using published databases available online and in print. The authors of the study gathered information on demographics and the history of psychiatric disorders, including symptoms of hallucination, delusions, and disorganization, as well as neurologic illness, substance abuse, legal history, and the type of weapon used (gun or other method). The study found that mass murderers who used firearms were less likely to have a lifetime history of psychosis, with only 8% of mass murderers having a lifetime history of psychotic disorder, compared to 18% of those who did not use guns. Furthermore, only 5% of mass murderers who used firearms had active symptoms of psychosis at the time of committing the crime.

These studies show that small fractions of individuals with psychotic disorders commit mass murder or use firearms in their violent acts.

Clinical Assessment Points

1. Assess the patient's history of past violence and threats of violence. We strongly recommend clinicians use a multi method approach, including the patient's self-report and collateral and record review. In constructing the patient's history of violence risk, it is crucial to understand what case-specific risk factors drive the patient to violence (Douglas & Reeves, 2010). In addition, it would be helpful to understand what role the patient's psychosis has played in episodes of past violence.
2. Assess positive symptoms of psychosis. Particular attention should be paid to the degree of anger that the patient may experience in response to psychotic symptoms. For example, some patients are highly distressed when they experience auditory hallucinations. For others, the nature and content of their delusional thinking may cause them to feel negative emotions. In addition, in a similar fashion to assessing suicide risk in psychosis, clinicians should explore the impact of delusions from the patient's perspective. In other words, what would happen if the delusional belief continues for the patient? For example, a patient with paranoid delusions that people are planning to harm him should be asked what he would do if he continues to be bothered by these "people." Clinicians should explore if there is a threshold past which the patient may consider violence as a solution to his hallucinations or delusions.
3. Assess for substance abuse. Given the strong association of alcohol and drugs with violence and the fact that certain drugs may exacerbate psychotic symptoms, substance abuse requires a careful assessment. In particular, attention should be paid to recent relapses, an increase in drug and alcohol use, as well as types of substance used and their role in inciting violence in the patient.
4. Assess the potential for suicide concurrently with violence risk assessment in individuals with psychosis. Recent studies show that there is a moderate relationship between violence and a history of past suicide attempts, although not with suicidal ideation (Witt et al., 2013). The authors of the study suggest that impulsivity may mediate the relationship between suicide attempts and violence.
5. Assess the level of insight and adherence to treatment and medication. Because impaired insight has been associated with violence, it is helpful to assess the patient's insight into her illness, violence, and need for treatment. When evaluating treatment adherence, the clinician should explore the degree of alliance and connection the patient

has with her treatment team or outpatient providers. Patients may feel connected and understood by their therapists or psychiatrists, but that does not necessarily translate into taking recommended medication; thus, medication adherence should be carefully assessed.

6. Conduct a violence risk assessment in individuals who are experiencing first-episode psychosis and are not receiving any treatment.
7. Assess protective factors. Although there is limited research identifying protective factors against violence in patients with a psychotic disorder, it is imperative to assess case-specific factors such as social support or a sense of responsibility to one's family that may be protective for the patient.
8. Finally, when possible, clinicians should receive training in the use of specialized violence risk assessment tools that have been developed. One instrument, the *Historical, Clinical, Risk management-20 Version 3* (HCR-20^{V3}, Douglas et al., 2013), utilizes a structured professional-judgment approach (SPJ) that assesses case-specific risk factors and provides individualized management strategies to reduce violence risk. It is a well-researched measure of violence risk (See De Vogel et al., 2022). More importantly, it has been used with civil and forensic psychiatric patients, including those diagnosed with psychotic disorders.

16

ASSESSING PSYCHOSIS IN CHILDREN AND ADOLESCENTS

Nine-year-old Jessie's mother brought him in for an evaluation because he had been hearing voices for several years. The taunting quality of these voices increased to the point that they began instructing him to hit other children. After he succumbed to these commands and struck a classmate, his symptoms reached a threshold requiring professional attention. A history of schizophrenia in a second-degree family member worried his pediatrician, who referred Jessie for a psychological evaluation. Jessie's response to items from a Scale to Measure Unusual Beliefs and Experiences Among Children and Adolescents, CUBESCALE (Child Unusual Belief Scale; Andersen, 2006; Viglione et al., 1994; Viglione & Senecal, 2014), a semi-structured instrument for assessing unusual beliefs in children, illustrated the bizarre nature of both his thoughts and how he communicated his ideas. The CUBESCALE, discussed later in this chapter, consists of 40 statements to which the child responds either "True" or "False." The interviewer follows up affirmative responses with additional clarifying questions. To the statement, "Sometimes, I don't have any insides," Jessie responded, "True," and explained his answer in the following way,

> I feel weightless, or if I am hungry, I feel my stomach disappear and everything having to do with the stomach. Everything that is linked or shares the same space. . . . Sometimes I feel weightless, and my bones are just missing, and I collapse. So if you think about sad things, normally you just turn sad.

Lucy had become increasingly withdrawn, to the point that she refused to go to school. She reluctantly accompanied her parents to meet with a clinician for an evaluation. Sitting next to her mother, she playfully grabbed her mother's hand and tapped her mother's face, chanting, "Why are you hitting yourself? Why are you hitting yourself? What are you hitting myself?" Further confusion between self-other boundaries was vividly reflected in her story about trying to give her parakeet a sunflower

DOI: 10.4324/9781003415206-21

seed. When her bird refused the seed and ate a piece of chicken instead, Lucy called it a *cannibird* and promptly added, "It thinks it's a human, and the bird threw it another piece of human." In this example, we first see Lucy's tendency to condense concepts in a playful manner (*cannibird*), but then her explanation became strained when she said, "It thinks it's a human, and the bird threw it another piece of human." Here, she seemed to conflate the concepts of "bird," "cannibal," and "human," leaving the listener confused.

Finally, there was Eddie, who, at the age of 16, had become increasingly confused and unable to concentrate at school. When given Card II of the Rorschach, Eddie demonstrated his peculiar way of thinking by giving the following overly embellished and idiosyncratic response, which went far beyond any of the objective features of the inkblot.

> I think I can see a rabbit if I look at it from the side. I think a rabbit who has or is either being slaughtered or has finished a race. Like there is some sort of fight or physical activity, like vomiting. Yes, it's definitely in some sort of physical pain. I feel that pain is . . . fake. I think it's just trying to show that it's in pain and it looks like a rabbit because it has resembling ears.

Each of these children was evaluated because the referring clinicians thought that their young patients had symptoms suggestive of psychosis. With each child, a more thorough evaluation was necessary to determine whether suspected hallucinations, odd beliefs, problematic behavior, and confused thinking reached a threshold for making a diagnosis of a psychotic disorder.

Identifying children and adolescents with psychotic-like features (PLEs) is a challenging diagnostic task because such symptom features can be placed along a continuum from developmentally normal to nonpathological presentations to psychotic spectrum disorders (House & Tyson, 2020). It is important to have an understanding of psychotic symptomatology in children and adolescents to provide an accurate assessment. Many might wonder what psychosis looks like in children, questioning whether psychotic disorders in children and adolescents are contiguous with adult forms and whether they present with the same set of core features. Others might question the prevalence of psychotic disorders in children and adolescents, and some might even doubt the existence of psychosis in young children.

Symptoms of Psychosis in Children and Adolescents

The DSM-5-TR does not have a separate section cataloging psychotic disorders in children and adolescents. Unless otherwise qualified, the diagnostic criteria are intended to apply to children, adolescents, and adults. Core symptoms such as hallucinations, delusions, thought disorders, and negative symptoms can be found in younger patients, just as they are found among adults.

As with adults, auditory hallucinations in children are more common than visual and tactile hallucinations; however, hallucinations in other sensory modalities are possible. Like adults, children (like Jessie) may hear one or multiple voices commenting on their behavior or issuing commands. It may even be more common for the young patient to hear sounds, noises, or muffled, unintelligible voices (Findling et al., 2001).

Delusional beliefs and overvalued ideas may also be present in child and adolescent patients; however, they are usually related to childhood themes and may be less complex and systematized than those of adults (Masi et al., 2006; Spencer & Campbell, 1994). Delusional content may involve false beliefs about popular games, toys, or animals. Paranoid and grandiose delusions are not unusual, whereas delusions of erotomania or jealousy are less common. First-rank Schneiderian symptoms (e.g., "Do you feel people can hear your thoughts out loud or put their thoughts into your mind?") may be found in children and adolescents with delusions. These first-rank symptoms may take the form of a child's belief that characters from his favorite television program are sending special communications intended only for him.

FTD, manifested in disorganized speech and illogical thinking, might also be characteristic of children and adolescents presenting with psychotic-like symptoms. All three of the youngsters described previously spoke in ways that were somewhat confusing for the listener and seemed to reflect idiosyncratic and illogical reasoning. In addition to reportedly hearing taunting voices, nine-year-old Jessie described his experiences about "not having any insides" in ways that were difficult to follow. Lucy demonstrated a collapse of boundaries between separate conceptual frames of reference (e.g., self–other and bird–human) and made strikingly illogical statements. Finally, Eddie displayed confused thinking while responding to Card II of the Rorschach, attributing highly specific, idiosyncratic, contradictory, and inappropriate meanings to an ambiguous stimulus.

We may address some of the questions about childhood psychosis by stating unequivocally that adolescents and children do present with psychotic symptoms that, with subtle differences, are similar to those found in adults. Additionally, as is the case with adults, children and adolescents with psychotic symptoms may present along a continuum, from nonpsychotic youngsters with psychotic-like features to those with more pronounced symptoms of a diagnosable psychotic disorder. However, there are developmental issues that can confound the diagnostic picture, especially with children. Unlike their adult counterparts, children and adolescents are unfinished products from an ontological perspective. Developmental forces are in flux during childhood, making it impossible to determine whether a child is psychotic without first considering the child's level of cognitive and linguistic development.

The Confounding Role of Development

The psychological functions that are compromised in psychotic conditions have normative developmental lines in childhood. For example, one cannot conclude that a young child is delusional without first understanding how children play and when they are able to distinguish reality from fantasy. For example, when does an imaginary friend reflect the normal child's fluid grasp of what is real and what is imagined, and when does it begin to suggest a belief that shades into the delusional realm? Similarly, how can we determine when a youngster is thinking illogically if we do not understand something about when and how children develop the capacity to reason, think symbolically, and form stable concepts? Finally, we cannot conclude that a child's speech is abnormal without understanding something about the development of language in children. Without this developmental perspective, we run the risk of concluding that a child's thinking is disordered or his sense of reality is impaired when the actual issue is one relating to the development of cognitive and linguistic abilities. Somewhere between the ages of five and seven, there are profound cognitive shifts that enable the developing child to form stable concepts, manage symbolic media, distinguish the real from the imaginary, understand the perspective of the listener, and make cohesive links from one idea to the next in their expressive speech. Thus, we cannot confidently determine the presence of psychotic symptoms in a child before she has developed the cognitive and language structures that make reality-testing and mature communication of their ideas possible. According to Piaget (1928, 1929, 1955, 1962), preoperational children have yet to grasp the stability of concepts or take the listener's perspective. Sullivan's term "parataxic distortion" (1947) describes this period of development when children think in magical, prelogical ways. Magical thinking may lead a young child to confuse coincidence with causality. Consequently, preoperational children may reach erroneous conclusions about sounds in the house or shadows in the room, which leads to the perception of threat and the construction of the belief that they are in danger.

Investigations of disturbances in thought and speech in children should include samples of normal children at different age levels. Such studies have demonstrated that normal children younger than ten years of age received higher scores on the TDI than older children (Arboleda & Holzman, 1985). Caplan et al. (1989; see also Caplan et al., 1990; Caplan,

1994; Caplan et al., 2000) found that normal children younger than seven years of age scored above the cut-off point for pathology on indices of illogical thinking and loose associations on their measure of formal thought disorder, K-FTD (Caplan et al., 1989).

Approaching the study of thought disorder in children from a developmental-discourse perspective, Caplan (1994, 1996) also concluded that from early childhood through adolescence, children gradually acquire the cognitive, linguistic, and social-pragmatic skills that enable them to utilize language cohesion devices to link their utterances together in ways that make their speech more understandable. At the level of the word and sentence, the child is developing linguistic cohesive devices such as conjunctions and referential cohesion (use of pronouns and articles that refer back to people or objects in the preceding spoken text). These linguistic devices enable the child to link objects, events, and ideas within and across sentences. At the paragraph level, the child then needs to develop the ability to connect her ideas and facts in a logical manner so that they form a coherent message that the listener can comprehend.

Once children have achieved the requisite cognitive, linguistic, and social-pragmatic abilities to comprehend reality, express themselves coherently, and understand the perspective of the listener, then we can determine the presence of deficits in their reality-testing and thought organization. However, even if a child has reached a chronological age when a sense of reality, logical reasoning, and coherent communication are developmentally expected, we must also be aware of the impact of delays in development, which may be mistaken for psychotic symptoms. For example, a child with intellectual deficits may lack the cognitive resources to form cohesive and stable concepts that support their appreciation for the constraints of reality. Similar delays or deficits in language development may lead to abnormal communication in what the child understands or attempts to express. Deficits in auditory perception, decoding, comprehension, storage, retrieval, or encoding and arranging words syntactically may result in confusion for the child and listener. Deficiencies in these linguistic processes may contribute to problems in how the child understands and reacts emotionally to himself and the world at large. Sometimes, the compensatory mechanisms employed by language-disordered children to avoid their deficits may appear peculiar and suggest the presence of an FTD. For example, such children may attempt to approximate or find inappropriate substitutes for words they are not able to encode or retrieve, which sound like neologisms. Likewise, efforts to express an idea by talking around it or stringing together related ideas when unable to think of precise terminology may sound like tangential thinking (Hassibi & Breuer, 1980).

Finally, impairment in a child's social-pragmatic language development may include the use of repetitive verbalizations and inappropriate comments and questions without regard for social context or relevant cues. Additionally, odd affect, lack of eye contact, and repetitive behavior may mislead clinicians to prematurely conclude that the child is psychotic and presents with both negative symptoms and catatonia. Delays and deficits in social language-processing skills define a key aspect of functioning within the autism spectrum, which may be mistaken for psychosis.

Differential Diagnosis

In addition to thinking developmentally, clinicians should view psychotic symptoms along a continuum of severity and remain aware of high-risk prodromal criteria, much as they do with adults. From a categorical perspective, practitioners will encounter the same group of diagnostic syndromes that they find with adult patients. However, there are some important caveats, qualifications, and issues to keep in mind when considering these diagnoses in children and adolescents.

First, psychotic conditions are generally quite rare in children. Clinicians need to be aware of base rates in their particular setting. For example, the chances of a school psychologist encountering a psychotically ill child are much less than they would be for the therapist in outpatient practice. Furthermore, the chances of an outpatient therapist making this diagnosis are much lower than they would be for the clinician in a hospital setting.

Second, along with having an understanding of how normative or delayed cognitive and language development may complicate and confuse the clinical picture, it is important for all clinicians to be cognizant of possible medical conditions that could present with psychotic symptomatology. As we describe later, clinicians need to be aware of the distinction between acute disruptions in brain functioning associated with delirium and psychosis.

Additionally, young children with psychosis may present with a broad array of symptoms and behavioral problems that are not, at first, suggestive of psychosis. For example, intense fears, obsessions and compulsive rituals, social withdrawal, anger, agitation, inattentiveness, sleep, and appetite disturbances may all be associated with an underlying psychosis. Recall how severe separation anxiety was the initial presenting symptom for Lucy, whose fears of losing her mother became so severe that she could not attend school. Thus, when a child presents with disruptive behaviors, crippling anxiety and fear, intense anger, social isolation, and suicidal/self-injurious behavior, the clinician should be mindful that any of these symptoms could conceivably be associated with delusions or hallucinations, which may be more difficult for the child to talk about.

In our review of the better-known and more common conditions that clinicians may encounter in children and adolescents, we begin with schizophrenia. Although a rare condition in children, it is considered to be the most severely debilitating psychotic disorder. The other categories included may or may not be classified among primary psychotic disorders. Some are not regarded as psychotic disorders but may occasionally include psychotic features, whereas other conditions may present in ways that mimic other psychotic conditions. In any case, the following are among the conditions that diagnosticians and clinicians need to consider when their young patients are referred for psychotic-like symptoms.

Child-Onset Schizophrenia and Spectrum Disorders

The onset of schizophrenia typically occurs between ages 16 and 30, with the rate increasing during adolescence and peaking before the age of 30 (Mueser & McGurk, 2004). When onset occurs prior to age 18, it is frequently considered early onset, with either an acute or gradual beginning. Onset before the age of 13 is considered childhood onset. Childhood-onset schizophrenia is rare (occurring in approximately one out of 10,000 children under the age of 13 years) and almost always has an insidious onset with a more guarded prognosis (Alaghband-Rad et al., 1995; Kodish & McClellan, 2008; McClellan & Werry, 2001). It is further estimated that only 4% of cases of schizophrenia appear before the age of 15 and only 1% before the age of ten. Although it is extremely rare, there are reports of cases in children as young as five (Findling et al., 2001). In light of the developmental factors described previously, such diagnoses in five-year-old children should be considered very carefully. Males appear to have an earlier age of onset: Slightly fewer than half of the males who carry this diagnosis experienced their symptoms prior to the age of 19.

Findling and colleagues (2001) noted the similarity of symptoms of schizophrenia in children, teenagers, and adults. Consistent with the adult literature, the vulnerable young person who develops schizophrenia may have had a history of social isolation and inadequacy. A review of early history may also reveal delays in motor, verbal, and social development, as well as poor academic performance. Among developmental vulnerabilities, low childhood IQ and motor dysfunction are the most significant antecedents of schizophrenia (Matheson et al., 2013).

Children with schizophrenia have a high incidence of language-processing problems, which contribute to their disorganized thinking and communication. Caplan and her team of researchers (Caplan et al., 1992, 2000) found that children with schizophrenia tended to use fewer linguistic devices to connect ideas than children without schizophrenia. In addition to decreased use of conjunctions, clarifying words, and referential cohesions, children with schizophrenia divert their speech from the context of the conversation and associate it with off-topic ideas. As a result, they have difficulty organizing their thinking, reasoning effectively, and preparing the listener for changes in topics of conversation.

Lewis and Lieberman (2000) charted the developmental course of schizophrenia, identifying signs from gestation to puberty of a premorbid stage that includes mild impairments in motor activity, social adjustment, and cognition. They divide the ensuing prodrome into early and late phases, prior to the onset of psychosis in late adolescence or early adulthood. Early adolescence is a time when subtle alterations in drive, affect, speech, perception, and thought may manifest, leading to vegetative symptoms and difficulties with peers and school. Mood symptoms and anxiety follow, along with increased withdrawal. Later in adolescence, attenuated symptoms may occur as the young person becomes clinically at risk for a first episode of psychosis.

A combination of genetic, environmental, and behavioral variables are considered to be causal factors of schizophrenia. Compared to the general population, the risk of developing schizophrenia is up to 15 times higher for those with first-degree family members and five times higher for second-degree relatives (Carpenter, 2004). Environmental factors include maternal malnutrition, infections during critical periods of fetal development, obstetric complications, and fetal hypoxia. Behavioral risk factors include trauma. Children who have been abused or bullied at a younger age are nearly twice as likely to develop psychotic symptoms. Child abuse may be a risk factor for childhood or early-onset schizophrenia in genetically vulnerable children (Spauwen et al., 2006). As indicated in Chapter 11, a growing body of literature has shown that traumatic experiences in childhood increase the risk for psychotic symptoms (Bendall et al., 2011; van Nierop et al., 2014).

Schizoaffective disorder is uncommon in children; however, clinicians may encounter it in adolescents presenting with affective and psychotic symptoms. As with adults, diagnosis requires that psychotic symptoms not be a function of or occur only in the presence of depression or mania. Some have indicated that manic symptoms are more common in adolescents and young adults, and depressive symptoms are found more frequently among older patients with schizoaffective disorder (Findling et al., 2001). As with childhood-onset schizophrenia, earlier occurring schizoaffective disorder has a poor prognosis and is associated with chronic psychosocial and cognitive impairment.

At the outer edge of the schizophrenia spectrum lies schizotypal disorder, which cannot decide where to find its home in current diagnostic taxonomies. The DSM-5-TR includes it in the family of schizophrenias and also nests it among personality disorders. As we have noted in previous chapters, schizotypal individuals may live on the fringe of psychosis without ever converting to a full psychotic disorder. They may exhibit any of the core features of psychosis at a subthreshold level. As discussed in Chapter 11, knowing which of these individuals is at high risk for conversion to psychosis is a major area of interest among researchers.

One difficulty in diagnosing schizotypal personality in children and adolescents is the fluidity of developmental factors discussed previously. There are age criteria in the DSM for making various diagnoses because it makes little sense to speak of stable personality configurations during a period when personality development is in flux. Thus, it seems to us that using the diagnosis of schizotypal personality in a young child is probably not the best way to capture pre-psychotic symptoms and behaviors.

Finally, there is the diagnosis of delusional disorder, another condition with some features similar to those of schizophrenia. There is very little literature on whether children or adolescents present with circumscribed delusions that reflect this disorder. This is most likely because it is not a disorder we expect to find in either children or even adolescents.

Affective Psychosis

Bipolar disorders were previously believed to develop during adolescence, with little incidence of childhood onset. However, there has been increasing interest in childhood bipolar disorder, which can be a severe and disabling condition (Findling et al., 2001). Symptoms of pediatric bipolar disorder may mimic those of severe ADHD at one extreme and paranoid schizophrenia at the other. According to Geller and Luby (1997), pediatric bipolar disorders often present initially with either mixed states or rapid cycling symptoms. Childhood and adolescent mania presents much the same as it does in adulthood. Manic youngsters may demonstrate pressured, distractible, and loud speech, racing thoughts, and elevated mood. Children under the age of nine may show a slightly different face of mania, characterized more by irritability, aggression, and emotional instability. Older children and adolescents may exhibit more euphoria and grandiosity. Grandiosity in younger children may appear more oppositional than overtly grandiose. Children and adolescents with bipolar disorders may also appear to be daredevils who seek excitement and demonstrate increased risk-taking activities.

Some studies have found that adults with bipolar disorders did not show the severe cognitive and social impairment during childhood that adults with schizophrenia showed (Cannon et al., 2002; Koenen et al., 2009). However, a recent review of neurodevelopmental similarities in early-onset psychotic bipolar disorders and schizophrenia concluded that they share a number of similarities (Arango et al., 2014). As with childhood schizophrenia, males with bipolar disorders seem to have an earlier age of onset. Yet, contrary to other studies, children with both conditions who become psychotic at an early age show similar levels of cognitive impairment and academic decline. Rates of language abnormalities and academic decline were equal in both disorders. However, children and adolescents with bipolar disorders demonstrate less social withdrawal and impoverished relationships than their childhood counterparts who develop schizophrenia. Clinical symptoms that signal a greater likelihood of juvenile bipolar disorder include early onset with psychotic symptoms, episodic aggression, and depression with atypical features (hypersomnia, increased appetite, lowered energy, and rejection sensitivity).

Major depression with psychotic features occurs more frequently than either bipolar or schizophrenia-spectrum disorders. Before puberty, boys may be more affected; however, by adolescence, girls receive the diagnosis of major depression with psychotic features more than twice as often as boys (Findling et al., 2001). Loss of energy, inattention to appearance, and social withdrawal may mimic negative or prodromal signs of schizophrenia. A much smaller number of depressed youngsters may present with psychotic symptoms, which are similar in nature to the mood-congruent delusions or hallucinations seen in adults. Hallucinations are most typically auditory and include critical or derogatory content. Delusions are less common in depressed children but may occur in psychotically depressed adolescents. As is the case with adults, delusions typically reflect depressive themes of guilt, nihilism, inadequacy, emptiness, decay, disease, and death. The psychotically depressed child may believe that he is the cause of all badness in the world. Similarly, the manically psychotic youngster may believe that she has superpowers. In contrast, the hallucinatory and delusional content in a child with schizophrenia may make little sense. Absurd beliefs with bizarre content are more characteristic of psychosis in these children. Thus, the youngster with schizophrenia may not hold himself responsible for his belief that the world is empty but instead may attribute this delusion to some alien or mechanical force.

Detecting Children and Adolescents at Clinical High Risk

Studies have applied early detection and intervention strategies to children and adolescents (Bearden et al., 2011; Schimmelmann et al., 2013). Bearden et al.'s study explored whether subtle disturbances in thinking and communication could predict conversion to psychosis in vulnerable young people. Using Caplan et al.'s Story Game and Kiddie Formal Thought Disorder Scale (K-FTDS, Caplan et al., 1989), researchers found that adolescents identified at clinical high risk who subsequently converted to psychosis showed higher rates of illogical thinking and poverty of content in their speech. High-risk youth who converted to psychosis also made less reference to people, objects, and events in their speech (lower rates of referential cohesion), providing the listener with less information on what or whom they were talking about. Of all variables, measures of illogical thinking were most predictive of subsequent conversion to psychosis, whereas a combination of poverty of thought content and lower referential cohesion significantly predicted poorer social and role functioning.

Autism Spectrum Disorders

Autism Spectrum Disorders (ASD) used to be conflated with childhood schizophrenia but is now well recognized as a distinct neurodevelopmental spectrum of symptoms varying in level of severity. Still, recent studies suggest a shared genetic risk (Skuse, 2022). However, there may be some overlap in clinical features and genetic risk factors; hallucinations, delusions, and formally disordered thinking are not typical features of children within the autism spectrum.

One exception might be a smaller group of children that have been diagnosed as having "multiple complex developmental disorders" or "multiplex developmental disorders" (Kumra et al., 1998; Zalsman & Cohen, 1998). These children with multiple social, emotional, and cognitive developmental delays are generally subsumed under the umbrella of the autism spectrum. However, what distinguishes these youngsters is the presence of more pronounced psychotic symptoms. In these cases, a comorbid diagnosis of psychosis is warranted, in addition to a diagnosis of an autism spectrum disorder.

Those unfamiliar with the spectrum of autism may mistake some superficial similarities as signs of psychosis. In both schizophrenia and autism spectrum disorders, children may demonstrate unusual speech patterns and express odd ideas and interests. With both disorders, children also may exhibit social withdrawal and flat affect. For example, abnormalities in pragmatic language – such as poor topic maintenance, difficulties with coherence, and lack of reciprocity – may first strike the evaluating clinician as evidence of an FTD rather than autism. Additionally, overfocusing on unusual interests may make one think about the possibility of delusions. Odd sensory interests or hypersensitivities might suggest hallucinations. Furthermore, poor mentalizing skills and impairments in social perception may lead diagnosticians to view the youngster as paranoid, not autistic. Executive deficits in initiation, activation, and motivation may present in a similar manner to negative symptoms of schizophrenia.

In a recent study of children and adolescents with ASD and psychosis, the authors discuss the clinical manifestations of psychosis in this group of individuals (Chandrasekhar et al., 2020). They note the appearance of catatonia in the ASD population and the overlapping features of catatonia and ASD.

Trauma and Dissociation

Earlier, we discussed the significant link between childhood trauma and later psychosis. Childhood trauma increases psychosis risk, symptom severity, and the number of comorbid conditions (Stanton et al., 2020).

Distinguishing primary psychotic disorders from psychotic-like symptoms in traumatized children and adolescents who dissociate may be challenging. In particular, these youngsters may present with hallucinatory experiences that reflect aspects of the traumatic events with which they are trying to cope. Such sensory-perceptual phenomena, which resemble psychotic hallucinations, can also be understood as extreme manifestations of re-experiencing phenomena. In the presence of a trigger, the child may react as if the traumatic event is recurring. At such times, ego functioning is compromised, and the child's capacity to distinguish a terrifying internal event from external reality disappears.

The term "dissociative hallucinosis" refers to the presence of hallucinations in the context of traumatogenic dissociation (Findling et al., 2001). Such hallucinations may be either visual or auditory in nature. However, other hallmark features of psychosis – such as FTD and bizarre and delusional beliefs – are not typically present. Additionally, compared to schizophrenia-spectrum disorders, children and adolescents presenting with psychotic-like symptoms in the context of trauma and dissociation usually demonstrate affect that is consistent with their terror. In contrast, a child with schizophrenia or a schizotypal pattern may appear socially detached and exhibit an odd or inappropriate affect. Moreover, trauma-based hallucinosis has a more abrupt, instead of insidious, onset.

Clinicians may also encounter a subset of traumatized young children who may present with fantastic and bizarre-sounding stories about their abuse. However, in many cases, aspects of the abuse situation are intermingled with fantasy that can be exploited by overly zealous interviewers and prospectors. The infamous McMartin preschool trial of the 1980s is a compelling example of how initial allegations of sexual abuse at the preschool by child witnesses seemed to mushroom into outlandish stories of sodomy, witches flying, sex in underground tunnels, orgies in car washes, and children being flushed down toilets (Reinhold, 1990). The case became a textbook example of how not to conduct interviews with childhood victims of alleged sexual abuse. Many interviewers of the alleged child witnesses and victims seemed to ignore factors relating to the children's level of cognitive development, their capacity to comprehend questions being asked, and their desire to please adults by answering as expected. Subsequent reviewers of interview transcripts demonstrated how coercive, suggestive, and leading interview techniques were used to instill false memories in these children.

In addition to highlighting improper techniques for interviewing children who were suspected victims of abuse, the case raised questions about whether some of these children might have had delusions. Taken at face value, the bizarre allegations were either initially mistakenly accepted as literal depictions of bizarre and evil acts perpetrated on innocent children or as indications that some of these children were psychotic. Either of these conclusions seemed to be suspect.

Personality Disorders

As noted previously, we are hesitant to posit the presence of personality disorders in individuals whose personality is in the process of developing. This is clearly the case in children and perhaps to a lesser extent in older adolescents. In all cases, it seems that it is better to speak of behaviors, traits, or patterns before prematurely establishing these features as a stable disorder.

Certain clusters of personality patterns include psychotic-like features. This is evident with schizotypal personality, in which a full range of attenuated psychotic symptoms may exist. In addition to perceptual anomalies and magical, sometimes outré beliefs, schizotypal children have been found to demonstrate similar kinds of communication deficits, which disrupt the flow and coherence of conversation, as found in children with schizophrenia (Caplan et al., 1992).

Similarly, one cannot speak of psychotic symptoms and personality disorders without also considering the occasional occurrence of such symptoms in young people with features of borderline personality. When psychotic-like symptoms occur, they may have a sudden onset and include lapses in reality testing associated with transient hallucinatory phenomena, ideas of reference, and paranoid thinking. Symptoms are typically transient and induced by stressful circumstances that may include painful separations and abandonment experiences or heightened affective turmoil.

When considering psychotic-like symptoms in children with personality difficulties, one common diagnostic question concerns the child who tells severe lies that lead parents, teachers, and therapists to wonder whether the youngster is delusional. These children often present for diagnostic consultations after they have told lies that they appear to be convinced are true. The lies, which distinguish them in some way, may include the death of family members, claims of having had unique life experiences, or knowing famous people. Somehow, they convince those around them that they believe their stories. Hence, the question arises, "Are they suffering from delusions?" When severe lying is the presenting symptom, clinicians will often understand lying in the context of the child or adolescent's immature personality development, narcissistic vulnerability, social inadequacy, and wish for interpersonal impact or gain. Just as delusions may serve an explanatory purpose for an individual who encounters frightening stress, a youngster's severe lies may also serve multiple functions. For these children and adolescents, external reality can be shaped in such a way as to compensate for painful feelings of inadequacy and clung to as if they were real. A nugget of truth can be stretched and manipulated in order to protect the self, which is more important to the youngster than fidelity to what is objectively real. However, these manipulations of the truth rarely reach the level of being true delusions; rather, they exist along the boundary of what is developmentally normal, developmentally immature, and a maladaptive way of trying to solve and avoid problems.

Medical, Neurological, and Adverse Reactions to Medication

Psychotic symptoms may be secondary to medical conditions. Merritt et al. (2020) reviewed genetic, metabolic, endocrinological, autoimmune, infectious, nutritious, and neurological conditions that may present with psychotic-like symptoms that include disordered thinking, delusions, and hallucinations. Additionally, an adverse reaction to medication can cause abrupt changes in behavior, perception, and thinking. A major differential diagnosis involves whether the child is delirious or psychotic. Delirium is an acute brain dysfunction resulting from a broad range of primary medical and neurological disorders. It is characterized by its sudden onset, marked confusion, severe distractibility, agitation, anxiety, and fluctuating mental status. The child may be disoriented by time, place, and person. Delirium may include disruptions in expressive and receptive language. Speech may be jumbled and disorganized. Visual hallucinations may be more common than auditory hallucinations. Somatic or tactile hallucinations may also occur, including the feeling of bugs on one's body. Delusions of formication describe the belief that bugs are crawling on one's skin. Caplan and Bursch (2012) note how a delirious child's mumbling, picking, and laughter might be mistaken for auditory hallucinations of a psychotic child.

Adolescents may induce psychotic episodes after using substances. As with adult patients, the challenge is distinguishing a substance-induced psychosis from a primary psychotic disorder (Beckmann et al., 2020).

Approaches to Assessment

In assessing psychosis in children and adolescents, diagnosticians encounter similar approaches as well as limitations of the methods that have been described in the assessment of adults. Structured and semi-structured interview methods have been developed to serve as the gold standard for establishing criteria validity in research studies. However, with children, as with their adult counterparts, structured interviews and rating-scale techniques are typically too time-consuming and require extensive training. As a result, they are not diagnostic tools typically employed by clinical practitioners.

Formal psychological assessment instruments are utilized by clinicians, but, as we have seen with adults, they can be rather blunt instruments that have higher sensitivity than specificity. Many standard personality assessment instruments yield findings that suggest the presence of psychotic symptoms and attenuated psychotic symptoms alike. It is then the task of the clinician to sift through the data and make distinctions between psychotic-like phenomena and the actual presence of a diagnosable psychotic condition.

Interview Methods: Unstructured, Semi-Structured, and Structured

We assume that most clinicians will use an unstructured clinical interview when conducting initial interviews with children suspected of having psychotic symptoms. Caplan and Bursch's book *How Many More Questions?* (2012) is essential reading for anyone working with children. In this masterful book, they present a developmentally attuned approach to interviewing children with major psychiatric and medical problems. Beginning with a practical review of dos and don'ts when interviewing young children, the authors provide a guide to assessing hallucinations, delusions, and thought disorders in children. They focus on matching the questions to youngsters' developmental capacity to understand and express themselves. Questions need to be clear and concise, nondiscursive, formulated in simple sentences asking about the "what" and "how" of the child's experiences, as opposed to the "why" and "when." Their book includes ample transcripts of interviews, examples of interview questions, and attention to differential diagnosis.

Cepeda (2007, 2012) provided several practical steps in assessing psychosis in children, beginning with a thorough history-taking and clinical interview. He stressed the importance of routine physical and neurological consultations to rule out medical, neurological, and drug-related conditions that may produce psychotic symptoms. Cepeda also recommended psychological testing.

The examiner should always pay attention to the child's demeanor, eye contact, language, behavior, thought processes, and affect. Language is a key factor in interviewing children. Cepeda advocated including parents as active participants in the interview process, acting as the questioners under the clinician's guidance. Sleep is a sensitive time for the emergence of fears, and the interviewer asks the parents to query their child about whether he is scared at night. Follow-up questions such as "What are you afraid of?" would naturally follow any positive answer to the first question. The interviewer can guide the parent to ask questions about perceptual anomalies and unusual beliefs. In keeping with Caplan and Bursch's recommendations, the interviewer can also help parents craft their questions in more open-ended ways.

With the interviewer present, the parent can ask such questions as:

- What kinds of noises do you hear at night? How do they scare you?
- Can you tell me if you hear voices or people talking when no one is around?
- Can you say if you have seen monsters, ghosts, or shadows?
- Do you feel that someone is touching you when no one is around?
- Do you feel people saying bad things about you or watching you?

Psychometrically sound structured and semi-structured diagnostic interviews and rating scales are available tools for determining whether criteria for various psychotic symptoms are present. The most well-known among these is the Kiddie Schedule for Affective Disorders and Schizophrenia for School-Aged Children, Present and Lifetime Version (K-SADS-PL; Kaufman et al., 2000). The K-SADS-PL assesses current and lifetime symptoms and is based on summary scores from separate interviews with the parent and child. A more specialized version of the K-SADS, developed at Washington University (WASH-U-K-SADS), focuses on diagnosing manic manifestations in early adolescents and prepubertal children (Geller et al., 1998). The Diagnostic Interview Schedule for Children and Adolescents (DICA; Reich et al., 1991) is another instrument with clinician-rated interviews for both the child and the parents. The DICA has been used in research studies on child and adolescent schizophrenia.

Caplan et al. (1989) developed an alternate approach to assess more directly FTD in children and adolescents. Caplan observed that because of developmental factors, children might have difficulty responding to questions posed by interviewers who used the structured and semi-structured methods described previously. To address this problem, she developed a method to elicit a free sample of the child's speech. Her method begins with a structured storytelling technique, the Story Game (SG), to elicit free speech samples, which are transcribed and scored with the Kiddie Formal Thought Disorder rating scale, K-FTDS (Caplan et al., 1989). The SG consists of a three-part audiotape. In the first and third portions, the child listens to an audiotaped story and is asked to retell it, then answer a set of open-ended questions about the story. In the middle part, the child is asked to select one of four thematically charged topics (e.g., an unhappy child). The recorded speech samples are scored according to criteria from the K-FTDS. The scores are based on frequency counts of illogical thinking, loose associations, incoherence, and poverty of content of speech divided by the number of utterances made by the subject. Caplan defined illogical thinking as a failure to present the listener with appropriate causal reasoning or contradicting oneself. Loose associations are characterized by unpredictable changes in the topic of conversation without preparing the listener for the diversion. Instances of the child speaking with scrambled syntax are scored as incoherence. Finally, the child with a poverty of content speaks in unelaborated ways, expressing minimal content. Caplan developed a manual with scoring examples and anchor points to aid in coding examples of thought disorder.

Unlike the K-FTD, the CUBESCALE focuses more on the content of a youngster's thoughts and qualities of perceptual experience rather than on qualities of formal thought disorder. A semi-structured set of questions with recommended prompts for certain affirmative responses, the CUBESCALE, has been shown to be a valid measure of psychotic-like experiences. The items range from mildly aberrant beliefs (e.g., "I know secrets about scary things that no one else would ever know") to more bizarre ideas (e.g., "Sometimes, I think I don't have any insides") to floridly psychotic delusions and hallucinations (e.g., "I worry sometimes that people could steal my thoughts" and "Sometimes I think I hear voices or sounds that no one else can hear"). Affirmative responses to most of these items prompt queries from the interviewer to clarify whether the child's response truly signifies a psychotic experience.

The CUBESCALE can be used with children between the ages of eight and 18. Preliminary research with this instrument has established this as a reliable and valid measure of psychotic experiences in children and adolescents. However, as the name of the instrument implies, this is a scale about unusual beliefs and perceptual experiences. What is missing from this approach is a direct measurement of the formal features of the child's thinking or communication. Children like Jessie may give more elaborate responses to prompts, which allow us to evaluate the formal qualities of their focusing, filtering, and coherence; however, it is likely that many children will not provide sufficient samples of their speech for us to determine the presence of an FTD.

Rating Scales

Popular rating scales used in research studies include the BPRS and the children's version of the PANSS, or Kiddie Version of the Positive and Negative Symptoms of Schizophrenia, K-PANSS (Fields et al., 1994). Both scales have been factor-analyzed with dimensions identifying positive and negative symptoms, depression, cognitive-conceptual disorganization, mania, and depression.

Use of the K-PANSS and BPRS, though they may be gold standards in establishing accurate diagnoses, are less likely to be used routinely in clinical settings. When used outside of research settings, these scales may be utilized in inpatient settings where establishing diagnoses and assessing response to medication are joint responsibilities of various members of the nursing staff and clinical treatment team. Rank-and-file clinicians in outpatient practice settings are even less likely to use these diagnostic scales or structured and semi-structured interview methods. Despite their impressive psychometric properties and citations in the literature, most of these instruments are often too lengthy and time-consuming to be used routinely. Additionally, most require specialized training in order for the clinician to establish an acceptable level of reliability as an interviewer and accuracy as a coder/rater.

More accessible instruments for clinicians include rating scales used for screening purposes. The Behavior Assessment System for Children, Second Edition (BASC-3; Reynolds & Kamphaus, 2006) is a multi-scale instrument that includes parent, teacher, and self-report forms. The Atypicality Scale is made up of 13 items covering major dimensions of psychotic experience. Items can be answered along a four-point Likert scale (Never, Sometimes, Often, Almost Always). The following sampling of items demonstrates their face validity for identifying possible symptom dimensions of psychosis:

- Acts confused (disorganization)
- Seems out of touch with reality (general psychosis; positive symptoms – delusions)
- Hears sounds that are not there (positive symptoms – hallucinations)
- Sees things that are not there (positive symptoms – hallucinations)
- Says things that make no sense (disorganization, positive symptoms – thought disorder)
- Seems unaware of others (negative symptoms)

In discussing the relative validity of ratings from parents, teachers, or self-report scales in identifying pediatric bipolar disorder, Youngstrom (2007) reported that parent ratings are generally more valid indicators than either self-report or teacher forms.

The CBCL is another popular broadband instrument used to assess behavioral and emotional problems in children and adolescents (Achenbach, 1991). The CBCL has a Thought Problem scale (TP) that includes items relating to hallucinations and strange thoughts and behavior (including obsessive-compulsive symptoms). The CBCL has also been described as a useful screening instrument for identifying possible bipolar disorders in children and adolescents (Biederman et al., 2009). In particular, a positive CBCL pediatric bipolar-disorder profile (CBCL-PBD), which is based on elevations on scales of attention problems, aggressive behavior, and anxiety/depression, may help identify children with bipolar disorder.

A children's version of The Prodromal Questionnaire (PQ, Loewy et al., 2005) was developed as a screening measure of PLEs in children aged nine to ten (Karcher et al., 2018). The Prodromal Questionnaire–Brief Child Version (PQ-BC) was shown to have adequate psychometric properties and correlate with a family history of non-affective psychosis, internalizing symptoms, cognitive deficits, and developmental delays. The authors conclude that the PQ–BC may be a useful screening tool to identify early risk in children.

Personality Inventories

Both the MMPI and PAI have forms for adolescents, with scales and subscales that address a range of psychotic and attenuated psychotic symptoms. The PAI-A includes the same scales as the adult version. The MMPI-A-RF also has many of the same special scales and subscales used to identify unusual thoughts and perceptions in the MMPI-3.

Performance and Projective Measures: TAT and Rorschach Test

In Chapter 8, we presented an example of a CAT response given by a nine-year-old patient we called "Shelly," which reflected severe problems with logic and discourse coherence. Here, we give another example of the illogical combination of figures and actions in the following story to Card 10 of the TAT, related by 14-year-old Teresa. The card depicts a shadowy close-up of two heads together in what looks like an embrace.

> Okay . . . um, it kind of looks like they're eating each other. I don't know why. Kind of in a dark room and they're just eating each other, and then they just eat each other until there is nothing left. It already looks like she took a pretty good chunk off his face. It's really weird. I don't know why I thought of that. It's strange. People shouldn't eat each other.

Teresa was actually demonstrating emergent borderline personality features. In her graphic concretization, we see several things worth noting. First, the fact that this was her only TAT story that showed such regressively bizarre thematic material suggests that she was triggered by the stimulus. In this case, the stimulus had to do with closeness and physical contact. We surmise that this idea precipitated an abrupt shift in her ability to maintain a realistic narrative. The other thing to note is how Teresa appeared to be cognizant, after the fact, of her strange and inappropriate response. Although she could not filter this beforehand, she demonstrated some awareness afterward that her ideas had been peculiar.

While a number of projective tests can be used to assess psychotic phenomena (Kleiger, 2000, 2003), the Rorschach stands alone as the most powerful psychological assessment tool for directly evaluating thought organization and reality testing in children and adolescents. Arboleda and Holzman (1985) demonstrated that psychotically vulnerable children and adolescents had significantly elevated scores on the TDI. Unfortunately, the TDI is not widely used by psycho diagnosticians, who prefer the Rorschach because of the unique method of administering on which the TDI is based. Most clinicians follow procedures of the Comprehensive Rorschach System (Exner & Weiner, 1982) or the newer Rorschach Performance Assessment System (R-PAS; Meyer et al., 2012). Both systems include scoring rubrics for identifying forms of disordered thinking and loss of reality testing. However, recent studies have raised questions about the adequacy of the norms for children and adolescents in the CS (Meyer et al., 2007). Authors of the R-PAS have begun to address these concerns by developing new sets of norms for children and adolescents.

Clinical Assessment Points

1. The onset of psychosis in adolescence is well recognized, but psychosis is rare in children. Clinicians need to consider the base rates of their particular settings when weighing the diagnosis of psychosis in children.
2. The presence of psychotic features in a child who is seven years of age or older is diagnostically meaningful, whereas their occurrence in a younger child may be confounded by normal developmental factors.
3. Cognitive, language, and social-emotional developmental factors, as well as medical, toxic, and neurological conditions, must be considered when assessing psychotic-like symptoms in children. Thus, if psychosis is suspected, the young patient should be referred to her pediatrician or family doctor for an initial consultation to rule out a primary medical basis for psychotic-like symptoms. Additionally, consultation with a speech and language therapist to rule out a language-processing disorder is important when puzzling over the question of thought disorder in a younger patient.
4. The use of multiple methods trumps single-instrument approaches when assessing psychosis in children and adolescents.

5. As with adults, a clinical interview is the best method for assessing hallucinations and delusions in children. Testing can be helpful in assessing disordered thinking, problems with logic, and concept formation.
6. Assessments for psychosis in children should begin with a careful interview of parents to obtain a thorough developmental history.
7. When interviewing young children, use developmentally attuned questions, as suggested by Caplan and Bursch (2012). For example:

   - Speak in short, simple, and concrete sentences.
   - Use action language close to the child's physical, emotional, and sensory experience.
   - Avoid lengthy sentences with embedded clauses.
   - Use "what" and "how" questions while staying away from "why" questions, which may be cognitively inappropriate for a younger child.
   - Avoid asking about chronology and causality.
   - Prompt open-ended questions instead of close-ended yes/no questions.

8. Additionally, parents can be primed for the kinds of questions they will be asking during the conjoint clinical interview with the child, as recommended by Cepeda (2012). Meet first with parents and review the kinds of questions that you want them to ask their child during the clinical interview.
9. If you have the time and proper training and there is a need for an unassailable diagnosis, use of gold-standard structured and semi-structured interviews like the K-SADS or K-PANSS will help establish a valid diagnosis.
10. The K-FTDS/SG and/or TDI are exceptional instruments for assessing thought disorders in children. They are empirically valid and conceptually rich instruments that have furthered the study of disordered thinking in adults, adolescents, and children. Unfortunately, nothing that is worthwhile is easy. Both instruments require extensive training for evaluators to learn anchor points for scoring variables. Furthermore, unlike the Rorschach, the K-FTDS has been used primarily as a research instrument.
11. Even if one does not use an instrument like the K-FTDS/SG, it is useful to obtain a sample of the child or adolescent's spontaneous speech when evaluating thought disorder. Caplan and Bursch (2012) recommend obtaining speech samples of adequate length – i.e., short paragraphs of several sentences for children. For adolescents, we recommend asking the patient to speak for one to two minutes in response to a prompt such as, "What do you think about legalizing drugs?" or "What are your thoughts about parents monitoring their

children's social media?" After obtaining permission, the interviewer can record the adolescent's free speech sample and examine it for aberrations in logic, focusing, coherence, and adequate elaboration.

12. Finally, caution should be exercised in making a diagnosis of a psychotic disorder in either a child or adolescent when the developmental unfolding of personality functioning is taking place. The most that assessment techniques can offer is a set of inferences about the presence of psychotic-like phenomena. As we have seen throughout this book, psychotic-like symptoms by themselves do not constitute a formal diagnosis of a psychotic disorder. Positive signs on assessment measures tell us that this *might* be a vulnerable young person who will need to be further evaluated by a psychiatrist and followed by a skilled psychotherapist who can provide necessary treatment for the child and educational information for parents. Ignoring early signs of psychotic-like phenomena or prematurely offering reassurance (e.g., "Your child will grow out of this") is as much of a mistake as prematurely diagnosing a child with a serious psychotic disorder.
13. We stress again that differential diagnosis requires multiple methods, including a comprehensive developmental history. One common diagnostic question is whether a child's peculiar cognitive and social behavior reflects a disorder on the schizophrenia or autism spectrum. An important clue in making this distinction is to see if features consistent with autism are present before the child's third birthday (Deprey & Ozonoff, 2009). Prodromal signs of schizophrenia are rarely present during preschool and develop more insidiously during childhood.

Appendix A

PSYCHOLOGICAL TESTING VARIABLES ASSOCIATED WITH PSYCHOTIC DIMENSIONS

A number of scales, subscales, and combinations of scales from the MMPI-3 (Ben-Porath & Tellegen, 2020; Nichols, 2011), MMPI-2-RF (Ben-Porath & Tellegen, 2008), and PAI (Morey, 1991) can be used to help clinicians assess various dimensions of psychosis, including psychosis proneness, acute risk, and levels of insight. The following tables organize scales, subscales, and scoring variables from personality inventories and performance measures along some of the dimensions of psychosis described in Chapters 8 and 11.

Table A1 Personality inventory and Rorschach variables possibly suggesting psychosis proneness and psychosis-risk syndromes

Attenuated Symptom Dimension	*Psychological Testing Variables: Personality Inventories*	*Psychological Testing Variables: Rorschach*
Unusual Beliefs: Strained reasoning, Suspiciousness, Overvalued ideas, Ideas of reference, Weak reality testing	Moderate elevations (T scores 60–65) on scales from personality inventories associated with delusions, suspiciousness, strained reasoning, and unusual thought content	Moderate levels of disordered thinking, hypervigilance, and weak reality testing: • CS & R-PAS System Special/Cognitive Scores of Level 1 & 2 severity, including • Incongruous and fabulized combinations • TDI scores at.25–75 level of severity • Indications of hypervigilance (HVI) • Elevated number of FQ-responses

(*Continued*)

Table A1 (Continued)

Attenuated Symptom Dimension	*Psychological Testing Variables: Personality Inventories*	*Psychological Testing Variables: Rorschach*
Expansiveness	Moderate Elevations MMPI-2 Scales: • *Ma2* MMPI-3 Scales: • *RC9; ACT* PAI Scales: • *MAN-G* MCMI-IV Scales: • Bipolar Spectrum • Narcissistic	• Elevated number of whole responses (Ws) and combination of blot details (combinatory responses) • Themes of birth, growth, control, grandiosity, connections, power
Perceptual Abnormalities	Moderate elevations on scales from personality inventories associated with hallucinations (see Chapter 8)	Elevated FQ- and lower FQo suggest inaccuracies in visually perceiving and forming impressions of external stimuli, although this may have no relationship to hallucinatory phenomena
Discursive Speech and Peculiar Word Usage	Moderate elevations on personality inventory scales associated with cognitive problems and disorganization (see Chapter 8)	Mild to moderate degrees of looseness and deviant verbalizations on Rorschach • Level I Deviant verbalizations • Level I Deviant responses
Maintenance of Some Insight	Lower scores on scales associated with lack of insight and self-reflection	Spontaneous comments which reflect that response was given in a fantasy context or that it could not actually be real. For example, comments during inquiry which show that the patient retains a critical perspective regarding the response (e.g., "It really doesn't look like that")

(*Continued*)

Table A1 (Continued)

Attenuated Symptom Dimension	*Psychological Testing Variables: Personality Inventories*	*Psychological Testing Variables: Rorschach*
Level of Stability and Distress	Indications of coping, stability, and distress • MMPI-3 *K*, *Ego Strength* • MMPI-3 distress scales *(EID, RCd, RC2)* • PAI distress scales *(ANX, DEP, ARD)*	Signs of stress and distress • Elevated inanimate movement and diffuse shading (psychosis-risk syndromes)

Table A2 Test variables associated with a general psychosis dimension

MMPI-2 scores • Goldberg Index • MMPI-2 *PSYC* > *NEGE* by 10T • *Scale 8* > 70T & *Sc3* > *D4 or DisOrg* > *CogProb* • *BIZ1*	Rorschach TDI scores • .75 level • 1.0 level
CS Rorschach scores • PTI > 3 • Level 2 scores • WSUM6	
MMPI-3 • *RC8* PAI • *SCZ1*	R-PAS Rorschach scores • EII-3 > 110 • TP-COMP>110 • SevCog>110

Table A3 Test variables associated with positive symptoms

Positive Symptom	*Personality Inventories*	*Performance Measures*
Delusions	MMPI-2 Scales: • *Codetype 86/68* • *Pal (Ideas of External Influence)* • *Pf (Paranoid Factors)* Nichols and Crowhurst (2006) • *Pf2 (Ideas of Reference)* • *Pf3 (Delusions of Control)* • *Pf4 (Persecutory Ideas & Delusions)* • *BIZ1 (Psychotic Symptomatology)* MMPI-3 Scales: • *RC6 (Ideas of Persecution)* • *RC8 (Aberrant Experiences)* PAI Scales: • *PAR-P (Persecutory Delusions)* • *SCZI (Schizophrenia) + MAN-G (Manic-Grandiosity) = Delusions of Grandeur* *SCZI (Schizophrenia) + SOM-C (Somatic-Complaints) or SOM-H (Somatic-Health) = Somatic Delusions*	Rorschach variables suggesting predisposition: • Level 2 Special Scores o *ALOG* • Hypervigilance Index • Focus on small and unusual details • Paranoid Thematic Content • Eyes • Protection, helmets, weapons • Judges, police, hooded figures
Hallucinations	MMPI-2 Scales: • *Codetype 86/68* • *BIZ1 (Psychotic Symptomatology)* MMPI-3 Scales: • *RC8 (Aberrant Experiences)* • *PSYC (Psychoticism)* PAI Scales • *SZC-P (Psychotic Experience)*	Rorschach variables possibly suggesting predisposition: • Elevated FQ-%

Table A4 Test variables associated with cognitive disorganization

Positive Symptom	*Personality Inventories*	*Performance Measures*
DISORGANIZED SPEECH: Problems with focusing and filtering	MMPI-2 Scales: • *D2 (Cognitive Infirmity)* • *Sc3 (Lack of Ego Mastery-Cognitive)* MMPI-3 Scales • *THD (Thought Dysfunction)* • *RC8 (Aberrant Experiences)* • *COG (Cognitive Problems)* PAI Scales: • *SCZ-T (Schizophrenia: Thought Disorder)*	Rorschach Variables: • Comprehensive System (CS) & R-PAS Scores • Deviant responses (DR Level 2) • Deviant verbalizations (DV Level 2) • Thought Disorder Index (TDI) Scores • Loose responses (TDI.50) • Peculiar and queer responses (TDI.25 & .50) • Wechsler Comprehension Subtest • Look for loose and disorganized verbalizations
ERRORS IN REASONING: Problems with conceptual and abstract thinking	MMPI-2 & 3 Scales: • *DisOrg (Cognitive Disorganization)* • *BIZ (Bizarre Mentation)* • *PSYC (Psychoticism)* • *Sc6 (Sensorimotor Dissociation)* MMPI-3: • *RC8 (Aberrant Experiences)* • *THX (Thought Dysfunction)* PAI Scales: • *SCZ-T (Schizophrenia-Thought Disorder)*	Rorschach Variables: • CS, R-PAS, & TDI Scores • Incongruous combinations INC Level 2 (TDI.25) • Fabulized combinations FAB Level 2 (TDI.50) • Autistic logic (ALOG) • CS & TDI (.75) • Peculiar logic (R-PAS) • Confabulation (TDI.75) • Contamination (CS, R-PAS, TDI 1.0) • Object Sorting Test • Loose or illogical conceptual groupings • Wechsler Similarities Subtest • Idiosyncratic responses • Proverbs Test • Idiosyncratic or inappropriately abstract interpretations

Table A5 Test variables associated with negative symptoms

Negative Symptom	*Personality Inventories*	*Performance Measures*
BLUNTED AFFECT: Emotional withdrawal	MMPI-2 Scales: • *Codetypes 28/82 & 20/02* • *DEP1 (Lack of Drive)* • *D2* • *Dr-2 (Inhibition of Aggression)* • *Sc2* • *Sc4* MMPI-3 Scales: • *RC2 (Low Positive Emotions)*	Rorschach Variables: • Low number of responses • Little or no use of color or shading • Dominant use of form features to justify responses
AVOLITIONALITY: Asociality, Anhedonia, Disengagement, Avoidance	*MMPI-2 Scales:* • *SOD1 (Introversion)* • *TRT1 (Low Motivation)* • *Si2 (Social Avoidance)* • *INTR (Introversion)* • *Sc4 (Lack of Ego Mastery-Conative)* MMPI-3 Scales: • *RC2 (Low Positive Emotions)* PAI Scales: • *SCZ-S (Social Detachment)*	Rorschach Variables: • Short, contracted responses • Vague verbalizations or confused responses • Excessive use of form features of inkblot to justify responses • Little or no human content or responses reflecting relationship themes • Perseverated content or verbalizations

Table A6 Test variables associated with depression

Depressive Symptom	*Personality Inventories*	*Performance Measures*
COGNITIVE COMPONENT: Helplessness, Inadequacy, Problems with concentration, decision-making, and memory	MMPI-2 Scales: • *D4 (Mental Dullness)* • *Dr4* • *Sc3* MMPI-3 Scales: • *RCd (Demoralization)* • *RC2 (Low Positive Emotions)* PAI Scales: • *DEP-C (Depression-Cognitive)*	Rorschach Variables: • Lower number of responses • Dominant use of form features to justify responses • Short, contracted responses • Expressions of incompetence or inability to do the task • Limited turning of the Rorschach card
AFFECTIVE COMPONENT: Sadness, Tearfulness, Guilt, Irritability	MMPI-2 Scales: • *D1 (Depressed Mood)* • *D5 (Brooding)* • *DEP2* • *DEP3*	Rorschach Variables: • Little or no use of color • Use of achromatic features of the inkblot • Attributing sadness or damage to the image
PHYSIOLOGICAL COMPONENT: Neurovegetative symptoms, Fatigue, Diminished energy and drive	MMPI-2 Scales: • *D2* • *D3* • *DEP1 (Lack of Drive)* MMPI-2 Scales • *Hy3 (Lassitude & Malaise)* PAI Scales: • *DEP-P (Depression-Physiological)*	MMPI-2-RF: • RC1

Table A7 Test variables associated with mania

Manic Symptoms	*Personality Inventories*	*Performance Measures*
ACTIVATION	MMPI-2 Scales: • *Scale 9 (Mania)* • *Ma1 (Psychomotor Acceleration)* MMPI-3 Scales: • *RC9 (Hypomanic Activation)* • *ACT (Activation)* PAI Scales: • *MAN-A (Mania-Activation)*	Rorschach Variables: • Elevated number of responses • Increased number of responses on colored cards
IRRITABILITY & HOSTILITY	MMPI-3 Scales: • *RC9* • *RC7* *ANP (Extreme Irritability)* PAI Scales: • *MAN-I (Mania-Irritability)*	Rorschach Variables: • Hostility manifest in patient-examiner relationship • Aggressive content, movement, and themes
EXPANSIVENESS & GRANDIOSITY	MMPI-2 Scales: • *Ma2* • *Low LSE* MMPI-3 Scales: • *RC9* • *SFI (Increased Self-Esteem/Grandiosity)* PAI Scales: • *MAN-G (Mania-Grandiosity)*	Rorschach Variables: • Over-striving and strained combinatory responses • Thematic content reflecting grandiosity, fame, power, and special abilities • Combinative responses CS, R-PAS, and TDI scores: • Fabulized combinations • Incongruous combinations
DISINHIBITION & DYSCONTROL	MMPI-2 Scales: • *Sc5, DISC (PSY-5)* MMPI-3 Scales: • *RC4* • *RC9* • *DISC* • *ACT*	Rorschach Variables: • Color-dominated responses • Explosions, blood, fire • Flippant responses

Table A8 Test variables associated with insight

Insight Dimension	*Personality Inventories*	*Performance Measures*
PSYCHOLOGICAL MINDEDNESS VERSUS POOR INSIGHT	MMPI-2 Scales: • *Scales 1, 3,9* suggest lack of insight or psychological mindedness MMPI-3 Scales: • *RC9, ACT, BXD* suggests lack of insight or psychological mindedness	Rorschach Variables: • Psychological mindedness may be associated with a high number of blends, with adequate form quality • Both Form Dimension and Vista responses (use of form or shading to produce perspective or depth), if given with good form level, no indications of thought disorder, and appropriate content, may reflect the capacity for insight and self-reflection
OPENNESS TO EXPERIENCE	MMPI-2 Scales: • Extremely low scores on *Scale 8* might suggest a lack of imaginative capacity • Elevations on *L scale* may reflect close-mindedness and lack of curiosity	Rorschach Variables: • Adequate number of responses • Moderate to Low Lambda (reflecting sensitivity to multiple aspects of the inkblot)
SOCIAL PERCEPTION (MENTALIZATION THEORY OF MIND)		Rorschach • Human Movement Response
	NEPSY-II • Affect Recognition • Theory of Mind	

Appendix B

RESEARCH INTERVIEW AND RATING INSTRUMENTS

The scales listed under each dimension in the following table are by no means exhaustive. We have chosen to present a variety of instruments using different formats (structured interview and self-report) without intending to endorse their clinical utility or extent of empirical support. As with the tables in Appendix A, we organize the scales according to a multidimensional model.

Table Bl Structured interview, clinician-rated, and self-report scales

Aspects of Psychotic Experience	*Instruments*
PSYCHOSIS PRONENESS	1. **Wisconsin Schizotypy Scales** (WSS or WMAPLE; Chapman & Chapman, 1980; Wisconsin Manual for Assessing Psychotic-Like Experiences (Kwapil et al., 1999) a. ***Perceptual Aberrations*** (PerAb; Chapman & Chapman, 1978) b. ***Magical Ideation*** (Magld; Eckblad & Chapman, 1983) c. ***Social Anhedonia*** (SocAnh; Chapman & Chapman, 1978) d. ***Physical Anhedonia*** (PhyAnh; Chapman & Chapman, 1978) 2. **Schizotypal Personality Questionnaire** (SPQ; Raine, 1991) 3. **Structured Clinical Interview for Psychotic Spectrum Disorders** (SCI-PSY; Sbrana et al., 2005) 4. **Structured Interview for Schizotypy** (SIS; Kendler et al., 1989)

(*Continued*)

Table Bl (Continued)

Aspects of Psychotic Experience	*Instruments*
PSYCHOSIS-RISK SYNDROMES (PRODROME)	1. **Bonn Scale for the Assessment of Basic Symptoms** (BSABS; Gross et al., 1987) 2. **Schizophrenia Proneness Instrument for Adults** (SPI-A; Klosterkotter, 2001) 3. **Comprehensive Assessment of At-Risk Mental States** (CAARMS; Yung et al., 2005) 4. **Structured Interview for Prodromal Symptoms/Scale of Prodromal Symptoms** (SIPS/SOPS; Miller et al., 2002, 2003) 5. **Community Assessment of Psychic Experiences** (CAPE-42; Konings et al., 2006) 6. **Prodromal Questionnaire (PQ;** Loewy et al., 2005) 7. **Prodromal Questionnaire** (PQ-16; Ising et al., 2012)
HALLUCINATIONS	1. **Beliefs About Voices** (BAVQ; Chadwick & Birchwood, 1995) 2. **Beliefs About Voices, Revised** (BAVQ-R; Chadwick et al., 2000) 3. **Cardiff Anomalous Perceptions Scale** (CAPS; Bell et al., 2006b) 4. **Child Unusual Belief Scale** (CUBESCALE; Andersen, 2006; Viglione, 1994, 2014) 5. **Delusion Assessment Scale** (DAS; Meyers et al., 2006) 6. **Launay-Slade Hallucination Scale** (LSHS-R; Launay & Slade, 1981) 7. **Psychotic Symptoms Rating Scales** (PSYRATS; Haddock et al., 1999) 8. **Unusual Perceptions Schedule** (MUPS; Carter et al., 1995) 9. **Clinical Characteristics of Auditory Hallucinations** (CCAH; Oulis et al., 1995)
DELUSIONAL THINKING	1. **Brown Assessment of Beliefs Scale** (BABS; Eisen et al., 1998) 2. **Child Unusual Belief Scale** (CUBESCALE; Andersen, 2006; Viglione, 1994, 2014) 3. **Delusions – Symptoms – State Inventory** (DSSI; Bedford & Dreary, 1999) 4. **Details of Threat Questionnaire** (DoT; Freeman & Garety, 2004) 5. **Delusion Assessment Scale** (DAS; Meyers et al., 2006)

(*Continued*)

Table Bl (Continued)

Aspects of Psychotic Experience	*Instruments*
	6. **Green Paranoid Thought Scales** (GPTS; Green et al., 2008) 7. **Maudsley Assessment of Delusions** (MADS; Wessely et al., 1993) 8. **Persecutory Ideation Questionnaire (PIQ;** McKay et al., 2006) 9. **Peters Delusion Inventory** (PDI; Peters et al., 2004) 10. **Psychotic Symptoms Rating Scales** (PSYRATS; Haddock et al., 1999) 11. **Safety Behaviors Questionnaire** (SBQ; Freeman & Garety, 2004)
THOUGHT DISORDER	1. **Bizarre-Idiosyncratic Thinking Index** (BIT; Marengo et al., 1986) 2. **Formal Thought Disorder Scale** (FTDS; Barrera et al., 2008) 3. **Scale for the Assessment of Thought, Language, and Communication** (TLC; Andreasen, 1978) 4. **Thought Disorder Questionnaire** (TDQ; Waring et al., 2003) 5. **Thought and Language Index** (TLI; Liddle, Ngan, Caissie et al., 2002)
NEGATIVE SYMPTOMS	1. **Scale for Assessing Negative Symptoms** (SANS; Andreasen, 1987) 2. **Negative Symptom Assessment** (NSA; Alphs et al., 1989) 3. **Negative Symptom Assessment** (NSA-16; Axelrod et al., 1993) 4. **Physical Anhedonia** (PhysAnh; Chapman & Chapman, 1978) 5. **Schedule for the Deficit Syndrome** (SDS; Kirkpatrick et al., 1989) 6. **Social Anhedonia** (SocAnh; Chapman & Chapman, 1978) 7. **Brief Negative Symptom Scale** (BNSS; Kirkpatrick et al., 2011) 8. **Clinical Assessment Interview for Negative Symptoms** (CNSS; Horan et al., 2011)

(*Continued*)

Table Bl (Continued)

Aspects of Psychotic Experience	*Instruments*
DEPRESSION	1. **Beck Depression Inventory-II** (Beck et al., 1996) 2. **Calgary Depression Scale** (Addington et al., 1993) 3. **Hamilton Psychiatric Rating Scale for Depression** (HRSD; Hamilton, 1960) 4. **Carroll Depression Scales** (CDS; Carroll et al., 1981) 5. **Major Depression Rating Scale** (MDS; Bech et al., 1977)
MANIA	1. **Altman Self-Rating Mania Scale** (ASRM; Altman et al., 1997) 2. **Young Mania Rating Scale** (YMRS; Young et al., 1978) 3. **Internal State Scale** (ISS; Cooke et al., 1996) 4. **Self-Report Manic Inventory** (SRMS: Cooke et al., 1996)
INSIGHT	1. **Insight Scale-Birchwood** (IS-B; Birchwood et al., 1994) 2. **Insight Interview** (II; Buchanan et al., 1992) 3. **Beck Cognitive Insight Scale** (BCIS; Beck et al., 2004) 4. **Insight and Treatment Attitude** Questionnaire (ITAQ; McEvoy et al., 1981) 5. **Scale to Assess Unawareness of Mental Disorder** (SUMD; Amador et al., 1994)

REFERENCES

Abramovitch, A., Short, T., & Schweiger, A. (2021). The C factor: Cognitive dysfunction as a transdiagnostic dimension in psychopathology. *Clinical Psychology Review*, *86*, 102007.

Achenbach, T. M. (1991). *Integrative guide for the 1991 CBCL/4–18, YSR and TRF profiles*. Department of Psychiatry, University of Vermont.

Acklin, M. W. (2017). Madness, Mayhem and Murder: A comparative Rorschach case study of methamphetamine psychosis and paranoid schizophrenia. In R. E. Erard & F. B. Evans (Eds.), *The Rorschach in multi-method forensic assessment*. Routledge.

Acklin, M. W. (2021). Forensic considerations in the assessment of disordered thought and perception. In I. B. Weiner & J. H. Kleiger (Eds.), *Psychological assessment of disordered thinking and perception* (pp. 243–270). American Psychological Association. https://doi.org/10.1037/0000245-015

Addington, D., Addington, J., & Maticka-Tyndale, E. (1993). Assessing depression in schizophrenia: The Calgary depression scale. *British Journal of Psychiatry*, *63*(Suppl. 22), 39–44.

Addington, J., & Addington, D. (1998). Effect of substance misuse in early psychosis. *The British Journal of Psychiatry*, *172*(Suppl. 33), 134–136.

Addington, J., Cadenhead, K. S., Cannon, T. D., Cornblatt, B., McGlashan, T. H., Perkins, D. O., Seidmen, L. J., Tsuang, M., Walker, E. F., Woods, S. W., & Heinssen, R. (2007). North American prodrome longitudinal study: A collaborative multisite approach to prodromal schizophrenia research. *Schizophrenia Bulletin*, *33*, 665–672.

Aggarwal, N. K., Jarvis, G. E., Gómez-Carrillo, A., Kirmayer, L. J., & Lewis-Fernández, R. (2020). The Cultural Formulation Interview since DSM-5: Prospects for training, research, and clinical practice. *Transcultural Psychiatry*, *57*(4), 496–514.

Alaghband-Rad, J., McKenna, K., Gordon, C. T., Albus, K. E., Hamburger, S. D., Rumsey, J. M., Frazier, J. A., Lenane, M. C., & Rapoport, J. L. (1995). Childhood-onset chizophrenia: The severity of premorbid course. *Journal of the American Academy of Child and Adolescent Psychiatry*, *34*, 1273–1283.

Aleman, A., Agrawal, N., Morgan, K. D., & David, A. S. (2006). Insight in psychosis and neuropsychological function: Meta-analysis. *The British Journal of Psychiatry*, *189*(3), 204–212.

Aleman, A., & Larøi, F. (2008). *Hallucinations: The science of idiosyncratic perception*. American Psychological Association.

Ali, S., Patel, M., Avenido, J., Bailey, R. K., Jabeen, S., & Riley, W. J. (2011). Hallucinations: Common features and causes. *Current Psychiatry*, *10*(11), 22–29.

Alphs, L. D., Summerfelt, A., Lann, H., & Muller, R. J. (1989). The negative symptom assessment: A new instrument to assess negative symptoms of schizophrenia. *Psychopharmacology Bulletin*, *25*, 159–163.

Altman, E. G., Hedeker, D., Peterson, J. L., & Davis, J. M. (1997). The Altman self-rating mania scale. *Biological Psychiatry*, *42*, 948–955.

Álvarez, A., Guàrdia, A., González-Rodríguez, A., Betriu, M., Palao, D., Monreal, J. A., . . . Labad, J. (2022). A systematic review and meta-analysis of suicidality in psychotic disorders: Stratified analyses by psychotic subtypes, clinical setting and geographical region. *Neuroscience & Biobehavioral Reviews*, *143*, 104964.

Amador, X. F., & David, A. S. (Eds.). (1998). *Insight and psychosis*. Oxford University Press.

Amador, X. F., & David, A. S. (2004). *Insight and psychosis: Awareness of illness in schizophrenia and related disorders*. Oxford University Press.

Amador, X. F., Flaum, M., Andreasen, N. C., Strauss, D. H., Yale, S. A., Clark, S. C., & Gorman, J. M. (1994). Awareness of illness in schizophrenia and schizoaffective and mood disorders. *Archives of General Psychiatry*, *51*(10), 826–836.

Amador, X. F., & Kronengold, H. (2004). Understanding and assessing insight. In X. F. Amador & A. S. David (Eds.), *Insight and psychosis* (2nd ed., pp. 3–30). Oxford University Press.

Amador, X. F., Strauss, D., Yale, S., Flaum, M., Endicott, J., & Gorman, J. M. (1993). Assessment of insight in psychosis. *American Journal of Psychiatry*, *150*, 873–879.

Amador, X. F., Strauss, D., Yale, S., & Gorman, J. (1991). Awareness of illness in schizophrenia. *Schizophrenia Bulletin*, *17*, 113–130.

Ambizas, E. M. (2014). Non-psychotropic medication-induced psychosis. *US Pharm*, *39*(11), Hs-8-Hs-15.

American Psychiatric Association. (1980). *Diagnostic and statistical manual of mental disorders* (3rd ed.). American Psychiatric Association.

American Psychiatric Association. (1987). *Diagnostic and statistical manual of mental disorders* (3rd ed., text Rev.). American Psychiatric Association.

American Psychiatric Association. (1994). *Diagnostic and statistical manual of mental disorders* (4th ed.). American Psychiatric Association.

American Psychiatric Association. (2000). *Diagnostic and statistical manual of mental disorders* (4th ed., text revision). American Psychiatric Association.

American Psychiatric Association. (2003). Practice guideline for the assessment and treatment of patients with suicidal behaviors. In *Practice guidelines for the treatment of psychiatric disorders compendium*. American Psychiatric Publishing, Inc.

American Psychiatric Association. (2013). *Diagnostic and statistical manual of mental disorders* (5th ed.). American Psychiatric Association.

American Psychiatric Association. (2022). *Diagnostic and statistical manual of mental disorders* (5th ed., text Rev.). American Psychiatric Association.

Andersen, L. M. (2006). *The child unusual beliefs scale: A preliminary validation study* (Doctoral dissertation). Pace University.

Andreasen, N. C. (1978). *The scale for the assessment of thought, language, and communication (TLC)*. University of Iowa.

Andreasen, N. C. (1979). Thought, language, and communication disorders: I. Clinical assessment, definitions of terms, and evaluation of their reliability. *Archives of General Psychiatry*, *36*, 1315–1321.

Andreasen, N. C. (1982). Negative symptoms in schizophrenia: Definition and reliability. *Archives of General Psychiatry*, *39*(7), 784–788.

Andreasen, N. C. (1983a). The clinical differentiation of affective and schizophrenic disorders. In M. R. Zales (Ed.), *Affective and schizophrenic disorders: New approaches to diagnosis and treatment*. Brunner/Mazel.

Andreasen, N. C. (1983b). *Scale for the assessment of negative symptoms (SANS)*. Department of Psychiatry, University of Iowa College of Medicine.

Andreasen, N. C. (1984). *Scale for the assessment of positive symptoms (SAPS)*. Department of Psychiatry, University of Iowa College of Medicine.

Andreasen, N. C. (1985). *Comprehensive assessment of symptoms and history (CASH)*. University of Iowa Hospitals & Clinics.

Andreasen, N. C. (1987). The diagnosis of schizophrenia. *Schizophrenia Bulletin*, *13*(1), 9–22.

Andreasen, N. C. (1990). Positive and negative symptoms: Historical and conceptual aspects. In T. A. Ban, A. M., Freedman, C. G. Gottfries, R. Levy, P. Pichot, & W. Pöldinger (Eds.), *Modern problems of pharmacopsychiatry. Positive and negative symptoms and syndromes* (pp. 1–42). Karger.

Andreasen, N. C., Arndt, S., Alliger, R., Miller, D., & Flaum, M. (1995). Symptoms of schizophrenia: Methods, meanings, and mechanisms. *Archives of General Psychiatry*, *52*(5), 341–351.

Andreasen, N. C., & Black, D. W. (2006). *Introductory textbook of psychiatry* (4th ed.). American Psychiatric Publishing, Inc.

Andreasen, N. C., Flaum, M., & Arndt, S. (1992). The comprehensive assessment of symptoms and history (CASH). An instrument for assessing diagnosis and psychopathology. *Archives of General Psychiatry*, *49*(8), 615–623.

Andreasen, N. C., & Grove, W. M. (1986a). Evaluation of positive and negative symptoms in schizophrenia. *Psychiatric Biology* (1), 108–121.

Andreasen, N. C., & Grove, W. M. (1986b). Thought, language, and communication in schizophrenia: Diagnostic and prognostic significance. *Schizophrenia Bulletin*, *12*, 348–359.

Andrews, G., Goldberg, D. P., Krueger, R. F., Carpenter, W. T., Hyman, S. E., Sachdev, P., & Pine, D. S. (2009). Exploring the feasibility of a meta-structure for DSM-V and ICD-11: Could it improve utility and validity? *Psychological Medicine*, *39*(12), 1993–2000.

Appelbaum, P. S., Robbins, P. C., & Monahan, J. (2000). Violence and delusions: Data from the MacArthur violence risk assessment study. *American Journal of Psychiatry*, 157, 566–572.

Appelbaum, P. S., Robbins, P. C., & Roth, L. H. (1999). Dimensional approach to delusions: comparison across types and diagnoses. *American Journal of Psychiatry*, *156*(12), 1938–1943.

Arango, C., Fraguas, D., & Parellada, M. (2014). Differential neurodevelopmental trajectories in patients with early-onset bipolar and schizophrenia disorders. *Schizophrenia Bulletin* (Suppl. 2), S138–S146.

Arboleda, C., & Holzman, P. S. (1985). Thought disorder in children at risk for psychosis. *Archives of General Psychiatry*, *42*(10), 1004–1013.

Astrup, C., & Noreik, K. (1966). *Functional psychoses – diagnostic and prognostic models*. CC Thomas.

Axelrod, B. N., Goldman, R. S., & Alphs, L. D. (1993). Validation of the 16-item negative symptoms assessment. *Journal of Psychiatric Research*, *27*(3), 253–258.

Axelrod, S. R., Grilo, C. M., Sanislow, C., & McGlashan, T. H. (2001). Schizotypal personality questionnaire-brief: Factor structure and convergent validity in inpatient adolescents. *Journal of Personality Disorders*, *15*(2), 168–179.

Baier, M., DeShay, E., Owens, K., Robinson, M., Lasar, K., Peterson, K., & Bland, R. S. (2000). The relationship between insight and clinical factors for persons with schizophrenia. *Archives of Psychiatric Nursing*, *14*(6), 259–265.

Banerjee, A. (2012). Cross-cultural variance of schizophrenia in symptoms, diagnosis and treatment. *Georgetown University Journal of Health Sciences*, *6*(2), 18–24.

Barch, D. M. (2005). The cognitive neuroscience of schizophrenia. *Annual Review of Clinical Psychology*, *1*, 321–353.

Barch, D. M., Bustillo, J., Gaebel, W., Gur, R., Heckers, S., Malaspina, D., Owen, M. J., Schultz, S., Tandon, R., Tsuang, M., van Os, J., & Carpenter, W. (2013). Logic and justification for dimensional assessment of symptoms and related clinical phenomena in psychosis: Relevance to DSM-5. *Schizophrenia Research*, *150*(1), 15–20.

Barnes, A. (2004). Race, schizophrenia, and admission to state psychiatric hospitals. *Administration and Policy in Mental Health*, *31*(3), 241–252.

Barrera, Á., Handel, A., Kondel, T. K., & Laws, K. R. (2015). Formal thought disorder: Self-report in non-clinical populations. *International Journal of Psychology and Psychological Therapy*, *15*(1), 155–167.

Barrera, A., McKenna, P. J., & Berrios, G. E. (2008). Two new scales of formal thought disorder in schizophrenia. *Psychiatry Research*, *157*(1–3), 225–234.

Bartko, D., Herczeg, J., & Zador, G. (1988). Clinical symptomatology and drug compliance in schizophrenic patients. *Acta Psychiatrica Scandinavica*, *77*, 74–76.

Bearden, C. E., Wu, K. N., Caplan, R., & Cannon, T. D. (2011). Thought disorder and communication deviance as predictors of outcome in youth at clinical high risk for psychosis. *Journal of the American Academy of Child and Adolescent Psychiatry*, *50*(7), 669–680.

Beavan, V., Read, J., & Cartwright, C. (2011). The prevalence of voice-hearers in the general population: A literature review. *Journal of Mental Health*, *20*(3), 281–292.

Bech, P., Stage, K. B., Nair, N. P. V., Larsen, J. K., Kragh-Sorensen, P., & Gjerris, A. (1977). The major depression rating scale (MDS). Inter-rater reliability and validity across different settings in randomized moclobemide trials. *Journal of Affective Disorders*, *42*, 39–48.

Bechdolf, A., Thompson, A., Nelson, B., Cotton, S., Simmons, M. B., Amminger, G. P., Leicester, S., Francey, S. M., McNab, C., Krstev, H., Sidis, A., McGorry, P. D., & Yung, A. R. (2010). Experience of trauma and conversion to psychosis in an ultra-high-risk (prodromal) group. *Acta Psychiatrica Scandinavica, 121*(5), 377–384.

Beck, A. T., Baruch, E., Balter, J. M., Steer, R. A., & Warman, D. M. (2004). A new instrument for measuring insight: The beck cognitive insight scale. *Schizophrenia Research, 68*(2), 319–329.

Beck, A. T., Steer, R. A., & Brown, G. K. (1996). *Beck depression inventory manual* (2nd ed.). Psychological Corporation.

Beck, J. C., & van der Kolk, B. A. (1987). Reports of childhood incest and current behavior of chronically hospitalized psychotic women. *American Journal of Psychiatry, 144*, 1474–1476.

Beck, K., Andreou, C., Studerus, E., Heitz, U., Ittig, S., Leanza, L., & Riecher-Roessler, A. (2019). Clinical and functional long-term outcome of patients at clinical high risk (CHR) for psychosis without transition to psychosis: A systematic review. *Schizophrenia Research, 210*, 39–47.

Beckmann, D., Lowman, K. L., Nargiso, J., McKowen, J., Watt, L., & Yule, A. M. (2020). Substance-induced psychosis in youth. *Child and Adolescent Psychiatric Clinics, 29*(1), 131–143.

Bedford, A., & Dreary, I. J. (1999). The delusions-symptoms-states inventory (DSSI): Construction, application and structural analyses. *Personality and Individual Differences, 26*, 397–424.

Beiser, M., Erickson, D., Fleming, J. A., & Iacono, W. G. (1993). Establishing the onset of psychotic illness. *American Journal of Psychiatry, 150*(9), 1349–1354.

Bell, V., Halligan, P. W., & Ellis, H. D. (2006a). Diagnosing delusions: A review of inter-rater reliability. *Schizophrenia Research, 86*(1), 76–79.

Bell, V., Halligan, P. W., & Ellis, H. D. (2006b). The Cardiff anomalous perceptions scale (CAPS): A newly validated measure of perceptual experience. *Schizophrenia Bulletin, 32*(2), 366–377.

Bell, V., Halligan, P. W., & Ellis, H. D. (2006c). Explaining delusions: A cognitive perspective. *Trends in Cognitive Sciences, 10*(5), 219–226.

Bendall, S., Jackson, H. J., & Hulbert, C. A. (2011). What self-generated speech is externally misattributed in psychosis? Testing three cognitive models in a first-episode sample. *Schizophrenia Research, 129*(1), 36–41.

Benjamin, J. (1944). A method for distinguishing and evaluating formal thinking disorders in schizophrenia. In J. Kasanin (Ed.), *Language and thought in schizophrenia* (p. 65). University of California Press.

Benjamin, L. S. (1989). Is chronicity a function of the relationship between the person and the auditory hallucination? *Schizophrenia Bulletin, 15*(2), 291–310.

Ben-Porath, Y. S., & Tellegen, A. (2008). *Minnesota multiphasic personality inventory-2-RF (MMPI-2-RF).* University of Minneapolis Press.

Ben-Porath, Y. S., & Tellegen, A. (2020). *MMPI manual for administration, scoring, and interpretation.* University of Minnesota Press.

Bentall, R. P. (2003). *Madness explained: Psychosis and human nature.* Penguin Group.

Bentall, R. P., Corcoran, R., Howard, R., Blackwood, N., & Kinderman, P. (2001). Persecutory delusions: A review and theoretical integration. *Clinical Psychology Review, 21*(8), 1143–1192.

Bentall, R. P., & Taylor, J. L. (2006). Psychological processes and paranoia: Implications for forensic behavioural science. *Behavioral Sciences & the Law*, *24*(3), 277–294.

Bentall, R. P., Claridge, G. S., & Slade, P. D. (1989). The multidimensional nature of schizotypal traits: A factor analytic study with normal subjects. *British Journal of Clinical Psychology*, *28*(4), 363–375.

Berenbaum, H., & Barch, D. (1995). The categorization of thought disorder. *Journal of Psycholinguistic Research*, *24*(5), 349–376.

Berrios, G. E., & Beer, D. (1994). The notion of unitary psychosis: A conceptual history. *History of Psychiatry*, *5*(17), 13–36.

Berrios, G. E., & Brook, P. (1984). Visual hallucinations and sensory delusions in the elderly. *The British Journal of Psychiatry*, *144*(6), 662–664.

Bianchi, R., & Verkuilen, J. (2021). Green et al. Paranoid thoughts scale: French validation and development of a brief version. *Personality and Individual Differences*, *171*, 110554.

Biagiarelli, M., Roma, P., Comparelli, A., Andraos, M. P., Di Pompinio, I., Corigliano, V., Curto, M., Masters, G. A., & Ferracuti, S. (2015). Relationship between the rorschach perceptual thinking index (PTI) and the positive and negative syndrome scale (PANSS) in psychotic patients: A validity study. *Psychiatry Research*, *3*(225), 315–321.

Biederman, J., Petty, C. R., Monuteaux, M. C., Evans, M., Parcell, T., Faraone, S. V., & Wozniak, J. (2009). The child behavior checklist-pediatric bipolar disorder profile predicts a subsequent diagnosis of bipolar disorder and associated impairments in ADHD youth growing up: A longitudinal analysis. *Journal of Clinical Psychiatry*, *70*(5), 732–740.

Birchwood, M., Meaden, A., Trower, P., Gilbert, P., & Plaistow, J. (2000). The power and omnipotence of voices: Subordination and entrapment by voices and significant others. *Psychological Medicine*, *30*(2), 337–344.

Birchwood, M., Smith, J., Drury, V., Healy, J., McMillan, F., & Slade, M. A. (1994). A self-report insight scale for psychosis: Reliability, validity and sensitivity to change. *Acta Psychiatrica Scandinavica*, *89*, 62–67.

Black, D. W., & Grant, J. E. (2014). *DSM-5 guidebook: The essential companion to the diagnostic and statistical manual of mental disorders*. American Psychiatric Publishing.

Blanchard, J. J., & Cohen, A. S. (2006). The structure of negative symptoms within schizophrenia: Implications for assessment. *Schizophrenia Bulletin*, *32*(2), 238–245.

Bleuler, E. (1950). *Dementia praecox or the group of schizophrenias*. International Universities Press. (Original work published 1911)

Bonnie, R. J. (1992). The competence of criminal defendant: A theoretical reformulation. *Behavioral Science and the Law*, *10*, 291–316.

Bonta, J., Law, M., & Hanson, K. (1998). The prediction of criminal and violent recidivism among mentally disordered offenders: A meta-analysis. *Psychological Bulletin*, *123*, 123–142.

Bornstein, R. F. (2021). The importance of multimethod psychological assessment in assessing disordered thought and perception. In I. B. Weiner & J. H. Kleiger (Eds.), *The psychological assessment of disordered thinking and perception* (pp. 17–32). American Psychological Association.

Borum, R. (2014). Psychological vulnerabilities and propensities for involvement in violent extremism. *Behavioral Sciences & the Law*, *32*(3), 286–305.

Bowden, C. L. (2001). Strategies to reduce misdiagnosis of bipolar depression. *Psychiatric Services*, *52*(1), 51–55.

Boyette, L. L., & Noordhof, A. (2021). *A commentary on "developments in the Rorschach assessment of disordered thinking and communication" (Kleiger & Mihura, 2021)*. Rorschachiana.

Braff, D. L. (1993). Information processing and attention dysfunctions in schizophrenia. *Schizophrenia Bulletin*, *19*(2), 233–259.

Braff, D. L., & Geyer, M. A. (1990). Sensorimotor gating and schizophrenia: Human and animal model studies. *Archives of General Psychiatry*, *47*(2), 181–188.

Braff, D. L., Grillon, C., & Geyer, M. A. (1992). Gating and habituation of the startle reflex in schizophrenic patients. *Archives of General Psychiatry*, *49*(3), 206–215.

Braff, D. L., & Saccuzzo, D. P. (1981). Slowness of information processing in schizophrenia: A two factor deficit theory. *American Journal of Psychiatry*, *138*, 1051–1056.

Braff, D. L., Saccuzzo, D. P., & Geyer, M. A. (1991). Information processing dysfunctions in schizophrenia: Studies of visual backward masking, sensorimotor gating, and habituation. In S. R. Steinhauer, J. H. Gruzelier, & J. Zubin (Eds.), *Handbook of schizophrenia, Neuropsychology and information processing* (Vol. 5). Elsevier.

Bram, A. D., & Peebles, M. J. (2014). *Psychological testing that matters: Creating a road map for effective treatment*. American Psychological Association.

Breier, A., & Astrachan, B. M. (1984). Characterization of schizophrenic patients who commit suicide. *American Journal of Psychiatry*, *141*(2), 206–209.

Brener, A. (2014). *The connection between impairments in the development of self-other representations and risk markers for the development of disturbances along the schizophrenia spectrum: A cross-sectional, correlative study of non-psychotic adolescents* (Masters thesis). University of Haifa.

Bromberg, P. M. (2011). The gorilla did it: Some thoughts on dissociation, the real, and the really real. *Psychoanalytic Dialogues*, *11*, 385–404.

Broome, M. R., Woolley, J. B., Tabraham, P., Johns, L. C., Bramon, E., Murray, G. K., Pariante, C., Mcguire, P. K., & Murray, R. M. (2005). What causes the onset of psychosis? *Schizophrenia Research*, *79*, 23–34.

Brucato, G., Appelbaum, P. A., Lieberman, J. A., Wall, M. M., Feng, T., Masucci, M. D., Altschuler, R. A., & Girgis, R. R. (2018). A longitudinal study of violent behavior in a psychosis-risk cohort. *Neuropsychopharmacology*, *43*(2), 264–271.

Brucato, G., Appelbaum, P. A., Masucci, M. D., Rolin, S., Wall, M. M., Levin, M., Altschuler, R. A., First, M. B., Lieberman, J. A., & Girgis, R. R. (2019). Prevalence and phenomenology of violent ideation and behavior among 200 young people at clinical high-risk for psychosis: An emerging model of violence and psychotic illness. *Neuropsychopharmacology*, *44*(5), 907–914.

Brucato, G., First, M. B., Dishy, G. A., Samuel, S. A., Xu, Q., Wall, M. M., Small, S. A., Masucci, M. D., Lieberman, J. A., & Girgis, R. R. (2021). Recency and intensification of positive symptoms enhance prediction of conversion to syndromal psychosis in clinical high-risk patients. *Psychological Medicine*, *51*(1), 112–120.

Brucato, G., Masucci, M. D., Arndt, L. Y., Ben-David, S., Colibazzi, T., Corcoran, C. M., Crumbley, A. H., Crump, F. M., Gill, K. E., Kimhy, D. and Lister, A. Girgis, R. R. (2017). Baseline demographics, clinical features and predictors of conversion among 200 individuals in a longitudinal prospective psychosis-risk cohort. *Psychological Medicine*, *47*(11), 1923–1935.

Buchanan, A., Reed, A., & Almeida, O. (1992). The assessment of insight in schizophrenia. *British Journal of Psychiatry*, *161*, 599–602.

Buchanan, A., Reed, A., Wessely, S., Garety, P., Taylor, P., Grubin, D., & Dunn, G. (1993). Acting on delusions. II. The phenomenological correlates of acting on delusions. *British Journal of Psychiatry*, *163*, 77–81.

Bush, G., Fink, M., Petrides, G., Dowling, F., & Francis, A. (1996). Catatonia I. Rating scale and standardized examination. *Acta Psychiatrica Scandinavia*, *93*, 129–136.

Bushra, A., Khadivi, A., & Frewat-Nikowitz, S. (2007). History, custom, and the Twin Towers: Challenges in adapting psychotherapy to Middle Eastern culture in the United States. In M. J. Christopher (Ed.), *Dialogues on difference: Studies of diversity in the therapeutic relationship* (pp. 221–235). American Psychological Association.

Butcher, J. N., Dahlstrom, W. G., Graham, J. R., Tellegen, A. M., & Kreammer, B. (1989). *The Minnesota multiphasic personality inventory-2* (MMPI-2) *manual for administration and scoring*. University of Minneapolis Press.

Cannon, T. D., Cadenhead, K., Cornblatt, B., Woods, S. W., Addington, J., Walker, E., Seidman, L. J., Perkins, D., Tsuang, M., McGlashan, T., & Heinssen, R. (2008). Prediction of psychosis in youth at high clinical risk: A multisite longitudinal study in North America. *Archives of General Psychiatry*, *65*, 28–37.

Cannon, M., Caspi, A., Moffitt, T. E., Murray, R., Harrington, H., & Poulton, R. (2002). Evidence for early-childhood, pan-developmental impairment specific to adult schizophreniform disorder: Results from a longitudinal birth cohort. *Archives of General Psychiatry*, *59*, 449–456.

Caplan, R. (1994). Discourse deficits in children with schizophrenia spectrum disorder. *Schizophrenia Bulletin*, *20*, 671–684.

Caplan, R. (1996). Communication deficits in childhood schizophrenia spectrum disorder. In J. H. Beichtman, N. Cohen, M. Konstantareas, & R. Tannock (Eds.), *Language, learning, and behavioral disorders* (pp. 156–177). Cambridge University Press.

Caplan, R., & Bursch, B. (2012). *How many more questions?* Oxford University Press.

Caplan, R., Foy, J. G., Asarnow, R. F., & Sherman, T. (1990). Information processing deficits of schizophrenic children with formal thought disorder. *Psychiatry Research*, *31*, 169–177.

Caplan, R., Guthrie, D., Fish, B., Tanguay, P. E., & David-Lando, G. (1989). The kiddie formal thought disorder rating scale: Clinical assessment, reliability, and validity. *Journal of the American Academy of Child & Adolescent Psychiatry*, *28*(3), 408–416.

Caplan, R., Guthrie, D., & Foy, J. G. (1992). Communication deficits and formal thought disorder in schizophrenic children. *Journal of the American Academy of Child and Adolescent Psychiatry*, *31*, 151–159.

Caplan, R., Guthrie, D., Tang, B., Komo, S., & Asarnow, R. F. (2000). Thought disorder in childhood schizophrenia: Replication and update of concept. *Journal of the American Academy of Child & Adolescent Psychiatry*, *39*, 771–778.

Carlin, P., Gudjonsson, G., & Rutter, S. (2005). Persecutory delusions and attributions for real negative events: A study in a forensic sample. *Journal of Forensic Psychiatry & Psychology*, *16*(1), 139–148.

Caton, C. L., Samet, S., & Hasin, D. S. (2000). When acute-stage psychosis and substance use co-occur: Differentiating substance-induced and primary psychotic disorders. *Journal of Psychiatric Practice®*, *6*(5), 256–266.

Carlson, G. A., & Goodwin, F. K. (1973). The stages of mania: A longitudinal analysis of the manic episode. *Archives of General Psychiatry*, *28*, 221–228.

Carpenter, W. T. (2004). What causes schizophrenia? *ACP Medicine*, *27*. http://www.acpmedicine.com/wnim/acp_0604.htm#L6

Carpenter, W. T., Bartko, J. J., Carpenter, C. L., & Strauss, J. S. (1976). Another view of schizophrenia subtypes: A report from the international pilot study of schizophrenia. *Archives of General Psychiatry*, *33*(4), 508–516.

Carpenter, W. T., Bustillo, J. R., Thaker, G. K., van Os, J., Krueger, R. F., & Green, M. J. (2009). The psychoses: Cluster 3 of the proposed meta-structure for DSM-V and ICD-11. *Psychological Medicine*, *39*(12), 2025–2042.

Carpenter, W. T., Heinrichs, D. W., & Wagman, A. M. (1988). Deficit and nondeficit forms of schizophrenia: The concept. *American Journal of Psychiatry*, *145*, 578–583.

Carpenter, W. T., & Strauss, J. S. (1973). Are there pathognomonic symptoms in schizophrenia? An empiric investigation of Schneider's first-rank symptoms. *Archives of General Psychiatry*, *27*, 847–852.

Carpenter, W. T., Strauss, J. S., & Bartko, J. J. (1973). Flexible system for the diagnosis of schizophrenia: Report from the WHO international pilot study of schizophrenia. *Science*, *182*(4118), 1275–1278.

Carroll, B. J., Feinberg, M., Smouse, P. E., Rawson, S. G., & Greden, J. F. (1981). The Carroll rating scale for depression. I. Development, reliability and validation. *British Journal of Psychiatry*, *138*, 194–200.

Carter, D. M., Mackinnon, A., Howard, S., Zeegers, T., & Copolov, D. L. (1995). The development and reliability of the mental health research institute unusual perceptions schedule (MUPS): An instrument to record auditory hallucinatory experience. *Schizophrenia Research*, *16*(2), 157–165.

Castillo, R. J. (2006, December 01). *Effects of culture on recovery from transient psychosis*. http://www.psychiatrictimes.com/articles/effects-culture-recovery-transient-psychosis.

Cepeda, C. (2007). *Psychotic symptoms in children and adolescents*. Routledge/Taylor & Francis Group.

Cepeda, C. (2012, December 21). *Diagnosing psychosis in children and adolescents*. Psychiatric News, American Psychiatric Association from the Experts.

Cermolacce, M., Sass, L., & Parnas, J. (2010). What is bizarre in bizarre delusions? A critical review. *Schizophrenia Bulletin*, *36*(4), 667–679.

Cervellione, K. L., Burdick, K. E., Cottone, J. G., Rhinewine, J. P., & Kumra, S. (2007). Neurocognitive deficits in adolescents with schizophrenia: Longitudinal stability and predictive utility for short-term functional outcome. *Journal of the American Academy of Child & Adolescent Psychiatry*, *46*(7), 867–878.

Chadwick, P. K. (2014). Peer-professional first person account: Before psychosis – Schizoid personality from the inside. *Schizophrenia Bulletin*, *40*(3), 483–486.

Chadwick, P. K., Barnbrook, E., & Newman-Taylor, K. (2007). Responding mindfully to distressing voices: Links with meaning, affect and relationship with voice. *Tidsskrift for Norsk Psykologforening*, *44*(5), 581–587.

Chadwick, P. K., & Birchwood, M. (1994). The omnipotence of voices. A cognitive approach to auditory hallucinations. *British Journal of Psychiatry*, *164*(2), 190–201.

Chadwick, P. K., & Birchwood, M. (1995). The omnipotence of voices: II. The beliefs about voices questionnaire (BAVQ). *British Journal of Psychiatry*, *166*(6), 773–776.

Chadwick, P. K., Lees, S., & Birchwood, M. (2000). The revised beliefs about voices questionnaire (BAVQ-R). *British Journal of Psychiatry*, *177*, 229–232.

Chaika, E. O. (1990). *Understanding psychotic speech: Beyond Freud and Chomsky*. Charles C Thomas Publisher Ltd.

Chandrasekhar, T., Copeland, J. N., Spanos, M., & Sikich, L. (2020). Autism, psychosis, or both? Unraveling complex patient presentations. *Child and Adolescent Psychiatric Clinics*, *29*(1), 103–113.

Chapman, J. P., Chapman, L. J., & Kwapil, T. R. (1995). Scales for the measurement of Schizotypy. In A. Raine, T. Lencz, & S. A. Mednick (Eds.), *Schizotypal personality* (pp. 79–109). Cambridge University Press.

Chapman, L. J., & Chapman, J. P. (1978). *Revised physical anhedonia scale*. Department of Psychology, University of Wisconsin.

Chapman, L. J., & Chapman, J. P. (1980). Scales for rating psychotic and psychotic-like experiences as continua. *Schizophrenia Bulletin*, *6*, 476–489.

Chapman, L. J., Chapman, J. P., Kwapil, T. R., Eckblad, M., & Zinser, M. C. (1994). Putatively psychosis-prone subjects 10 years later. *Journal of Abnormal Psychology*, *103*, 171–183.

Chapman, L. J., Chapman, J. P., & Raulin, M. L. (1978). Body-image aberration in schizophrenia. *Journal of Abnormal Psychology*, *87*, 399–407.

Chapman, L. J., Day D., & Burstein, A. (1961). The process-reactive distinction and prognosis in schizophrenia. *The Journal of Nervous and Mental Disease*, *133*(5), 383–391.

Chen, E. Y. H., Lam, L. C. W., Kan, C. S., Chan, C. K. Y., Kwok, C. L., Nguyen, D. G. H., & Chen, R. Y. L. (1996). Language disorganisation in schizophrenia: Validation and assessment with a new clinical rating instrument. *Hong Kong Journal of Psychiatry*, *6*, 4–13.

Chen, W. J., Hsiao, C. K., & Lin, C. (1997). Schizotypy in community samples: The three-factor structure and correlation with sustained attention. *Journal of Abnormal Psychology*, *106*(4), 649–654.

Cheung, P., Schweitzer, I., Crowley, K., & Tuckwell, V. (1997). Violence in schizophrenia: Role of hallucinations and delusions. *Schizophrenia Research*, *26*(2–3), 181–190.

Cheyne, J. A., Newby-Clark, I. R., & Rueffer, S. D. (1999). Relations among hypnagogic and hypnopompic experiences associated with sleep paralysis. *Journal of Sleep Research*, *8*(4), 313–317.

Christopher, P. P., Foti, M. E., Roy-Bujnowski, K., & Appelbaum, P. S. (2007). Consent form readability and educational levels of potential participants in mental health research. *Psychiatric Services*, *58*, 227–232.

Claridge, G., McCreery, C., Mason, O., Bentall, R., Boyle, G., Slade, P., & Popplewell, D. (1996). The factor structure of 'schizotypal' traits: A large replication study. *British Journal of Clinical Psychology*, *35*(1), 103–115.

Clark, S. M., & Harrison, D. A. (2012). How to care for patients who have delusions with religious content – To improve outcomes, look beyond delusion content and enlist spiritual care experts. *Current Psychiatry*, *11*(1), 47–51.

Cohen, A. S., Matthews, R. A., Najolia, G. M., & Brown, L. A. (2010). Toward a more psychometrically sound brief measure of schizotypal traits: Introducing the SPQ-Brief Revised. *Journal of Personality Disorders*, *24*(4), 516–537.

Coleman, M., Levy, D., Lezenweger, M., & Holzman, P. S. (1996). Thought disorder, perceptual aberrations, and schizotypy. *Journal of Abnormal Psychology*, *105*, 469–473.

Corcoran, R., Mercer, G., & Frith, C. D. (1995). Schizophrenia, symptomatology and social inference: Investigating 'theory of mind' in people with schizophrenia. *Schizophrenia Research*, *17*(1), 5–13.

Cooke, R. G., Kruger, S., & Shugar, G. (1996). Comparative evaluation of two self-report mania rating scales. *Biological Psychiatry*, *40*, 279–283.

Correll, C. U., Penzner, J. B., Frederickson, A. M., Richter, J. J., Auther, A. M., Smith, C. W., Kane, J. M., & Cornblatt, B. A. (2007). Differentiation in the preonset phases of schizophrenia and mood disorders: Evidence in support of a bipolar mania prodrome. *Schizophrenia Bulletin*, *33*(3), 703–714.

Crow, T. J. (1980). Positive and negative schizophrenic symptoms and the role of dopamine: II. *British Medical Journal*, 66–68.

Crow, T. J., MacMillan, J. F., Johnson, A. L., & Johnstone, E. C. (1986). The Northwick Park study of first episodes of schizophrenia. II: A controlled trial of prophylactic neuroleptic treatment. *British Journal of Psychiatry*, *148*, 120–127.

Crump, F. M., Arndt, L., Grivel, M., Horga, G., Corcoran, C. M., Brucato, G., & Girgis, R. R. (2018). Attenuated first-rank symptoms and conversion to psychosis in a clinical high-risk cohort. *Early Intervention in Psychiatry*, *12*(6), 1213–1216.

Cuesta, M. J., Peralta, V., & Zarzuela, A. (1998). Psychopathological dimensions and lack of insight in schizophrenia. *Psychological Reports*, *83*(3), 895–898.

Cullberg, J. (2006). *Psychoses: An integrative perspective*. Routledge.

Cummings, J. L., & Mega, M. S. (2003). *Neuropsychiatry and behavioral neuroscience*. Oxford University Press.

Cunningham, M. (2010). *Evaluation for capital sentencing*. Oxford University Press.

Cunningham, M. D. (2018). Differentiating delusional disorder from the radicalization of extreme beliefs: A 17-factor model. *Journal of Threat Assessment and Management*, *5*(3), 137–154. https://doi.org/10.1037/tam00001

Curran, H. V., Freeman, T. P., Mokrysz, C., Lewis, D. A., Morgan, C. J., & Parsons, L. H. (2016). Keep off the grass? Cannabis, cognition and addiction. *Nature Reviews Neuroscience*, *17*(5), 293–306.
David, A. S. (1990). Insight and psychosis. *The British Journal of Psychiatry*, *156*(6), 798–808.
David, A. S. (1999). To see ourselves as others see us: Aubrey Lewis's insight. *British Journal of Psychiatry*, *175*, 210–216.
David, A. S. (2004). The cognitive neuropsychiatry of auditory verbal hallucinations: An overview. *Cognitive Neuropsychiatry*, *9*(1–2), 107–123.
David, A. S. (2010, February 11). Why we need more debate on whether psychotic symptoms lie on a continuum with normality. *Psychological Medicine*, 1–8.
David, A. S., Buchanan, A., Reed, A., & Almeida, O. (1992). The assessment of insight in psychosis. *The British Journal of Psychiatry*, *161*(5), 599–602.
David, A. S., van Os, J., Jones, P., Harvey, I., Foerster, A., & Fahy, T. (1995). Insight and psychotic illness. Cross-sectional and longitudinal associations. *British Journal of Psychiatry*, *167*, 621–628.
Delis, D. C., Kaplan, E., & Kramer, J. H. (2001). *Delis-Kaplan executive function system (D-KEFS)*. The Psychological Corporation.
Demjaha, A., Morgan, K., Morgan, C., Landau, S., Dean, K., Reichenberg, A., Sham, P., Fearon, P., Hutchinson, G., Jones, P. B., Murray, R. M., & Dazzan, P. (2009). Combining dimensional and categorical representation of psychosis: The way forward for DSM-V and ICD-11? *Psychological Medicine*, *39*(12), 1943–1955.
De Pablo, G. S., Besana, F., Arienti, V., Catalan, A., Vaquerizo-Serrano, J., Cabras, A., Pereira, J., Soardo, L., Coronelli, F., Kaur, S., & Da Silva, J. (2021). Longitudinal outcome of attenuated positive symptoms, negative symptoms, functioning and remission in people at clinical high risk for psychosis: A meta-analysis. *EClinicalMedicine*, *36*.
De Pablo, G. S., Radua, J., Pereira, J., Bonoldi, I., Arienti, V., Besana, F., & Fusar-Poli, P. (2021). Probability of transition to psychosis in individuals at clinical high risk: An updated meta-analysis. *JAMA Psychiatry*, *78*(9), 970–978.
Deprey, L., & Ozonoff, S. (2009). Assessment of psychiatric conditions in autism spectrum disorders. In S. Goldstein, J. Naglieri, & S. Ozonoff (Eds.), *Assessment of autism spectrum disorders* (pp. 290–317). Guilford Press.
DeRosse, P., & Karlsgodt, K. H. (2015). Examining the psychosis continuum. *Current Behavioral Neuroscience Reports*, *2*, 80–89.
Desai, P. R., Lawson, K. A., Barner, J. C., & Rascati, K. L. (2013). Estimating the direct and indirect costs for community-dwelling patients with schizophrenia. *Journal of Pharmaceutical Health Services Research*, *4*(4), 187–194.
De Vogel, V., De Beuf, T., Shepherd, S., & Schneider, R. D. (2022). Violence risk assessment with the HCR-20V3 in legal contexts: A critical reflection. *Journal of personality assessment*, *104*(2), 252–264.
Dingman, C. W., & McGlashan, T. H. (1986). Discriminating characteristics of suicide. Chesnut Lodge study follow-up sample including patients with affective disorder, schizophrenia and schizoaffective disorder. *Acta Psychiatrica Scandinavia*, *74*(1), 91–97.
Dzamonja-Ignjatovic, T., Smith, B. L., Djuric Jocic, D., & Milanovic, M. (2013). A comparison of new and revised Rorschach measures of schizophrenic

functioning in a Serbian clinical sample. *Journal of Personality Assessment*, *95*(5), 471–478.

Doody, G. A., Götz, M., Johnstone, E. C., Frith, C. D., & Cunningham Owens, D. G. (1998). Theory of mind and psychoses. *Psychological Medicine*, *28*(2), 397–405.

Douglas, K. S., Guy, L. S., & Hart, S. D. (2009). Psychosis as a risk factor for violence to others: A meta-analysis. *Psychological Bulletin*, *135*(5), 679–706.

Douglas, K. S., Hart, S. D., Webster, C. D., & Belfrage, H. (2013). *HCR-20V3: Assessing risk of violence user guide*. Mental Health, Law, and Policy Institute, Simon Fraser University.

Douglas, K. S., & Reeves, K. A. (2010). Historical-clinical-risk management-20 (HCR-20) violence risk assessment scheme: Rationale, application, and empirical overview. In R. K. Otto & K. S. Douglas (Eds.), *Handbook of violence risk assessment* (pp. 147–185). Routledge/Taylor & Francis Group.

Drake, R. J., Kinderman, P., Bentall, R. P., Dunn, G., & Lewis, S. W. (2000). Insight, attribution and symptoms in first episode schizophrenia. *Schizophrenia Research*, *41*(1), 50.

Drury, V. M., Robinson, E. J., & Birchwood, M. (1998). 'Theory of mind' skills during an acute episode of psychosis and following recovery. *Psychological Medicine*, *28*(5), 1101–1112.

Dutta, R., & Murray, R. (2010). A life course approach to psychoses: Outcome and cultural variation. In T. Millon, R. F. Krueger, & E. Simonsen (Eds.), *Contemporary directions in psychopathology*. Guilford Press.

East-Richard, C., R-Mercier, A., Nadeau, D., & Cellard, C. (2020). Transdiagnostic neurocognitive deficits in psychiatry: A review of meta-analyses. *Canadian Psychology/Psychologie canadienne*, *61*(3), 190.

Eckblad, M., & Chapman, L. J. (1983). Magical ideation as an indicator of schizotypy. *Journal of Consulting and Clinical Psychology*, *51*, 215–225.

Eckblad, M., Chapman, L. J., Chapman, J. P., & Mishlove, M. (1982). *The revised social anhedonia scale* (Unpublished manuscript). University of Wisconsin.

Edell, W. (1987). Role of structure in disordered therapy in borderline and schizophrenia disorders. *Journal of Personality Assessment*, *51*, 23–41.

Egeland, J. A., Hostetter, A. M., Pauls, D. L., & Sussex, J. N. (2000). Prodromal symptoms before onset of manic-depressive disorder suggested by first hospital admission histories. *Journal of the American Academy of Child & Adolescent Psychiatry*, *39*(10), 1245–1252.

Eisen, J. L., Phillips, K. A., Baer, L., Beer, D. A., Atala, K. D., & Rasmussen, S. A. (1998). The brown assessment of beliefs scale: Reliability and validity. *American Journal of Psychiatry*, *155*, 102–108.

Elvevag, B., & Goldberg, T. E. (2000). Cognitive impairment in schizophrenia is the core of the disorder. *Current Reviews in Neurobiology*, *14*(1), 1–21.

Emsley, R., Rabinowitz, J., & Torreman, M. (2003). The factor structure for the positive and negative syndrome scale (PANSS) in recent-onset psychosis. *Schizophrenia Research*, *61*(1), 47–57.

Erkwoh, R., Willmes, K., Eming-Erdmann, A., & Kunert, H. J. (2002). Command hallucinations: Who obeys and who resists when? *Psychopathology*, *35*(5), 272–279.

Esterberg, M. L., & Compton, M. T. (2009). The psychosis continuum and categorical versus dimensional diagnostic approaches. *Current Psychiatry Reports, 11*(3), 179–184.

Evans III, F. B. (2024). *Harry Stack Sullivan: Interpersonal theory and psychotherapy*. Routledge.

Exner, J. E. (1986). Some Rorschach data comparing schizophrenics with borderlines and schizotypal personality disorders. *Journal of Personality Assessment, 50*, 455–471.

Exner, J. E., & Weiner, I. B. (1982). *The Rorschach: A comprehensive system, assessment of children and adolescents* (Vol. 3). Wiley & Sons.

Eysenck, H. J. (1952). Schizothymia-cyclothymia as a dimension of personality. *Journal of Personality, 20*(3), 345–384.

Eysenck, H. J. (1960). Description and measurement of abnormal behaviour: Classification and the problem of diagnosis. In H. J. Eysenck (Ed.), *Handbook of abnormal psychology* (pp. 1–31). Pitman Medical Publishing.

Eysenck, H. J., & Eysenck, S. B. G. (1976). *Psychoticism as a dimension of personality*. Hodder and Stoughton.

Falloon, I. R. H. (1992). Early intervention for first episodes of schizophrenia: A preliminary exploration. *Psychiatry, 55*, 4–15.

Fazel, S., Gulati, G., Linsell, L., Geddes, J. R., & Grann, M. (2009). Schizophrenia and violence: Systematic review and meta-analysis. *PLOS Medicine, 6*, 1–15.

Fear, C. F., & Healy, D. (1997). Probabilistic reasoning in obsessive–compulsive and delusional disorders. *Psychological Medicine, 27*(1), 199–208.

Fein, R. A., & Vossekuil, B. (1999). Assassination in the United States: An operational study of recent assassins, attackers, and near-lethal approachers. *Journal of Forensic Sciences, 44*(2), 321–333.

Fenton, W. S., & McGlashan, T. H. (1987). Prognostic scale for chronic schizophrenia. *Schizophrenia Bulletin, 13*(2), 277–286.

Fenton, W. S., & McGlashan, T. H. (1991). Natural history of schizophrenia subtypes: I. Longitudinal study of paranoid, hebephrenic, and undifferentiated schizophrenia. *Archives of General Psychiatry, 48*, 969–977.

Fenton, W. S., & McGlashan, T. H. (1994). Antecedents, symptom progression, and long-term outcome of the deficit syndrome in schizophrenia. *American Journal of Psychiatry, 151*(3), 351–356.

Fenton, W. S., McGlashan, T. H., Victor, B. J., & Blyler, C. R. (1997). Symptoms, subtype, and suicidality in patients with schizophrenia spectrum disorders. *American Journal of Psychiatry, 154*(2), 199–204.

Fialko, L., Freeman, D., Bebbington, P. E., Kuipers, E., Garety, P. A., Dunn, G., & Fowler, D. (2006). Understanding suicidal ideation in psychosis: Findings from the Psychological Prevention of Relapse in Psychosis (PRP) trial. *Acta Psychiatrica Scandinavica, 114*(3), 177–186.

Fields, J. H., Grochowski, S., Lindenmeyer, J. P., Kay, S. R., Gross, D., Hyman, R. B., & Alexander, G. (1994). Assessing positive and negative symptoms in children and adolescents. *American Journal of Psychiatry, 15*, 249–253.

Findling, R. L., Schulz, S. C., Kashani, J. H., & Harlan Drewel, E. T. (2001). *Psychotic disorders in children and adolescents (developmental clinical psychology and psychiatry)*. SAGE Publications Ltd.

Fiorentini, A., Cantù, F., Crisanti, C., Cereda, G., Oldani, L., & Brambilla, P. (2021). Substance-induced psychoses: An updated literature review. *Frontiers in Psychiatry*, *12*, 694863.

First, M. B. (2006). *Dimensional aspects of psychiatric diagnosis*. Consultant to the American psychiatric institute for research and education (AIRE), a subsidiary of the American Psychiatric Association.

First, M. B. (2014). *DSM-5 handbook of differential diagnosis*. American Psychiatric Publishing.

First, M. B., Spitzer, R. L., Gibbon M., & Williams, J. B. W. (1996). *Structured clinical interview for DSM-IV Axis I disorders, clinician version (SCID-CV)*. American Psychiatric Press, Inc.

First, M. B., Spitzer, R. L., Gibbon, M., & Williams, J. B. W. (2002). *Structured clinical interview for DSM-IV-TR Axis I disorders, research version, patient version, patient edition with psychotic screen (SCID-I/P W/PSY SCREEN)*. Biometrics Research, New York State Psychiatric Institute.

First, M. B., Williams, J. B., Karg, R. S., & Spitzer, R. L. (2016). *User's guide for the SCID-5-CV Structured Clinical Interview for DSM-5® disorders: Clinical version*. American Psychiatric Publishing, Inc.

First, M. B., Williams, J. B. W., Spitzer, R. L., & Gibbon, M. (2007). *Structured clinical interview for DSM-IV-TR Axis I disorders, clinical trials version (SCID-CT)*. Biometrics Research, New York State Psychiatric Institute.

Flashman, L. A., & Roth, R. M. (2004). Neural correlates of unawareness of illness in psychosis. In X. F. Amador & A. S. David (Eds.), *Insight and psychosis: Awareness of illness in schizophrenia and related disorders* (2nd ed., pp. 157–176). Oxford University Press.

Folstein, M. F., Folstein, S. E., & McHugh, P. R. (1975). Mini-mental state: A practical method for grading the cognitive state of patients for the clinician. *Journal of Psychiatric Research*, *12*, 189–198.

Forgácová, L. (2008). Delusion assessment scales. *Neuropsychopharmacologia Hungarica*, *10*(1), 23–30.

Foulds, G. A., Bedford, A., & Csapo, K. G. (1975). Class change in the personal illness hierarchy. *British Journal of Psychiatry*, *127*, 316–319.

Fox, J. R. E., Gray, N. S., & Lewis, H. (2004). Factors determining compliance with command hallucinations with violent content: The role of social rank, perceived power of the voice and voice malevolence. *The Journal of Forensic Psychiatry & Psychology*, *15*(3), 511–531.

Frances, A. (2013). *Essentials of psychiatric diagnosis: Responding to the challenge of DSM-5* (1st ed.). Guilford Press.

Francis, J. L., & Penn, D. L. (2001). The relationship between insight and social skill in persons with severe mental illness. *The Journal of Nervous and Mental Disease*, *189*(12), 822–829.

Frederick, J. A., & Killeen, M. R. (1998). Instruments for assessment of auditory hallucinations. *Archives of Psychiatric Nursing*, *12*(5), 255–263.

Freeman, D. (2007). Suspicious minds: The psychology of persecutory delusions. *Clinical Psychology Review*, *27*(4), 425–457.

Freeman, D. (2010). Cognitive and social processes in psychosis: Recent developments. In W. F. Gattaz & G. Busatto (Eds.), *Advances in schizophrenia research 2009* (pp. 283–298). Springer.

Freeman, D., & Garety, P. (2006). Helping patients with paranoid and suspicious thoughts: A cognitive-behavioural approach. *Advances in Psychiatric Treatment, 12*, 404–415.

Freeman, P., & Garety, P. A. (2004). *Paranoia: The psychology of persecutory delusions*. Psychology Press.

Freeman, S. A. (2012). Suicide assessment: Targeting acute risk factors. Focus on time-sensitive factors that may respond to treatment. *Current Psychiatry, 11*(1), 52–57.

Freud, S. (1958). Psychoanalytic notes on an autobiographical account of a case of paranoia (dementia paranoides). In J. Strachey (Ed.), *Standard edition of the complete psychological works of Sigmund Freud* (Vol. 12, pp. 1–82). Hogarth Press. (Original work published 1911)

Frith, C. D. (1992). *The cognitive neuropsychology of schizophrenia*. Psychology Press.

Frith, C. D., & Frith, U. (1999). Interacting minds--a biological basis. *Science, 286*(5445), 1692–1695.

Fuji, D., & Ahmed, I. (Eds.). (2007). *The spectrum of psychotic disorders: Neurobiology, etiology, and pathogenesis*. Cambridge University Press.

Fusar-Poli, P., Bonoldi, I., Yung, A. R., Borgwardt, S., Kempton, M. J., Valmaggia, L., Barale, F., Caverzasi, E., & McGuire, P. (2012). Predicting psychosis: Meta-analysis of transition outcomes in individuals at high clinical risk. *Archives of General Psychiatry, 69*(3), 220–229.

Fusar-Poli, P., De Pablo, G. S., Rajkumar, R. P., López-Díaz, Á., Malhotra, S., Heckers, S., Lawrie, S. M., & Pillmann, F. (2022). Diagnosis, prognosis, and treatment of brief psychotic episodes: A review and research agenda. *The Lancet Psychiatry, 9*(1), 72–83.

Fusar-Poli, P., McGuire, P., & Borgwardt, S. (2012). Mapping prodromal psychosis: A critical review of neuroimaging studies. *European Psychiatry, 27*(3), 181–191.

Fusar-Poli, P., Meneghelli, A., Valmaggia, L., Allen, P., Galvan, F., McGuire, P., & Cocchi, A. (2009). Duration of untreated prodromal symptoms and 12-month functional outcome of individuals at risk of psychosis. *The British Journal of Psychiatry, 194*(2), 181–182.

Gaebel, W. (2012). Status of psychotic disorders in ICD-11. *Schizophrenia Bulletin, 38*(5), 895–898. https://doi.org/10.1093/schbul/sbs104

Gallup, G. Jr., & Newport, F. (1991). Belief in paranormal phenomena among adult Americans. *Skeptical Enquirer, 15*, 137–146.

Garety, P. A., Freeman, D., Jolley, S., Ross, K., Walker, H., & Dunn, G. (2011). Jumping to conclusions: The psychology of delusional reasoning. *Advances in Psychiatric Treatment, 17*, 332–339.

Garety, P. A., & Hemsley, D. R. (1987). Characteristics of delusional experience. *European Archives of Psychiatry and Neurological Sciences, 236*(5), 294–298.

Gelder, M., Gath, D., Mayou, R., & Cowen, P. (1998). *Oxford textbook of psychiatry* (3rd ed.). Oxford University Press.

Geller, B., & Luby, J. (1997). Child and adolescent bipolar disorder: A review of the past 10 years. *Journal of the American Academy of Child and Adolescent Psychiatry, 36*, 1168–1176.

Geller, B., Warner, K., Williams, M., & Zimerman, B. (1998). Prepubertal and young adolescent bipolarity versus ADHD: Assessment and validity using the WASH-U-KSADS, CBCL, and TRF. *Journal of Affective Disorders, 51*, 91–100.

Geltman, D., & Chang, G. (2004). Hallucinations in Latino outpatients: A preliminary investigation. *General Hospital Psychiatry*, *26*, 153–157.

Gerretsen, P., Remington, G., Borlido, C., Quilty, L., Hassan, S., Polsinelli, G., Teo, C., Mar, W., Simon, R., Menon, M., Pothier, D., Nakajima, F., Cavavaggio, F., Mamo, D., Rajji, T. K., Mulsant, B., Deluca, H., Ganguli, R., Pollock, B. G., . . . Graff-Guerrero, A. (2014). The VAGUS insight into psychosis scale–self-report and clinician-rated versions. *Psychiatry Research*, *220*(3), 1084–1089.

Ghaemi, S. N., & Rosenquist, K. J. (2004). Is insight in mania state-dependent? A meta-analysis. *The Journal of Nervous and Mental Disease*, *192*(11), 771–775.

Ghaemi, S. N., Stoll, A. L., & Pope Jr., H. G. (1995). Lack of insight in bipolar disorder: The acute manic episode. *The Journal of Nervous and Mental Disease*, *183*(7), 464–467.

Gill, C., Weisburd, D., Telep, C. W., Vitter, Z., & Bennett, T. (2014). Community-oriented policing to reduce crime, disorder and fear and increase satisfaction and legitimacy among citizens: A systematic review. *Journal of Experimental Criminology*, *10*, 399–428.

Gill, P. (2015). *Lone-actor terrorists: A behavioural analysis*. Routledge.

Glancy, G. D., Ash, P., Bath, E. P., Buchanan, A., Fedoroff, P., Frierson, R. L., & Zonana, H. V. (2015). AAPL practice guideline for the forensic assessment. *The Journal of the American Academy of Psychiatry and the Law*, *43*(2 Suppl), S3–S53.

Gold, J. M., & Hurt, S. W. (1990). The effects of haloperidol on thought disorder and IQ in schizophrenia. *Journal of Personality Assessment*, *54*, 390–400.

Gold, J. M., Queern, C., Iannone, V. N., & Buchanan, R. W. (1999). Repeatable battery for the assessment of neuropsychological status as a screening test in schizophrenia, I: Sensitivity, reliability, and validity. *American Journal of Psychiatry*, *156*, 1944–1950.

Goldberg, T. E., & Weinberger, D. R. (2000). Thought disorder in schizophrenia: A reappraisal of older formulations and an overview of some recent studies. *Cognitive Neuropsychiatry*, *5*, 1–19.

Golding, S. L. (2007). Evaluations of adult adjudicative competency. In R. Jackson (Ed.), *Learning forensic assessment* (pp. 75–108). International Perspectives on Forensic Mental Health.

Goldstein, A. M., Morse, S. J., & Packer, I. K. (2013). Evaluation of criminal responsibility. In R. K. Otto & I. B. Weiner (Eds.), *Handbook of psychology: Volume 11: Forensic Psychology* (2nd ed., pp. 440–472). John Wiley & Son, Inc.

Goldstein, K. (1939). The significance of special tests for diagnosis and prognosis in schizophrenia. *American Journal of Psychiatry*, *96*, 575–588.

Goldstein, K., & Scheerer, M. (1941). Abstract and concrete behavior: An experimental study with special tests. *Psychological Monographs*, *53*(2), i–151.

Gorham, D. R. (1956). Use of the proverb test for differentiating schizophrenics from normals. *Journal of Consulting Psychology*, *20*(6), 435–440.

Grebb, J. A., & Cancro, R. (1989). Schizophrenia: Clinical features. In J. I. Kaplan & B. J. Sadock (Eds.), *Synopsis of psychiatry: Behavioral sciences, clinical psychiatry* (Vol. 5, pp. 757–777). Williams & Wilkins.

Green, C. E., Freeman, D., Kuipers, E., Bebbington, P., Fowler, D., & Dunn, G. (2008). Measuring ideas of persecution and social reference: The Green, et al. Paranoid thought scales (GPTS). *Psychological Medicine*, *38*(1), 101–111.

Green, M. F., Kern, R. S., & Heaton, R. K. (2004). Longitudinal studies of cognition and functional outcome in schizophrenia: Implications for MATRICS. *Schizophrenia Research*, *72*(1), 41–51.

Grimby, A. (1993). Bereavement among elderly people: Grief reactions, post-bereavement hallucinations and quality of life. *Acta Psychiatrica Scandinavica*, *87*(1), 72–80.

Grimby, A. (1998). Hallucinations following the loss of a spouse: Common and normal events among the elderly. *Journal of Clinical Gerontology*, *4*, 65–74.

Grivel, M., Leong, W., Masucci, M. D., Altschuler, R. A., Arndt, L. Y., Redman, S. L., Yang, L. H., Brucato, G., & Girgis, R. R. (2018). Impact of lifetime traumatic experiences on suicidality and likelihood of conversion in a cohort of individuals at clinical high-risk for psychosis. *Schizophrenia Research*, *195*, 549–553.

Gross, G. (1969). Prodrome und Vorpostensyndrome schizophrener Erkrankungen. In G. Huber (Ed.), *Schizophrenie und Zyklothymie. Ergebnisse und Probleme* (pp. 177–187). Thieme.

Gross, G. (1989). The 'basic' symptoms of schizophrenia. *British Journal of Psychiatry*, *155*(Suppl. 7), 21–25.

Gross, G., Huber, G., Klosterkötter, J., & Linz, M. (1987). *Bonner Skala für die Beurteilung von Basissymptomen* (BSABS; Bonn Scale for the Assessment of Basic Symptoms). Springer.

Grover, S., Dua, D., Chakrabarti, S., & Avasthi, A. (2018). Factor analysis of symptom dimensions (psychotic, affective and obsessive compulsive symptoms) in schizophrenia. *Asian Journal of Psychiatry*, *38*, 72–77.

Gruenewald, J., Chermak, S., & Freilich, J. D. (2013). Distinguishing "loner" attacks from other domestic extremist violence: A comparison of far-right homicide incident and offender characteristics. *Criminology & Public Policy*, *12*(1), 65–91.

Hacker, D., Birchwood, M., Tudway, J., Meaden, A., & Amphlett, C. (2008). Acting on voices: Omnipotence, sources of threat, and safety-seeking behaviors. *British Journal of Clinical Psychology*, *47*(2), 201–213.

Haddock, G., McCarron, J., Tarriere, N., & Faragher, E. B. (1999). Scales to measure dimensions of hallucinations and delusions: The psychotic symptom rating scales (PSYRATS). *Psychological Medicine*, *29*(4), 879–889.

Haeffel, G. J., Jeronimus, B. F., Fisher, A. J., Kaiser, B. N., Weaver, L. J., Vargas, I., Goodson, J. T., Soyster, P. D., & Lu, W. (2022). The hierarchical taxonomy of psychopathology (HiTOP) is not an improvement over the DSM. *Clinical Psychological Science*, *10*(2), 285–290.

Hafkenscheid, A. (1993). Reliability of a standardized and expanded brief psychiatric rating scale: A replication study. *Acta Psychiatrica Scandinavia*, *88*, 305–310.

Häfner, H., Maurer, K., Löffler, W., Bustamante, S., Van der Heiden, W., Riecher-Rössler, A., & Nowotny, B. (1995). Onset and early course of schizophrenia. In *Search for the causes of schizophrenia: Volume III* (pp. 43–66). Springer.

Häfner, H., Maurer, K., Löffler, W., Fätkenheuer, B., Der Heiden, W. A., Riecher-Rössler, A., Behrens, S., & Gattaz, W. F. (1994). The epidemiology of early schizophrenia: Influence of age and gender on onset and early course. *The British Journal of Psychiatry*, *164*(S23), 29–38.

Häfner, H., Riecher-Rossler, A., Maurer, K., Fatkenheuer, B., & Löffler, W. (1992). First onset and early symptomatology of schizophrenia: A chapter of epidemiological and neurobiological research into age and sex differences. *European Archives of Psychiatry and Clinical Neuroscience*, *242*(2–3), 109–118.

Hamilton, M. (1960). A rating scale for depression. *Journal of Neurology, Neurosurgery, and Psychiatry*, *23*, 56–62.

Hanfmann, E., & Kasanin, J. (1942). *Conceptual thinking in schizophrenia*. Nervous and Mental Disease Publishing Co.

Hardy, K. V., & Mueser, K. T. (2017). Trauma, psychosis and posttraumatic stress disorder. *Frontiers in Psychiatry*, *8*, 314459.

Harrow, M., Grossman, L. S., Silverstein, M. L., Meltzer, H. Y., & Kettering, R. L. (1968). A elongitudinal study of thought disorder in manic patients. *Archives of General Psychiatry*, *43*(8), 781–785.

Harrow, M., Herbener, E. S., Shanklin, A., Jobe, T., Rattenbury, F., & Kaplan, F. J. (2004). Follow up of psychotic outpatients: Dimensions of delusions and work functioning in schizophrenia. *Schizophrenia Bulletin*, *30*(1), 147–161.

Harrow, M., Lanin-Kettering, I., & Miller, J. G. (1989). Impaired perspective and thought pathology in schizophrenic and psychotic disorders. *Schizophrenia Bulletin*, *15*(4), 605–623.

Harrow, M., & Quinlan, D. M. (1977). Is disordered thinking unique to schizophrenia? *Archives of general psychiatry*, *34*, 15–21.

Harrow, M., & Quinlan, D. M. (1985). *Disordered thinking and schizophrenic psychopathology*. Gardner Press.

Harty, M. K. (1986). Action language in the psychological test report. *Bulletin of the Menninger Clinic*, *50*, 456–463.

Harvey, P. D., & Neale, J. M. (1983). The specificity of thought disorder to schizophrenia: Research methods in their historical perspective. *Progress in Experimental Personality Research*, *12*, 153–180.

Hassibi, M., & Breuer, H. (1980). *Disordered thinking and communication in children*. Springer.

Havens, L. (1996). *A safe place* laying-the-groundwork-of-psychotherapy. Harvard University Press.

Hawton, K., Sutton, L., Haw, C., Sinclair, J., & Deeks, J. J. (2005). Schizophrenia and suicide: Systematic review of risk factors. *British Journal of Psychiatry*, *187*, 9–20.

Heckers, S., Barch, D. M., Bustillo, J., Gaebel, W., Gur, R., Malaspina, D., Owen, M. J., Schultz, S., Tandon, R., Tsuang, M., van Os, J., & Carpenter, W. (2013). Structure of the psychotic disorders classification in DSM-5. *Schizophrenia Research*, *150*(1), 11–14.

Hedlund, J. L., & Vieweg, B. W. (1980). The brief psychiatric rating scale (BPRS): A comprehensive review. *Journal of Operational Psychiatry*, *11*, 48–65.

Heinrichs, R. W., Goldberg, J. O., Miles, A. A., & McDermid Vaz, S. (2008). Predictors of medication competence in schizophrenia patients. *Psychiatry Research*, *157*(1), 47–52.

Heinrichs, R. W., Miles, A. A., Ammari, N., & Muharib, E. (2013). Cognition as a central illness feature in schizophrenia. *Cognitive Impairment in Schizophrenia: Characteristics, Assessment and Treatment*, 1–23.

Heinz, A., & Schlagenhauf, F. (2010). Dopaminergic dysfunction in schizophrenia: Salience attribution revisited. *Schizophrenia Bulletin*, *36*(3), 472–485.

Hobart, M. P., Bratko, J. J., & Gold, J. M. (1999). Repeatable battery for the assessment of neuropsychological status as a screening test in schizophrenia, II: Convergent/discriminant validity and diagnostic group comparisons. *American Journal of Psychiatry*, *156*, 1951–1957.

Hoff, P. (2006). Delusion in general and forensic psychiatry—historical and contemporary aspects. *Behavioral Sciences & the Law*, *24*(3), 241–255.

Hoffman, D. D. (2012). The Construction of visual reality. In J. D. Bloom & I. E. C. Sommer (Eds.), *Hallucinations–research and practice* (pp. 7–15). Springer.

Hoffman, R. E., Gueorguieva, R., Hawkins, K. A., Varanko, M., Boutros, N. N., Wu, Y. T., Carroll, K., & Krystal, J. H. (2005). Temporoparietal transcranial magnetic stimulation for auditory hallucinations: Safety, efficacy and moderators in a fifty patient sample. *Biological Psychiatry*, *58*(2), 97–104.

Hoffman, R. E., Hawkins, K. A., Gueorguieva, R., Boutros, N. N., Rachid, F., Carroll, K., & Krystal, J. H. (2003). Transcranial magnetic stimulation of left temporoparietal cortex and medication-resistant auditory hallucinations. *Archives of General Psychiatry*, *60*(1), 49–56.

Holzman, P. S., Levy, D. L., & Johnston, M. H. (2005). The use of the Rorschach technique for assessing formal thought disorder. In R. F. Bornstein & J. M. Masling (Eds.), *Scoring the Rorschach – seven validated systems*. Routledge.

Holzman, P. S., Shenton, M. E., & Solovay, M. R. (1986). Quality of thought disorder in differential diagnosis. *Schizophrenia Bulletin*, *12*(3), 360–371.

Hor, K., & Taylor, M. (2010). Suicide and schizophrenia: A systematic review of rates and risk factors. *Journal of Psychopharmacology*, *24*(Suppl. 4), 81–90.

Horan, W. P., Kring, A. M., Gur, R. E., Reise, S. P., & Blanchard, J. J. (2011). Development and psychometric validation of the clinical assessment interview for negative symptoms (CAINS). *Schizophrenia Bulletin*, *132*, 140–145.

Horgan, J. (2005). The social and psychological characteristics of terrorism and terrorists. In *Root causes of terrorism: Myths, reality and ways forward* (pp. 44–53). Routledge.

Horgan, J. (2008). From profiles to pathways and roots to routes: Perspectives from psychology on radicalization into terrorism. *The ANNALS of the American Academy of Political and Social Science*, *618*(1), 80–94.

Hotchner, A. E. (2011, July 2). Hemingway, hounded by the feds. *The New York Times*, p. A19.

House, E. M., & Tyson, J. W. (Eds.). (2020). Psychosis in children and adolescents: A guide for clinicians. *An Issue of Child & Adolescent Psychiatric Clinics of North America*, *29*(1).

Huang, X., Fox, K. R., Ribeiro, J. D., & Franklin, J. C. (2018). Psychosis as a risk factor for suicidal thoughts and behaviors: A meta-analysis of longitudinal studies. *Psychological Medicine*, *48*(5), 765–776.

Huguelet, P., Mohr, S., Jung, V., Gillieron, C., Brandt, P. Y., & Borras, L. (2007). Effects of religion on suicide attempts in outpatients with schizophrenia or schizo-affective disorders compared with inpatients with non-psychotic disorders. *European Psychiatry*, *22*(3), 188–194.

Humpston, C. S. (2014). Perplexity and meaning: Toward a phenomenological 'core' of psychotic experiences. *Schizophrenia Bulletin*, *40*(2), 240–243.

Hunsley, J., & Mash, E. J. (2008). *A guide to assessments that work*. Oxford University Press.

Hurt, S. S., Holzman, P. S., & Davis, J. M. (1983). Thought disorder: The measurement of its changes. *Archives of General Psychiatry*, *40*, 1281–1285.

Illonen, T., Heinimaa, M., Korkeila, J., Svirskis, T., & Salokangas, R. K. R. (2010). Differentiating adolescents at clinical high risk for psychosis from psychotic and non-psychotic patients with the Rorschach. *Psychiatry Research*, *179*, 151–156.

Inoue, N., Yorozuya, Y., & Mizuno, M. (2014). *Identifying comorbidities of patients at ultra-high risk for psychosis using the Rorschach Comprehensive System*. Paper presented at the XXI International Congress of Rorschach and Projective Methods.

Ising, H. K., Veling, W., Loewy, R. L., Rietveld, M. W., Rietdijk, J., Dragt, S., Klaassen, R. M., Nieman, D. H., Wunderlink, L., Linszen, D. H., & van der Graag, M. (2012). The validity of the 16-item version of the prodromal questionnaire (PQ-16) to screen for ultra high risk of developing psychosis in the general help seeking population. *Schizophrenia Bulletin*, *38*(6), 1288–1296.

Jacobs, D. G., & Brewer, M. L. (2006). Application of the APA practice guidelines on suicide to clinical practice. *CNS Spectrums*, *11*(6), 447–454.

Jaeger, J., Bitter, I., Czobor, P., & Volavka, J. (1990). The measurement of subjective experience in schizophrenia: The subjective deficit syndrome scale. *Comprehensive Psychiatry*, *31*, 216–226.

Jaspers, K. (1913). *Allgemeine psychopathologie*. Springer.

Jaspers, K. (1963). *General psychopathology* (7th ed., J. Hoenig & M. W. Hamilton, Trans.). Manchester University Press.

Jeffries, J. J. (1977). The trauma of being psychotic: A neglected element in the management of chronic schizophrenia? *The Canadian Psychiatric Association Journal/La Revue de l'Association des Psychiatres du Canada*, *22*(5), 199–206.

Jenkins, S. R. (2023). Thematic apperception test (TAT) and other narrative assessments of bipolar spectrum disorders. In J. H. Kleiger & I. B. Weiner (Eds.), *The psychological assessment of bipolar spectrum disorders* (pp. 155–170). American Psychological Association.

Johnson, D. L. (2010). *A compendium of psychological measures*. Springer Publishing Company.

Johnston, M. H., & Holzman, P. S. (1979). *Assessing schizophrenic thinking*. Jossey-Bass.

Jones, S. R. (2010). Do we need multiple models of auditory verbal hallucinations? Examining the phenomenological fit of cognitive and neurological models. *Schizophrenia Bulletin*, *36*(3), 566–575.

Junginger, J. (2006). "Stereotypic" delusional offending. *Behavioral Sciences & the Law*, *24*(3), 295–311.

Kampman, O., Laippala, P., Vaanahen, J., Koivisto, E., Kiviniemi, P., Kilkku, N., & Lehtinen, K. (2002). Indicators of medication-compliance in first episode psychosis. *Psychiatry Research*, *110*(1), 39–48.

Kane, J. M., & Smith, J. M. (1982). Tardive dyskinesia: Prevalence and risk factors. *Archives of General Psychiatry*, *39*, 473–481.

Kaney, S., & Bentall, R. P. (1989). Persecutory delusions and attributional style. *British Journal of Medical Psychology*, *62*(2), 191–198.

Kaney, S., Bowen-Jones, K., Dewey, M. E., & Bentall, R. P. (1997). Two predictions about paranoid ideation: Deluded, depressed and normal participants' subjective frequency and consensus judgments for positive, neutral and negative events. *British Journal of Clinical Psychology*, *36*(3), 349–364.

Kapur, S. (2003). Psychosis as a state of aberrant salience: A framework linking biology, phenomenology, and pharmacology in schizophrenia. *American Journal of Psychiatry*, *160*(1), 13–23.

Karcher, N. R., Barch, D. M., Avenevoli, S., Savill, M., Huber, R. H., Simon, T. J., Leckliter, I. N., Sher, K. J., & Loewry, R. L. (2018). Assessment of the prodromal questionnaire–brief child version for measurement of self-reported psychoticlike experiences in childhood. *JAMA, Psychiatry*, *75*, 853–861. https://doi.org/10.1001/jamapsychiatry.2018.1334

Kasanin, J. (1933). The acute schizoaffective psychosis. *American Journal of Psychiatry*, *90*(1), 97–126.

Kaufman, J., Birmaher, B., Brent, D., Rao, U., Flynn, C., Moreci, P., Williamson, D., & Ryan, N. (2000). Schedule for affective disorders and schizophrenia for school-aged children present and lifetime version (K-SADS-PL): Initial reliability and validity data. *Journal of the American Academy of Child and Adolescent Psychiatry*, *36*, 980–988.

Kay, S. R., Fiszbein, A., & Opler, L. A. (1987). The positive and negative syndrome scale (PANSS) for schizophrenia. *Schizophrenia Bulletin*, *13*(2), 261–276.

Kay, S. R., Opler, L. A., Spitzer, R. L., Williams, J. B., Fiszbein, A., & Gorelick, A. (1991). SCID-PANSS: Two-tier diagnostic system for psychotic disorders. *Comprehensive Psychiatry*, *32*(4), 355–361.

Keefe, R. S., Poe, M., Walker, T. M., Kang, J. W., & Harvey, P. D. (2006). The schizophrenia cognition rating scale: An interview-based assessment and its relationship to cognition, real-world functioning, and functional capacity. *American Journal of Psychiatry*, *163*, 426.

Keers, R., Ullrich, S., DeStavola, B., & Coid, J. W. (2014). Association of violence with emergence of persecutory delusions in untreated schizophrenia. *American Journal of Psychiatry*, *171*(3), 332–339.

Kelly, J., & Murray, R. M. (2000). What risk factors tell us about the causes of schizophrenia and related psychoses. *Current Psychiatry Reports*, *2*(5), 378–385.

Kemp, R. A., & Lambert, T. J. (1995). Insight in schizophrenia and its relationship to psychopathology. *Schizophrenia Research*, *18*(1), 21–28.

Kendell, R. E. (1986). What are mental disorders? In A. M. Freedman, R. Brotman, I. Silverman, & D. Hutson (Eds.), *Issues in psychiatric classification: Science and social policy* (pp. 23–45). Human Science Press.

Kendler, K. S. (1990). Toward a scientific psychiatric nosology – Strengths and limitations. *Archives of General Psychiatry*, *47*(10), 969–973.

Kendler, K. S., Glazer, W. M., & Morgenstern, H. (1983). Dimensions of delusional experience. *American Journal of Psychiatry*, *140*, 466–469.

Kendler, K. S., Lieberman, J. A., & Walsh, D. (1989). The structured interview for Schizotypy (SIS): A preliminary report. *Schizophrenia Bulletin, 15*, 559–571.

Kennedy, L., Brucato, G., Lundgren, B., Califano, A., Dishy, G., Hesson, H., Masucci, M. D., Pia, T., Goldberg, P. H., Xu, Q., & Wall, M. M. (2021). Thematic content of obsessive and compulsive symptoms and conversion to psychosis in a clinical high-risk cohort. *Early Intervention in Psychiatry, 15*(5), 1423–1428.

Khadivi, A. (2017). The Rorschach in the differential diagnosis of psychotic conditions. In R. E. Erard & F. B. Evans (Eds.), *The Rorschach in multi-method forensic assessment*. Routledge.

Khadivi, A. (2021). Clinical Interview methods. In I. B. Weiner & J. H. Kleiger (Eds.), *Psychological assessment of disordered thinking and perception*. American Psychological Association Press.

Khadivi, A. (2023). Clinical interview methods. In J. H. Kleiger & I. B. Weiner (Eds.), *Psychological assessment of bipolar spectrum disorders*. American Psychological Association Press.

Khadivi, A., Wetzler, S., & Wilson, A. (1997). Manic indices on the Rorschach. *Journal of Personality Assessment, 69*, 365–375.

Killaspy, H., White, S., Lalvani, N., Berg, R., Thachil, A., Kallumpuram, S., Nasiruddin, O., Wright, C., & Mezey, G. (2014). The impact of psychosis on social inclusion and associated factors. *International Journal of Social Psychiatry, 60*(2), 148–154.

Kim, Y., Sakamoto, K., Kamo, T., Sakamura, Y., & Miyaoka, H. (1997). Insight and clinical correlates in schizophrenia. *Comprehensive Psychiatry, 38*(2), 117–123.

Kimhy, D., Corcoran, C., Harkavy-Friedman, J. M., Ritzler, B., Javitt, D. C., & Malaspina, D. (2007). Visual form perception: A comparison of individuals at high risk for psychosis, recent onset schizophrenia and chronic schizophrenia. *Schizophrenia Research, 97*, 25–34.

Kircher, T., Krug, A., Stratmann, M., Ghazi, S., Schales, C., Frauenheim, M., Turner, L., Fährmann, P., Hornig, T., Katzev, M., Grosvald, M., Müller-Isberner, R., & Nagels, A. (2014). A rating scale for the assessment of objective and subjective formal Thought and Language Disorder (TALD). *Schizophrenia Research*, 160(1–3), 216–221.

Kirkpatrick, B. (2014). Progress in the study of negative symptoms. *Schizophrenia Bulletin, 40*(Suppl. 2), S101–S106.

Kirkpatrick, B., Buchanan, R. W., McKenney, P. D., Alphs, L. D., & Carpenter, S. T. (1989). The schedule for the deficit syndrome: An instrument for research in schizophrenia. *Psychiatry Research* (30), 119–123.

Kirkpatrick, B., Strauss, G. P., Nguyen, L., Fischer, B. A., Daniel, D. G., Cienfuegos, A., & Marder, S. R. (2011). The brief negative symptoms scale: Psychometric properties. *Schizophrenia Bulletin, 37*(2), 300–305.

Kleiger, J. H. (1999). *Disordered thinking and the Rorschach*. The Analytic Press.

Kleiger, J. H. (2000). Projective testing with children and adolescents. In M. Roberts & G. Walker (Eds.), *The handbook of child clinical psychology*. Wiley.

Kleiger, J. H. (2003). Disordered thinking and projective testing. In M. Hilsenroth & D. Segal (Eds.), *The handbook of projective psychological assessment*. Wiley & Sons.

Kleiger, J. H. (2017). *Rorschach assessment of psychotic phenomena*. Routledge.

Kleiger, J. H. (2023). Rating scales and screening assessment of bipolar spectrum disorders. In J. H. Kleiger & I. B. Weiner (Eds.), *The psychological assessment of bipolar spectrum disorders* (pp. 107–122). APA.

Kleiger, J. H., & Mihura, J. L. (2021). Developments in the Rorschach assessment of disordered thinking and communication. *Rorschachiana*, *42*(2), 265–280. https://doi.org/10.1027/1192-5604/a000132

Kleiger, J. H., & Weiner, I. B. (2023). *Psychological assessment of bipolar spectrum disorders*. American Psychological Association.

Klosterkötter, J., Gross, G., Huber, G., Wienke, A., Steinmeyer, E. M., & Schultze-Lutter, F. (1997). Evaluation of the 'Bonn scale for the assessment of basic symptoms – BSABS' as an instrument for the assessment of schizophrenia proneness: A review of recent findings. *Neurology, Psychiatry and Brain Research*, *51*, 137–150.

Klosterkötter, J., Hellmich, M., Steinmeyer, E. M., & Schultze-Lutter, F. (2001). Diagnosing schizophrenia in the initial prodromal phase. *Archives of General Psychiatry*, *58*, 158–164.

Kodish, I., & McClellan, J. (2008). Early onset schizophrenia. In M. Hersen & D. Reitman (Eds.), *Handbook of psychological assessment, case conceptualization, and treatment, children and adolescents* ((Vol. 2, pp. 405–443). John Wiley & Sons.

Koenen, K. C., Moffitt, T. E., Roberts, A. L., Martin, L. T., Kubzansky, L., Harrington, H., Poulton, R., & Caspi, A. (2009). Childhood IQ and adult mental disorders: A test of the cognitive reserve hypothesis. *American Journal of Psychiatry*, *166*(1), 50–57.

Konings, M., Bak, M., Hanssen, M., van Os, J., & Krabbendam, L. (2006). Validity and reliability of the CAPE: A self-report instrument for the measurement of psychotic experiences in the general population. *Acta Psychiatrica Scandinavia*, *114*(1), 55–61.

Kotov, R., Cicero, D. C., Conway, C. C., DeYoung, C. G., Dombrovski, A., Eaton, N. R., First, M. B., Forbes, M. K., Hyman, S. E., Jonas, K. G., Krueger, R. F., Latzman, R. D., Li, J. J., Nelson, B. d., Regier, d., A., Rodriguez,-Seijas, C., Ruggero, C. J., Simms, L. J., Skodol, A. E., Waldman, I. d., Waszczuk, M. a., Watson, D., Widiger, T. a., Wilson, S., & Wright, A. G. C. (2022). The hierarchical taxonomy of psychopathology (HiTOP) in psychiatric practice and research. *Psychological Medicine*, *52*(9), 1666–1678.

Kotov, R., Foti, D., Li, K., Bromet, E. J., Hajcak, G., & Ruggero, C. J. (2016). Validating dimensions of psychosis symptomatology: Neural correlates and 20-year outcomes. *Journal of Abnormal Psychology*, *125*(8), 1103.

Kotov, R., Krueger, R. F., Watson, D., Achenbach, T. M., Althoff, R. R., Bagby, R. M., Kotov, R., Krueger, R. F., Watson, D., Achenbach, T. M., Althoff, R. R., Bagby, R. M., Brown, T. A., Carpenter, W. T., Caspi, A., Clark, L. A., Eaton, N. R., Forbes, M. K., Forbush, K. T., Goldberg, D., Hasin, D., Hyman, S. E., Ivanova, M. Y., Lynam, D. R., Markon, K., . . . Zimmerman, M. (2017). The hierarchical taxonomy of psychopathology (HiTOP): A dimensional alternative to traditional nosologies. *Journal of Abnormal Psychology*, *126*(4), 454.

Kraepelin, E. (1896). *Dementia praecox and paraphrenia*. Chicago Medical Book Co.

Kraepelin, E. (1921). Manic-depressive insanity and paranoia. In R. M. Barclay (Trans.), *Text-book of psychiatry*. E&S Livingstone.

Kruh, I., & Grisso, T. (2009). *Juveniles' competence to stand trial*. Oxford University Press.

Ksir, C., & Hart, C. L. (2016). Cannabis and psychosis: A critical overview of the relationship. *Current Psychiatry Reports*, *18*, 1–11.

Kumra, S., Jacobsen, L. K., Lenane, M., Zahn, T. P., Wiggs, E., Alaghband-Rad, J., Castellanos, F. X., Frazier, J. A., McKenna, K., Gordon, C. T., Smith, A., Hamburger, S., & Rapoport, J. L. (1998). 'Multidimensionally impaired disorder': Is it a variant of very early-onset schizophrenia? *Journal of the American Academy of Child and Adolescent Psychiatry*, *37*, 91–99.

Kwapil, T. R., Barrantes-Vidal, N., & Silvia, P. T. (2008). The dimensional structure of the Wisconsin Schizotypy scales: Factor identification and construct validity. *Schizophrenia Bulletin*, *34*(3), 444–457.

Kwapil, T. R., Chapman, L. J., & Chapman, J. (1999). Validity and usefulness of the Wisconsin manual for assessing psychotic-like experiences. *Schizophrenia Bulletin*, *22*(2), 371–382.

Lacoua, L., Koren, D., & Rothschild-Yakar, L. (2014). *The Rorschach and risk for psychosis: A correlational study among non-psychotic, hon-help seeking adolescents from the community*. Poster presented at the XXI International Congress of Rorschach and Projective Methods, Istanbul, TR.

Lacro, J. P., Dunn, L. B., Dolder, C. R., Leckband, S. G., & Jeste, D. V. (2002). Prevalence of and risk factors for medication nonadherence in patients with schizophrenia: A comprehensive review of recent literature. *The Journal of Clinical Psychiatry*, *63*(10), 892–909.

Lampshire, D. (2012). The sounds of a wounded world. In J. Geekie, P. Randal, D. Lampshire, & J. Read (Eds.), *Experiencing psychosis: Personal and professional perspectives* (pp. 139–145). Routledge.

Langdon, R., Michie, P. T., Ward, P. B., McConaghy, N., Catts, S. V., & Coltheart, M. (1997). Defective self and/or other mentalising in schizophrenia: A cognitive neuropsychological approach. *Cognitive Neuropsychiatry*, *2*(3), 167–193.

Langfeldt, G. (1960). Diagnosis and prognosis of schizophrenia. *Proceedings of the Royal Society of Medicine*, *53*, 1047–1052.

Large, M. M., & Nielssen, O. (2011). Violence in first-episode psychosis: A systematic review and meta-analysis. *Schizophrenia Research*, *125*, 209–220.

Large, M. M., Smith, G., & Nielssen, O. (2009). The relationship between the rate of homicide by those with schizophrenia and the overall homicide rate: A systematic review and meta-analysis. *Schizophrenia Research*, *112*, 123–129.

Larkin, W., & Morrison, A. P. (2006). *Trauma and psychosis: New directions for theory and therapy*. Routledge.

Larøi, F. (2006). The phenomenological diversity of hallucinations: Some theoretical and clinical implications. *Psychologica Belgica*, *46*(1–2), 163–183.

Larøi, F., & Aleman, A. (2010). *Hallucinations – A practical guide to treatment and management*. Oxford University Press.

Larøi, F., Luhrmann, T. M., Bell, V., Christian, W. A., Jr, Deshpande, S., Fernyhough, C., Jenkins, J., & Woods, A. (2014). Culture and hallucinations:

Overview and future directions. *Schizophrenia Bulletin*, *40*(Suppl. 4), S213–S220. https://doi.org/10.1093/schbul/sbu012

Larøi, F., Sommer, I. E., Blom, J. D., Fernyhough, C., Hugdahl, K., Johns, L. C., McCarthy-Jones, S., Preti, A., Raballo, A., Slotema, C. W., Stephane, M., & Waters, F. (2012). The characteristic features of auditory verbal hallucinations in clinical and nonclinical groups: State-of-the-art overview and future directions. *Schizophrenia Bulletin*, *38*(4), 724–733.

Launay, G., & Slade, P. D. (1981). The measurement of hallucinatory predisposition in male and female prisoners. *Personality and Individual Differences*, *2*, 221–234.

Lawrie, S. M. (2016). Whether "psychosis" is best conceptualized as a continuum or in categories is an empirical, practical and political question. *World Psychiatry*, *15*(2), 125.

Lawrie, S. M., Hall, J., McIntosh, A. M., Owens, D. G., & Johnstone, E. C. (2010). The 'continuum of psychosis': Scientifically unproven and clinically impractical. *The British Journal of Psychiatry*, *197*(6), 423–425.

Lehembre-Shiah, E., Leong, W., Brucato, G., Abi-Dargham, A., Lieberman, J. A., Horga, G., & Girgis, R. R. (2017). Distinct relationships between visual and auditory perceptual abnormalities and conversion to psychosis in a clinical high-risk population. *JAMA Psychiatry*, *74*(1), 104–106.

Lewis, D. A. (1934). The psychopathology of insight. *British Journal of Medical Psychology*, *14*, 332–348.

Lewis, D. A., & Lieberman, J. A. (2000). Catching up on schizophrenia: Natural history and neurobiology. *Neuron*, *28*(2), 325–334.

Lewis-Fernández, R., & Díaz, N. (2002). The cultural formulation: A method for assessing cultural factors affecting the clinical encounter. *Psychiatry Quarterly*, *73*(4), 27–295.

Liddle, P. F. (1987). The symptoms of chronic schizophrenia: A re-examination of the positive-negative dichotomy. *The British Journal of Psychiatry*, *151*(2), 145–151.

Liddle, P. F. (2019). The core deficit of classical schizophrenia: Implications for predicting the functional outcome of psychotic illness and developing effective treatments. *The Canadian Journal of Psychiatry*, *64*(10), 680–685.

Liddle, P. F., Ngan, E. T. C., Caissie, S. L., &erson, C. M., Bates, A. T., Quested, D. J., White, R., & Weg, R. (2002). Thought and language index: An instrument for assessing thought and language in schizophrenia. *The British Journal of Psychiatry*, *181*(4), 326–330.

Liddle, P. F., Ngan, E. T. C., Duffield, G., Kho, K., & Warren, A. (2002). Signs and symptoms of psychotic illness (SSPI): A rating scale. *The British Journal of Psychiatry*, *108*, 45–50.

Liemburg, E. J., van der Meer, L., Swart, M., Curcic-Blake, B., Bruggeman, R., Knegtering, H., & Aleman, A. (2012). Reduced connectivity in the self-processing network of schizophrenia patients with poor insight. *PloS One*, *7*(8), e42707.

Lin, A., Wood, S. J., Nelson, B., Beavan, A., McGorry, P., & Yung, A. R. (2015). Outcomes of nontransitioned cases in a sample at ultra-high risk for psychosis. *American Journal of Psychiatry*, *172*(3), 249–258.

Link, B. G., & Stueve, A. S. (1994). Psychotic symptoms and the violent/illegal behavior of mental patients compared to the community. In J. Monahan & H. Steadman (Eds.), *Violence and mental disorder: Development in risk assessment* (pp. 137–158). University of Chicago Press.

Link, B. G., Stueve, A. S., & Phelan, J. (1998). Psychotic symptoms and violent behaviors: Probing the components of 'threat/control-override' symptoms. *Social Psychiatry & Psychiatric Epidemiology*, *33*, S55–S60.

Linscott, R. J., & van Os, J. (2013). An updated and conservative systematic review and meta-analysis of epidemiological evidence on psychotic experiences in children and adults: On the pathway from proneness to persistence to dimensional expression across mental disorders. *Psychological Medicine*, *43*(6), 1133–1149. https://doi.org/10.1017/S0033291712001626

Liraud, F., Droulout, T., Parrot, M., & Verdoux, H. (2004). Agreement between self-rated and clinically assessed symptoms in subjects with psychosis. *Journal of Nervous and Mental Disease*, *192*(5), 352–356.

Loebel, A. D., Lieberman, J. A., Alvir, J. M. J., Mayerhoff, D. I., Geisler, S. H., & Szymanski, S. R. (1992). Duration of psychosis and outcome in first episode schizophrenia. *American Journal of Psychiatry*, *149*, 183–1188.

Loewy, R. L., Bearden, C. E., Johnson, J. K., Raine, A., & Cannon, T. D. (2005). The prodromal questionnaire (PQ): Preliminary validation of a self-report screening measure for prodromal and psychotic syndromes. *Schizophrenia Research*, *77/79*(1), 117–125, 141–149.

Long, J. D., & Brekke, J. S. (1999). Longitudinal factor structure of the brief psychiatric rating scale in schizophrenia. *Psychological Assessment*, *11*, 498–506.

Longden, E. (2012). Negative symptoms: More not less. In J. Geekie, P. Randal, D. Lampshire, & J. Read (Eds.), *Experiencing psychosis: Personal and professional perspectives* (pp. 179–186). Routledge.

Lukoff, D., Nuechterlein, K., & Ventura, A. (1986). Manual for the expanded brief psychiatric rating scale. *Schizophrenia Bulletin*, *13*, 261–276.

Luria, R. E., & Berry, R. (1979). Reliability and descriptive validity of the PSE syndromes. *Archives of General Psychiatry*, *36*, 1187–1195.

Lysaker, P. H., & Bell, M. (1994). Insight and cognitive impairment in schizophrenia performance on repeated administrations of the Wisconsin card sorting test. *The Journal of Nervous and Mental Disease*, *182*(11), 656–660.

Lysaker, P. H., Bryson, G. J., & Bell, M. D. (2002). Insight and work performance in schizophrenia. *The Journal of Nervous and Mental Disease*, *190*(3), 142–146.

Lysaker, P. H., Buck, K. D., Salvatore, G., Popolo, R., & Dimaggio, G. (2009). Lack of awareness of illness in schizophrenia: Conceptualizations, correlates and treatment approaches. *Expert Review of Neurotherapeutics*, *9*(7), 1035–1043.

MacKinnon, A., Copolov, D. L., & Trauer, T. (2004). Factors associated with compliance and resistance to command hallucinations. *The Journal of Nervous and Mental Disease*, *192*(5), 357–362.

Mantere, O., Suominen, K., Valtonen, H. M., Arvilommi, P., & Isometsä, E. (2008). Only half of bipolar I and II patients report prodromal symptoms. *Journal of Affective Disorders*, *111*(2), 366–371.

Marantz, A. (2013, September 16). Unreality Star. *The New Yorker*, 32.

Marengo, J. T., & Harrow, M. (1985). Thought disorder: A function of schizophrenia, mania, or psychosis? *The Journal of Nervous and Mental Disease*, *173*(1), 35–41.

Marengo, J. T., Lanin-Kettering, I., & Wilson, A. (1986). Evaluating bizarre-idiosyncratic thinking: A comprehensive index of positive thought disorder. *Schizophrenia Bulletin*, *12*, 497–511.

Margaro, P. A. (1981). The paranoid and schizophrenic: The case for distinctive cognitive style. *Schizophrenia Bulletin*, *7*, 632–661.

Maris, R. W. (2019). *Suicidology: A comprehensive biopsychosocial perspective*. The Guilford Press.

Marková, I. S. (2005). *Insight in psychiatry*. Cambridge University Press.

Marková, I. S., & Berrios, G. E. (1992). The assessment of insight in clinical psychiatry: A new scale. *Acta Psychiatrica Scandinavia*, *186*, 1185–1188.

Marshall, M., Lewis, S., Lockwood, A., Drake, R., Jones, P., & Croudace, T. (2005). Association between duration and untreated psychosis and outcome in cohorts of first episode patients – A systematic review. *Archives of General Psychiatry*, *62*, 975–983.

Masi, G., Mucci, M., & Pari, C. (2006). Children with Schizophrenia. *CNS Drugs, 20*(10), 841–866.

Matheson, S. L., Shepherd, A. M., Pinchbeck, R. M., Laurens, K. R., & Carr, V. J. (2013). Childhood adversity in schizophrenia: A systematic meta-analysis. *Psychological Medicine*, *4*(2), 225–238.

Mazza, M., De Risio, A., Surian, L., Roncone, R., & Casacchia, M. (2001). Selective impairments of theory of mind in people with schizophrenia. *Schizophrenia Research*, *47*(2), 299–308.

McCarthy-Jones, S., & Resnick, P. J. (2014). Listening to voices: the use of phenomenology to differentiate malingered from genuine auditory verbal hallucinations. *International Journal of Law and Psychiatry*, *37*(2), 183–189.

McCarthy-Jones, S., Trauer, T., Mackinnon, A., Sims, E., Thomas, N., & Copolov, D. L. (2014). A new phenomenological survey of auditory hallucinations: Evidence for subtypes and implications for theory and practice. *Schizophrenia Bulletin*, *40*(1), 231–235.

McClellan, J., & Werry, J. (2001). Practice parameter for the assessment and treatment of children and adolescents with schizophrenia. *Journal of the American Academy of Child and Adolescent Psychiatry*, *40*(Suppl. 7), 4S–23S.

McClure, M. M., Bowie, C. R., Leung, W. L., Siever, L. J., & Harvey, P. D. (2007). Functional capacity in schizotypal personality disorder: Evidence of impaired performance across the schizophrenia spectrum. *Schizophrenia Bulletin*, *33*(2), *596–597.*

McClure, M. M., Bowie, C. R., Patterson, T. L., Heaton, R. K., Weaver, C., Anderson, H., & Harvey, P. D. (2007). Correlations of functional capacity and neuropsychological performance in older patients with schizophrenia: Evidence for specificity of relationships? *Schizophrenia Research*, *89*(1), 330–338.

McCredie, M. N., Hopwood, C. J., & Morey, L. C. (2021). Personality assessment inventory (PAI) for assessing disordered thinking and perception. In

I. B. Weiner & J. H. Kleiger (Eds.), *The psychological assessment of disordered thinking and perception* (pp. 79–98). American Psychological Association.

McCredie, M. N., Hopwood, C. J., & Morey, L. C. (2023). Personality assessment inventory (PAI) assessment of bipolar spectrum disorders. In J. H. Kleiger & I. B. Weiner (Eds.), *Psychological assessment of bipolar spectrum disorders* (pp. 63–78). American Psychological Association. https://doi.org/10.1037/0000356-005

McEvoy, J. P., Aland, J., & Wilson, W. H. (1981). Measuring chronic schizophrenic patients' attitudes towards their illness and treatment. *Hospital and Community Psychiatry*, *32*, 856–858.

McEvoy, J. P., Apperson, L. J., Appelbaum, P. S., Ortlip, P., Brecosky, J., Hammill, K., Geller, J., & Roth, L. (1989). Insight in schizophrenia: Its relationship to acute psychopathology. *The Journal of Nervous and Mental Disease*, *177*(1), 43–47.

McGhie, A., & Chapman, J. (1961). Disorders of attention and perception in early schizophrenia. *British Journal of Medical Psychology*, *34*, 103–116.

McGlashan, T. H., & Carpenter, W. T. Jr. (1979). Affective symptoms and the diagnosis of schizophrenia. *Schizophrenia Bulletin*, *5*(4), 547–553.

McGlashan, T. H., & Fenton, W. S. (1993). Subtype progression and pathophysiologic deterioration in early schizophrenia. *Schizophrenia Bulletin*, *19*(1), 71–84.

McGlashan, T. H., Miller, T. J., Woods, S. W., Hoffman, R. E., & Davidson, L. (2001). A scale for the assessment of prodromal symptoms and states. In T. J. Miller, S. A. Mednick, T. H. McGlashan, J. Liberger, & J. O. Johannessen (Eds.), *Early intervention in psychotic disorders* (pp. 135–149). Kluwer Academic Publishers.

McGlashan, T. H., Walsh, B., & Woods, S. (2010). *The psychosis-risk syndrome: Handbook for diagnosis and follow-up*. Oxford University Press.

McKay, R., Langdon, R., & Coltheart, M. (2006). The persecutory ideation questionnaire. *Journal of Nervous and Mental Diseases*, *194*, 628–631.

Meehl, P. E. (1962). Schizotaxia, schizotypy, schizophrenia. *American Psychologist*, *17*(12), 827.

Meissner, W. W. (1981). The schizophrenic and the paranoid process. *Schizophrenia Bulletin*, *7*, 611–631.

Meloy, J. R., & Rahman, T. (2021). Cognitive-affective drivers of fixation in threat assessment. *Behavioral Sciences & the Law*, *39*(2), 170–189.

Mensi, M. M., Molteni, S., Iorio, M., Filosi, E., Ballante, E., Balottin, U., Fusar-Poli, P., & Borgatti, R. (2021). Prognostic accuracy of DSM-5 attenuated psychosis syndrome in adolescents: Prospective real-world 5-year cohort study. *Schizophrenia Bulletin*, *47*(6), 1663–1673.

Merritt, J., Tanguturi, Y., Fuchs, C., & Cundiff, A. W. (2020). Medical etiologies of secondary psychosis in children and adolescents. *Child and Adolescent Psychiatric Clinics*, *29*(1), 29–42.

Meyer, G. J., Erdberg, P., & Shaffer, T. (2007). Towards international normative reference data for the comprehensive system. *Journal of Personality Assessment*, *89*(Supp. 1), S201–S216.

Meyer, G. J., & Mihura, J. L. (2021). Rorschach performance assessment system (R-PAS) for assessing disordered thought and perception. In I. B. Weiner & J. H. Kleiger (Eds.), *Psychological assessment of disordered thinking and perception* (pp. 151–168). American Psychological Association.

Meyer, G. J., Viglione, D. J., Mihura, J. L., Erard, R. E., & Erdberg, P. (2012). *Rorschach performance assessment system: Administration, coding, interpretation, and technical manual.* Rorschach Performance Assessment System.

Meyers, B. S., English, J., Gabriele, M., Peasley-Miklus, C., Heo, M., Flint, A., Mulsant, B. H., Rothschild, A. J., & STOP-PD Study Group. (2006). A delusion assessment scale for psychotic major depression: Reliability, validity and utility. *Biological Psychiatry*, *60*, 1336–1342.

Michalakeas, A., Skoutas, C., Charalambous, A., Peristeris, A., Marinos, V., Keramari, E., & Theologou, A. (1994). Insight in schizophrenia and mood disorders and its relation to psychopathology. *Acta Psychiatrica Scandinavica*, *90*(1), 46–49.

Michel, P., Baumstarck, K., Auquier, P., Amador, X., Dumas, R., Fernandez, J., Lancon, C., & Boyer, L. (2013). Psychometric properties of the abbreviated version of the scale to assess unawareness in mental disorder in schizophrenia. *BMC Psychiatry*, *13*, 229.

Michels, R. (1984). First rebuttal. *American Journal of Psychiatry*, *141*(4), 548–551.

Mihura, J. L., Boyette, L.-L., Görner, K. J., Kleiger, J. H., Jowers, C. E., & Ales, F. (2023). *Helping HiTOP be the best it can be for conceptualizing psychosis: Requiring systematic review methodology and the correction of known errors* [Manuscript under review]. Department of Psychology, University of Toledo.

Mihura, J. L., Meyer, G. J., Dumitrascu, N., & Bombel, G. (2013). The validity of individual Rorschach variables: Systematic reviews and meta-analyses of the comprehensive system. *Psychological Bulletin*, *139*(3), 548–605.

Mihura, J. L., & Starin, M. (2023). An empirically informed framework for multimethod assessment with a focus on psychosis. In J. L. Mihura (Ed.), *The Oxford handbook of personality and psychopathology assessment* [Manuscript-in-progress]. Oxford University Press.

Miller, H. A. (2001). *M-FAST: Miller forensic assessment of symptom test professional manual.* Psychological Assessment Resources.

Miller, S. B. (1987). A comparison of methods of inquiry: Testing and interviewing contributions to the diagnostic process. *Bulletin of the Menninger Clinic*, *51*(6), 505–518.

Miller, T. J., & McGlashan, T. H. (2000). Early identification and intervention in psychotic illness. *Connecticut Medicine*, *64*, 339–341.

Miller, T. J., McGlashan, T. H., Rosen, J. L., Cadenhead, K., Ventura, J., McFarlane, W., Perkins, D. O., Pearlson, G. D., & Woods, S. (2003). Prodromal assessment with the structured interview for prodromal symptoms: Predictive validity, interrater reliability, and training to reliability. *Schizophrenia Bulletin*, *29*(4), 703–715.

Miller, T. J., McGlashan, T. H., Rosen, J. L., Somjee, L., Markovich, P. J., Stein, K., & Woods, S. W. (2002). Prospective diagnosis of the initial prodrome for schizophrenia based on the structured interview for prodromal syndromes:

Preliminary evidence of interrater reliability and predictive validity. *American Journal of Psychiatry*, *159*, 863–863.
Mintz, A. R., Dobson, K. S., & Romney, D. M. (2003). Insight in schizophrenia: A meta-analysis. *Schizophrenia Research*, *61*(1), 75–88.
Mitgang, H. (1983, March 11). Publishing F.B.I file on Hemingway. *New York Times on the Web*. http://www.nytimes.com/books/99/07/04/specials/hemingway-fbi.html.
Molnar, G., Feeney, M. G., & Fava, G. A. (1988). Duration and symptoms of bipolar prodromes. *The American Journal of Psychiatry*, *145*, 1576–1578.
Monahan, J., Steadman, H. J., Silver, E., Appelbaum, P. S., Robbins, P. C., Mulvey, E. P., Roth, L. H., Grisso, T., & Banks, S. (2001). *Rethinking risk assessment: The MacArthur study of mental disorder and violence*. Oxford University Press, Inc.
Montagnese, M., Leptourgos, P., Fernyhough, C., Waters, F., Larøi, F., Jardri, R., . . . Urwyler, P. (2021). A review of multimodal hallucinations: Categorization, assessment, theoretical perspectives, and clinical recommendations. *Schizophrenia Bulletin*, *47*(1), 237–248.
Moran, P. W., & Lambert, M. J. (1983). A review of current assessment tools for monitoring changes in depression. In M. S. Lambert, E. R. Christensen, & S. S. DeJulio (Eds.), *The assessment of psychotherapy outcome* (pp. 263–303). John Wiley & Sons.
Moreira-Almeida, A., & Cardeña, E. (2011). Differential diagnosis between non-pathological psychotic and spiritual experiences and mental disorder: A contribution from Latin American studies to the ICD-11. *Revista Brasileira de Psiquiatria*, *33*(Suppl. 1), S29–S36.
Morey, L. C. (1991). *The personality assessment inventory professional manual*. Psychological Assessment Resources.
Morgan, C., Dazzan, P., Lappin, J., Heslin, M., Donoghue, K., Fearon, P., Jones, P. B., Murray, R. M., Doody, G. A., & Reininghaus, U. (2022). Rethinking the course of psychotic disorders: Modelling long-term symptom trajectories. *Psychological Medicine*, *52*(13), 2641–2650.
Morgan, K. D., & David, A. S. (2004). Neuropsychological studies of insight in patients with psychotic disorders. In X. F. Amador & A. S. David (Eds.), *Insight and psychosis* (2nd ed., pp. 177–193. Oxford University Press.
Morrison, A. P., French, P., Walford, L., Lewis, S. W., Kilcommons, A., Green, J., Parker, S., & Bentall, R. (2004). Cognitive therapy for the prevention of psychosis in people at ultra-high risk: Randomised controlled trial. *British Journal of Psychiatry*, *185*, 291–297.
Morrison, A. P., Wells, A., & Nothard, S. (2000). Launay-slade hallucination scale – revised. *British Journal of Clinical Psychology*, *39*, 67–78.
Moskowitz, A., Read, J., Farrelly, S., Rudegeair, T., & Williams, O. (2009). Are psychotic symptoms traumatic in origin and dissociative in kind? In P. Dell & J. O'Neil (Eds.), *Dissociation and dissociative disorders: DSM-V and beyond*. Routledge.
Mueser, K. T., Curran, P. J., & McHugo, G. (1997). Factor structure of the brief psychiatric rating scale in schizophrenia. *Psychological Assessment*, *9*(3), 196–204.
Mueser, K. T., & McGurk, S. R. (2004). Schizophrenia. *Lancet*, *363*(9426), 2063–2072.

Mukherjee, S., Shukla, S., Woodle, J., Rosen, A. M., & Olarte, S. (1983). Misdiagnosis of schizophrenia in bipolar patients: A multiethnic comparison. *American Journal of Psychiatry*, *140*, 1571–1574.

Munro, A. (1995). The classification of delusional disorders. *Psychiatric Clinics of North America*, *18*(2), 199–212.

Murray, R. M., Englund, A., Abi-Dargham, A., Lewis, D. A., Di Forti, M., Davies, C., & D'Souza, D. C. (2017). Cannabis-associated psychosis: Neural substrate and clinical impact. *Neuropharmacology*, *124*, 89–104.

Nasreddine, Z. S., Phillips, N. A., Bedirian, V., Charbonneau, S., Whitehead, V., Collin, I., Cummings, J. L., & Chertkow, H. (2005). The montreal cognitive assessment, MoCA: A brief screening tool for mild cognitive impairment. *Journal of American Geriatric Society*, *53*(4), 695–699.

Nayani, T. H., & David, A. S. (1996). The auditory hallucination: A phenomenological survey. *Psychological Medicine*, *26*(1), 177–190.

Nichols, D. S. (2011). *Essentials of MMPI-2 assessment*. Wiley.

Nichols, D. S. (2021). Minnesota multiphasic personality inventory-2 (MMPI-2) for assessing disordered thinking and perception. In I. B. Weiner & J. H. Kleiger (Eds.), *The psychological assessment of disordered thinking and perception* (pp. 49–62). American Psychological Association Press.

Nichols, D. S., & Crowhurst, B. (2006). The use of the MMPI-2 in inpatient mental health settings. In J. N. Butcher (Ed.), *MMPI-2: The practitioner's handbook*. American Psychological Association.

Nickerson, R. S. (1998). Confirmation bias: A ubiquitous phenomenon in many guises. *Review of General Psychology*, *2*(2), 175.

Novak-Grubic, V., & Tavcar, R. (2002). Predictors of noncompliance in males with first-episode schizophrenia, schizophreniform and schizoaffective disorder. *European Psychiatry*, *17*(3), 148–154.

Nuechterlein, K. H., & Dawson, M. E. (1984). Information processing and attentional functioning in the developmental course of schizophrenic disorders. *Schizophrenia Bulletin*, *10*(2), 160–203.

Ohayon, M. M. (2000). Prevalence of hallucinations and their pathological associations in the general population. *Psychiatry Research*, *97*(2), 153–164.

Ohayon, M. M., Priest, R. G., Caulet, M., & Guilleminault, C. (1996). Hypnagogic and hypnopompic hallucinations: Pathological phenomena? *The British Journal of Psychiatry*, *169*(4), 459–467.

Olson, P. R., Suddeth, J. A., Peterson, P. J., & Egelhoff, C. (1985). Hallucinations of widowhood. *Journal of the American Geriatrics Society*, *33*(8), 543–547.

Oltmanns, T. F. (1998). Approaches to the definition and study of delusions. In T. F. Oltmanns & B. A. Maher (Eds.), *Delusional beliefs* (pp. 3–12). John Wiley & Sons.

Oltmanns, T. F., & Neale, J. M. (1978). Distractibility in relation to other aspects of schizophrenic disorder. In S. Schwartz (Ed.), *Language and cognition in Schizophrenia* (pp. 117–143). Lawrence Erlbaum Associates.

Oulis, P. G., Mavreas, V. G., Mamounas, J. M., & Stefanis, C. N. (1995). Clinical characteristics of auditory hallucinations. *Acta Psychiatrica Scandinavica*, *92*, 97–102.

Overall, J. E. (1974). The brief psychiatric rating scale in psychopharmacology research. In P. Pichot (Ed.), *Psychological measurements in psychopharmacology* (pp. 67–78). Krager.

Overall, J. E., & Gorham, D. R. (1962). The brief psychiatric rating scale. *Psychological Reports*, *10*, 799–812.

Packer, I. K. (2009). *Evaluation of criminal responsibility*. Oxford University Press.

Paris, J. (2013). *The intelligent clinician's guide to the DSM-5*. Oxford University Press.

Parker, G. F. (2014). Competence to stand trial evaluations of sovereign citizens: A case series and primer of odd political and legal beliefs. *Journal of the American Academy of Psychiatry and the Law Online*, *42*(3), 338–349.

Palmer, B. A., Pankratz, V. S., & Bostwick, J. M. (2005). The lifetime risk of suicide in schizophrenia: A reexamination. *Archives of General Psychiatry*, *62*(3), 247–253.

Parnas, J., & Henriksen, M. G. (2014). Disordered self in the schizophrenia spectrum: A clinical and research perspective. *Harvard Review of Psychiatry*, *22*(5), 251.

Penn, D. L., Sanna, L. J., & Roberts, D. L. (2008). Social cognition in schizophrenia: An overview. *Schizophrenia Bulletin*, *34*(3), 408–411.

Peralta, V., & Cuesta, M. J. (1998). Lack of insight in mood disorders. *Journal of Affective EDisorders*, *49*(1), 55–58.

Peters, E. R. (2010). Are delusions on a continuum? The case of religious and delusional beliefs. In I. Clarke (Ed.), *Psychosis and spirituality: Consolidating the new paradigm* (2nd ed., pp. 127–138). Wiley Ltd. http://dx.doi.org/10.1002/9780470970300.ch11

Peters, E. R., Joseph, S. A., Day, S., & Garety, P. (2004). Measuring delusional ideation: The 21-item Peters et al. delusions inventory (PDI). *Schizophrenia Bulletin*, *30*(4), 1005–1022.

Peters, E. R., Joseph, S. A., & Garety, P. A. (1999). Measurement of delusional ideation in the normal population: Introducing the PDI (Peters et al. Delusions inventory). *Schizophrenia Bulletin*, *25*(3), 553–576.

Piaget, J. (1928). *Judgment and reasoning in the child*. Routledge & Kegan Paul.

Piaget, J. (1929). *The child's conception of the world*. Routledge & Kegan Paul.

Piaget, J. (1955). *Growth of logical thinking* (with Bärbel Inhelder). Routledge & Kegan Paul.

Piaget, J. (1962). *Play, dreams, and imitation in childhood* (C. Gattegno & F. M. Hodgson, Trans.). Norton.

Picardi, A. (2019). The two faces of first-rank symptoms. *Psychopathology*, *52*(4), 221–231.

Pierre, J. M. (2001). Faith or delusion? At the crossroads of religion and psychosis. *Journal of Psychiatric Practice®*, *7*(3), 163–172.

Pinkham, A. E., Gloege, A. T., Flanagan, S., & Penn, D. L. (2004). Group cognitive behavioral therapy for auditory hallucinations: A pilot study. *Cognitive Behavioral Practice*, *11*, 93–98.

Pirelli, G., Zapf, P. A., & Gottdiener, W. H. (2011). Competency to stand trial research: Guidelines and future directions. *Journal of Forensic Psychiatry & Psychology*, 22(3), 340–370.

Pogue-Geile, M. F., & Harrow, M. (1984). Negative and positive symptoms in schizophrenia and depression. *Schizophrenia Bulletin*, *10*(3), 371–387.

Pope, H. G., Jr., & Lipinski, J. F., Jr. (1978). Diagnosis in schizophrenia and manic depressive illness: A reassessment of the specificity of 'schizophrenic' symptoms in the light of current research. *Archives of General Psychiatry, 35*(7), 811–828.

Powers, A. R., Addington, J., Perkins, D. O., Bearden, C. E., Cadenhead, K. S., Cannon, T. D., & Woods, S. W. (2020). Duration of the psychosis prodrome. *Schizophrenia Research, 216*, 443–449.

Powers, A. R., McGlashan, T. H., & Woods, S. W. (2021). Clinical phenomenology of the prodrome for psychosis. In C. A. Tamminga, E. I. Ivleva, U. Reininghaus, & J. Van Os (Eds.), *Psychotic disorders: Comprehensive conceptualization and treatments* (p. 106). Oxford University Press.

Pytyck, J., & Chaimowitz, G. A. (2013). The Sovereign Citizen Movement and fitness to stand trial. *International Journal of Forensic Mental Health, 12*(2), 149–153.

Quee, P. J., van der Meer, L., Bruggeman, R., de Haan, L., Cahn, W., Krabbendam, L., Mulder, N. C. L., Wiersma, D., & Aleman, A. (2010). Insight in psychosis: The role of neurocognition and the additional explained variance of social cognition and symptom dimensions. *Schizophrenia Research, 117*(2), 333.

Radomsky, E. D., Hass, G. L., Mann, J. J., & Sweeney, J. A. (1999). Suicidal behavior in patients with schizophrenia and other psychotic disorders. *American Journal of Psychiatry, 156*(10), 1590–1595.

Raffard, S., Madouini, C., Laraki, Y., Eisenblaetter, M., Broc, G., Capdevielle, D., & Bayard, S. (2023). Green et al. Paranoid thoughts scale-revised: Structural invariance and clinical utility of a brief version in schizophrenia. *Journal of Psychiatric Research, 163*, 9–13.

Rahman, T., Zheng, L., & Meloy, J. R. (2021). DSM-5 cultural and personality assessment of extreme overvalued beliefs. *Aggression and Violent Behavior, 60*, 101552.

Raine, A. (1991). A scale for the assessment of schizotypal personality based on the DSM-III-R criteria. *Schizophrenia Bulletin, 17*(4), 555–564.

Raine, A., & Benishay, D. (1995). The SPQ-B: A brief screening instrument for schizotypal personality disorder. *Journal of Personality Disorders, 9*(4), 346–355.

Raine, A., Reynolds, C., Lencz, T., Scerbo, A., Triphon, N., & Kim, D. (1994). Cognitive-perceptual, interpersonal, and disorganized features of schizotypal personality. *Schizophrenia Bulletin, 20*(1), 191–201.

Rapaport, D., Gill, M., & Shafer, R. (1946). *Diagnostic psychological testing* (Vol. 2). Year Book Publishers.

Ratcliff, K., Farhall, J., & Shawyer, F. (2010). Auditory hallucinations: A review of assessment tools. *Clinical Psychology & Psychotherapy, 18*, 524–534.

Read, J., van Os, J., Morrison, A. P., & Ross, C. A. (2005). Childhood trauma, psychosis and schizophrenia: A literature review with theoretical and clinical implications. *Acta Psychiatrica Scandinavia, 112*, 330–350.

Reese, W. D. (1971). The hallucinations of widowhood. *British Medical Journal, 4*(5778), 37–41.

Regier, D. A., Narrow, W. E., Clarke, D. E., Kraemer, H. C., Kuramoto, S. J., Kuhl, E. A., & Kupfer, D. J. (2013). DSM-5 field trials in the United States and

Canada, Part II: Test-retest reliability of selected categorical diagnoses. *American Journal of Psychiatry, 170*, 59–70.
Reich, W., Shayka, T., & Taibleson, C. (1991). *The diagnostic interview for children and adolescents – revised*. Washington University.
Reichenberg, A., Harvey, P. D., Bowie, C. R., Mojtabai, R., Rabinowitz, J., Heaton, R. K., & Bromet, E. (2009). Neuropsychological function and dysfunction in schizophrenia and psychotic affective disorders. *Schizophrenia Bulletin, 35*(5), 1022–1029.
Reinhold, R. (1990, January 24). The longest trial – a post-mortem; Collapse of child-abuse case: So much agony for so little. *The New York Times*. http://www.nytimes.com/1990/01/24/us/longest-trial-post-mortem-collapse-child-abuse-case-so-much-agony-for-so-little.html
Reininghaus, U., Priebe, S., & Bentall, R. P. (2013). Testing the psychopathology of psychosis: Evidence for a general psychosis dimension. *Schizophrenia Bulletin, 39*(4), 884–895.
Resnick, P. J. (2002). Recognizing that the suicidal patient views you as an adversary. *Current Psychiatry, 1*(1), 8.
Resnick, P. J., & Knoll, J. L. (2018). Malingered psychosis. In R. Rogers (Eds.), *Clinical assessment of malingering and deception* (4th ed., pp. 98–121). New York Guilford Press.
Reynolds, C. R., & Kamphaus, R. W. (2006). *BASC-2: Behavior assessment system for children* (2nd ed.). Pearson Education, Inc.
Riecher-Rössler, A. (2006). The FEPSY (Early detection of psychosis) study – transition rates and predictors of psychosis. *Schizophrenia Research, 86*(Suppl. S54).
Riedesser, P. (2004). Psychosis as traumatic event. In D. Buergin & H. Meng (Eds.), *Childhood and adolescent psychosis* (pp. 61–66). Krager.
Roessner, V., Ehrlich, S., Backhausen, L., Rempel, S., & Uhlmann, A. (2022). Heterogeneous courses of obsessive–compulsive disorders—better data on a lifetime perspective urgently needed. *European Child & Adolescent Psychiatry, 31*(8), 1–3.
Roger, R., Sewell, K. W., & Gillard, N. D. (2010). *Structured interview of reported symptoms (SIRS-2) and professional manual*. Psychological Assessment Resources.
Rogers, R., & Shuman, D. W. (2000). *Conducting insanity evaluations*. Guilford Press.
Rorschach, H. (1942). *Psychodiagnostik* (Hans Huber Verlag, Trans.). Bircher. (Original work published 1921)
Ross, C. A., & Joshi, S. (1992). Paranormal experiences in the general population. *Journal of Nervous and Mental Disease, 180*, 357–361.
Samamé, C., Cattaneo, B. L., Richaud, M. C., Strejilevich, S., & Aprahamian, I. (2022). The long-term course of cognition in bipolar disorder: A systematic review and meta-analysis of patient-control differences in test-score changes. *Psychological Medicine, 52*(2), 217–228.
Sanjuán, J., Aguilar, E. J., Olivares, J. M., Ros, S., Montejo, A. L., Mayoral, F., Gonzales-Torres, M. A., & Bousono, M. (2006). Subjective perception of cognitive deficit in psychotic patients. *Journal of Nervous and Mental Disease, 194*, 58–60.

Sanjuán, J., Prieto, R., Olivares, J. M., Montejo, M., Ferrer, F., Mayoral, F., Gonzalez-Torres, M. A., & Bousono, M. (2003). GEOPTE scale of social cognition for psychosis. *Actas Espanolas de Psiquiatria*, *31*, 120–128.

Sanz, M., Constable, G., Lopez-Ibor, I., Kemp, R., & David, A. (1998). A comparative study of insight scales and their relationship to psychopathological and clinical variables. *Psychological Medicine*, *28*, 437–446.

Sarfati, Y., Hardy-Baylé, M. C., Besche, C., & Widlöcher, D. (1997). Attribution of intentions to others in people with schizophrenia: A non-verbal exploration with comic strips. *Schizophrenia Research*, *25*(3), 199–209.

Sato, M., Numachi, Y., & Hamamura, T. (1992). Relapse of paranoid psychotic state in methamphetamine model of schizophrenia. *Schizophrenia Bulletin*, *18*, 115–122.

Sayers, S. L., Curran, P. J., & Mueser, K. T. (1996). Factor structure and construct validity of the scale for the assessment of negative symptoms. *Psychological Assessment*, *8*, 269–280.

Sbrana, A., Dell'Osso, L., Benvenuti, A., Rucci, P., Cassano, P., Banti, S., Gonnelli, C., Doria, M. R., Ravani, L., Spagnolli, S., Rossi, L., Raimondi, F., Catena, M., Endicott, J., Frank, E., Kupfer, D. J., & Cassano, G. B. (2005). The psychotic spectrum: Validity and reliability of the structured clinical interview for the psychotic spectrum. *Schizophrenia Research*, *75*(2), 375–387.

Schafer, R. (1976). *A new language for psychoanalysis*. Yale University Press.

Schilder, P. (1951). On the development of thoughts. In D. Rapaport (Ed. & Trans.), *Organization and pathology of thought* (pp. 497–518). Columbia University Press.

Schimmelmann, B. G., Walger, P., & Schultze-Lutter, F. (2013). The significance of at-risk symptoms for psychosis in children and adolescents. *Canadian Journal of Psychiatry*, *58*(1), 32–40.

Schlesinger, H. J. (2003). *Texture of treatment: On the matter of psychoanalytic technique*. The Analytic Press.

Schneider, K. (1950). Letter from Germany: Systematic psychiatry. *American Journal of Psychiatry*, *107*, 334.

Schneider, K. (1959). *Clinical psychopathology*. Grune and Stratton.

Schothorst, P. F., Emck, C., & van Engeland, H. (2006). Characteristics of early psychosis. *Comprehensive Psychiatry*, *47*(6), 438–442.

Schrank, F. A., McGrew, K. S., & Mather, N. (2014). *Woodcock–Johnson tests of cognitive abilities* (4th ed.). Riverside Publishing.

Schultze-Lutter, F., Ruhrmann, S., & Klosterkoetter, J. (2006). Can schizophrenia be predicted phenomenologically? In J. O. Johannessen, B. Martindale, & J. Cullberg (Eds.), *Evolving psychosis, different stages, different treatments* (pp. 104–123). Routledge.

Schultze-Lutter, F., Ruhrmann, S., Picker, H., Graf von Reventlow, Brockhaus-Dumke, A., & Klosterkötter, J. (2007). The schizophrenia proneness instrument (SPI-A) – a tool for the assessment of basic symptoms. *European Psychiatry*, *21*(Suppl. 1), s27.

Scott, C. L., & Resnick, P. J. (2009). Assessing potential for harm: Would your patient injure himself or others? *Current Psychiatry*, *8*(7), 24–33.

Scott, C. L., & Resnick, P. J. (2013). Evaluating psychotic patients' risk of violence: A practical guide. Investigating persecutory delusions and command hallucinations. *Current Psychiatry*, *12*(5), 29–32.

Seiler, N., Maguire, J., Nguyen, T., Sizer, H., McGorry, P., Nelson, B., & O'Donoghue, B. (2020). Prevalence of subthreshold positive symptoms in young people without psychotic disorders presenting to a youth mental health service. *Schizophrenia Research*, *215*, 446–448.

Selbom, M., & Whitman, M. R. (2023). Minnesota multiphasic personality inventory-3 (MMPI-3) assessment of bipolar spectrum disorders. In I. B. Weiner & J. H. Kleiger (Eds.), *The psychological assessment of disordered thinking and perception* (pp. 47–62). American Psychological Association.

Selten, J. P., Cantor-Graae, E., & Kahn, R. S. (2007). Migration and schizophrenia. *Current Opinions in Psychiatry*, *20*(2), 111–115.

Sendiony, M. F. (1976). Cultural aspects of delusions: A psychiatric study of Egypt. *Australian and New Zealand Journal of Psychiatry*, *10*, 201–207.

Shah, N., Grover, S., & Rao, G. P. (2017). Clinical practice guidelines for management of bipolar disorder. *Indian Journal of Psychiatry*, *59*(Suppl 1), S51–S66.

Shaner, A., Roberts, L., Eckman, T. A., Racenstein, M., Tucker, D., Tsuang, J. W., & Mintz, J. (1998). Sources of diagnostic uncertainty for chronically psychotic cocaine abusers. *Psychiatric Services*, *49*(5), 684–690.

Shankman, S. A., Funkhouser, C. J., Klein, D. N., Davila, J., Lerner, D., & Hee, D. (2018). Reliability and validity of severity dimensions of psychopathology assessed using the structured clinical interview for DSM-5 (SCID). *International Journal of Methods in Psychiatric Research*, *27*(1), e1590.

Shawyer, F., MacKinnon, A., Farhall, J., Sims, E., Blaney, S., Yardley, P., Daly, M., Mullen, P., & Copolov, D. (2008). Acting on harmful command hallucinations in psychotic disorders: An integrative approach. *Journal of Nervous & Mental Disease*, *196*(5), 390–398.

Shawyer, F., Ratcliff, K., Mackinnon, A., Farhall, J., Hayes, S. C., & Copolov, D. (2007). The voices acceptance and action scale (VAAS): Pilot data. *Journal of Clinical Psychology*, *63*(6), 593–606.

Shawyer, F., Thomas, N. A., Morris, E. M., & Farhall, J. (2013). 'Theory on voices'. In E. M. J. Morris, L. C. Johns, & J. E. Oliver (Eds.), *Acceptance and commitment therapy and mindfulness for psychosis* (pp. 12–32). John Wiley & Sons.

Shea, S. C. (2016). *Psychiatric interviewing: The Art of understanding a practical guide for the psychiatrist, psychologist, counselors, social workers, nurses and other mental professionals* (3rd ed.). Elsevier.

Shenton, M. E., Solovay, M. R., Holzman, P. S., Coleman, M., & Gale, H. J. (1989). Thought disorder in relatives of psychotic patients. *Archives of General Psychiatry*, *46*, 897–901.

Shergill, S. S., Murray, R. M., & McGuire, P. K. (1998). Auditory hallucinations: A review of psychological treatments. *Schizophrenia Research*, *32*(3), 137–150.

Shrivastava, A., McGorry, P. D., Tsuang, M., Woods, S. W., Cornblatt, B. A., Corcoran, C., & Carpenter, W. (2011). 'Attenuated psychosis symptoms syndrome' as a risk syndrome of psychosis, diagnosis in DSM-V: The debate. *Indiana Journal of Psychiatry*, *53*(1), 57–65.

Siddle, R., Haddock, G., Tarrier, N., & Faragher, E. B. (2002). Religious delusions in patients admitted to hospital with schizophrenia. *Social Psychiatry & Psychiatric Epidemiology*, *37*(3), 130–138.

Simon, R. I. (2004). *Assessing and managing suicide risk: Guidelines for clinically based risk management.* American Psychiatric Publishing, Inc.

Sims, A. (1995). *Symptoms in the mind.* Saunders.

Skodol, A. E. (1989). *Problems in differential diagnosis: From DSM-III to DSM-III-R in clinical practice.* American Psychiatric Press.

Skuse, D. H. (2022). Early-onset psychosis and autism spectrum disorder: Similar rates of deleterious copy n umber variants, yet diverse phenotypic manifestations. *American Journal of Psychiatry*, *179*(11), 798–799.

Smith, B. L. (2021). Cultural consideration in assessment of disordered thought and perception. In I. B. Weiner & J. H. Kleiger (Eds.), *Psychological assessment of disordered thinking and perception* (pp. 285–302). American Psychological Association. https://doi.org/10.1037/0000245-015

Smith, T. E., Hull, J. W., Goodman, M., Hedayat-Harris, A., Willson, D. F., Israel, L. M., & Munich, R. L. (1999). The relative influences of symptoms, insight, and neurocognition on social adjustment in schizophrenia and schizoaffective disorder. *The Journal of Nervous and Mental Disease*, *187*(2), 102–108.

Smith, T. E., Hull, J. W., Israel, L. M., & Willson, D. F. (2000). Insight, symptoms, and neurocognition in schizophrenia and schizoaffective disorder. *Schizophrenia Bulletin*, *26*(1), 193–200.

Smith, T. E., Hull, J. W., & Santos, L. (1998). The relationship between symptoms and insight in schizophrenia: A longitudinal perspective. *Schizophrenia Research*, *33*(1), 63–67.

Soares-Weiser, K., Maayan, N., Bergman, H., Davenport, C., Kirkham, A. J., Grabowski, S., & Adams, C. E. (2015). First rank symptoms for schizophrenia. *Cochrane Database of Systematic Reviews*, (1).

Solovay, M. R., Shenton, M. E., & Holzman, P. S. (1987). Comparative studies of thought disorder: I. Mania and schizophrenia. *Archives of General Psychiatry*, *44*, 13–20.

Spaaij, R. (2010). The enigma of lone wolf terrorism: An assessment. *Studies in Conflict & Terrorism*, *33*(9), 854–870.

Spauwen, J., Krabbendam, L., Lieb, R., Wittchen, H. U., & van Os, J. (2006). Impact of psychological trauma on the development of psychotic symptoms: Relationship with psychosis proneness. *British Journal of Psychiatry*, *188*, 527–533.

Spencer, E. K., & Campbell, M. (1994). Children with schizophrenia: Diagnosis, phenomenology and pharmacotherapy. *Schizophrenia Bulletin*, *20*, 713–725.

Spitzer, M. (1990). On defining delusions. *Comprehensive Psychiatry*, *31*(5), 377–397.

Spitzer, R. L., Endicott, J., & Robins, E. (1978). *Research diagnostic criteria (RDC) for a select group of functional disorders* (3rd ed.). Biometric Research, New York State Psychiatric Institute.

Spohn, H. E., Coyne, L., Larson, J., Mittlernan, E., Spray, J., & Hayes, K. (1986). Episodic and residual thought pathology in chronic schizophrenics: Effects of neuroleptics. *Schizophrenia Bulletin*, *12*, 394–407.

Stanton, K. J., Denietolis, B., Goodwin, B. J., & Dvir, Y. (2020). Childhood trauma and psychosis: An updated review. *Child and Adolescent Psychiatric Clinics*, *29*(1), 115–129.

Statham, V., Emerson, L. M., & Rowse, G. (2019). A systematic review of self-report measures of paranoia. *Psychological Assessment*, *31*(2), 139.

Steadman, H. J., Monahan, J., Pinals, D. A., Vesselinov, R., & Robbins, P. C. (2015). Gun violence and victimization of strangers by persons with a mental illness: Data from the MacArthur Violence Risk Assessment Study. *Psychiatric Services*, *66*(11), 1238–1241.

Steadman, H. J., Mulvey, E. P., Monahan, J., Robbins, P. C., Appelbaum, P. S., Grisso, T., Roth, L. H., & Silver, E. (1998). Violence by people discharged from acute psychiatric inpatient facilities and by others in the same neighborhoods. *Archives of General Psychiatry*, *55*, 393–401.

Stefanis, N. C., Hanssen, M., Smirnis, N. K., Avramopoulos, D. A., Evdokimidis, I. K., Stefanis, C. N., Verdoux, H., & van Os, J. (2018, January). Evidence that three dimensions of psychosis. *Psychiatry Research*, *259*, 95–103. https://doi.org/10.1016/j.psychres.2017.09.089 (Original work published 2002)

Stephane, M., Thuras, P., Nasrallah, H., & Georgopoulos, A. P. (2003). The internal structure of phenomenology of auditory verbal hallucinations. *Schizophrenia Research*, *61*, 185–193.

Stephens, J. H., Astrup, C., & Mangrum, J. C. (1966). Prognostic factors in recovery of deteriorated schizophrenics. *American Journal of Psychiatry*, *122*, 1116–1121.

Strakowski, S. M., McElroy, S. L., Keck, P. E. Jr., & West, S. A. (1996). Racial influence on diagnosis in psychotic mania. *Journal of Affective Disorders*, *39*(2), 157–162.

Straube, E. R., & Oades, R. D. (1992). *Schizophrenia: Empirical research and findings*. Academic Press.

Strauss, C., Hugdahl, K., Waters, F., Hayward, M., Bless, J. J., Falkenberg, L. E., Kråkvik, B., Asbjørnsen, A. E., Johnsen, E., Sinkevicuite, R. A., Kroken, E. L., & Thomas, N. (2018). The beliefs about voices questionnaire – revised: A factor structure from 450 participants. *Psychiatric Research*, *259*, 95–10. https://doi.org/10.1016/j.psychres.2017.09.089

Su, W-S., Viglione, D. J., Green, E. E., Wai-Cheong, C. T., Su, J-A., & Chang, Y-T. (2015). Cultural and linguistic adaptability of the Rorschach performance assessment system as a measure of psychotic characteristics and severity of mental disturbance in Taiwan. *Psychological Assessment*, *27*, 1273–1285. https://doi.org/10.1037/pas0000144.

Sullivan, H. S. (1994). The onset of schizophrenia. *American Journal of Psychiatry*, *151*(Suppl. 6), 134–139. (Original work published 1927)

Sullivan, H. S. (1947). *Conceptions of modern psychiatry*. William A. White Foundation.

Sussman, N., & Cancro, R. (1988). Differential diagnosis of manic depressive and schizophrenic illnesses. In G. Anastasios & R. Cranco (Eds.), *Depression and mania*. Elsevier.

Swanson, C. L. Jr., Freudenreich, O., McEnvoy, J. P., Nelson, L., Kamaraju, L., & Wilson, W. H. (1995). Insight in schizophrenia and mania. *The Journal of Nervous and Mental Disease*, *183*(12), 752–755.

Swanson, J. W., Borum, R., Swartz, M. S., & Monahan, J. (1996). Psychotic symptoms and disorders and the risk of violent behavior in the community. *Criminal Behavior and Mental Health*, *6*, 309–329.

Swanson, J. W., Swartz, M. S., van Dorn, R. A., Elbogen, E. B., Wagner, H. R., Rosenheck, R. A., Stroup, T. S., McEvoy, J. P., & Lieberman, J. A. (2006). A national study of violent behavior in persons with schizophrenia. *Archives of General Psychiatry*, *26*, 490–499.

Switaj, P., Anczewska, M., Chrostek, A., Sabariego, C., Cieza, A., Bickenbach, J., & Chatterji, S. (2012). Disability and schizophrenia: A systematic review of experienced psychosocial difficulties. *BMC Psychiatry*, *12*, 193.

Taiminen, T., Huttunen, J., Heila, H., Hendriksson, M., Isometsa, E., Kahkonen, J., Tuomemen, K., Lonnquist, J., Addington, D., & Helenious, H. (2001). The schizophrenia suicide risk scale (SSRS): Development and initial validation. *Schizophrenia Research*, *47*, 199–213.

Takai, A., Dematsu, M., Ueki, H., Sone, K., & Kaiya, H. (1992). Insight and its related factors in chronic schizophrenic patients: A preliminary study. *European Journal of Psychiatry*, 6, 159–170.

Tamburello, A. C., Bajgier, J., & Reeves, R. (2015). The prevalence of delusional disorder in prison. *Journal of the American Academy of Psychiatry and the Law*, *43*(1), 82–86.

Tandon, R., Keshavan, M. S., & Nasrallah, H. A. (2008). Schizophrenia, 'Just the facts': What we know in 2008, part 1: Overview. *Schizophrenia Research*, *100*, 4–19.

Tanenberg-Karant, M., Fennig, S., Ram, R., Krishna, J., Jandorf, L., & Bromet, E. J. (1995). Bizarre delusions and first-rank symptoms in a first-admission sample: A preliminary analysis of prevalence and correlates. *Comprehensive Psychiatry*, *36*(6), 428–434.

Tarescavage, A. M., & Selbom, M. (2021). Minnesota multiphasic personality inventory-2-RF (MMPI-2-RF) for assessing disordered thinking and perception. In I. B. Weiner & J. H. Kleiger (Eds.), *The psychological assessment of disordered thinking and perception* (pp. 63–78). American Psychological Association.

Taylor, M. A. (1981). *The neuropsychiatric mental status examination*. Spectrum.

Taylor, P. J. (2006). Delusional disorder and delusions: Is there a risk of violence in social interactions about the core symptom? *Behavioral Sciences & the Law*, *24*(3), 313–331.

Taylor, P. J., & Felthous, A. R. (2006). Introduction to this issue: International perspectives on delusional disorders and the law. *Behavioral Sciences & the Law*, *24*, 235–240. http://dx.doi.org/10.1002/bsl.716

Taylor, P. J., Garety, P., Buchanan, A., Reed, A., Wessely, S., Ray, K., Dunn, G., & Grubin, D. (1994). Delusions and violence. In J. Monahan & H. J. Steadman (Eds.), *Violence and mental disorder: Developments in risk assessment* (pp. 161–182). Chicago University Press.

Teglasi, H. (2021). Thematic Apperception Test (TAT) for assessing disordered thought and perception. In I. B. Weiner & J. H. Kleiger (Eds.), *The psychological assessment of disordered thinking and perception* (pp. 169–186). American Psychological Association.

Thompson, A. D., Nelson, B., Yuen, H. P., Lin, A., Amminger, G. P., McGorry, P. D., Wood, S. J., & Yung, A. R. (2014). Sexual trauma increases the risk of developing psychosis in an ultra high-risk "prodromal" population. *Schizophrenia Bulletin*, *40*(3), 697–706.

Thompson, J. L., Kelly, M., Kimhy, D., Harkavay-Friedman, J. M., Kahn, S., Messinger, J. W., Schobel, S., Goetz, R., Malaspina, D., & Corcoran, C. (2009). Childhood trauma and prodromal symptom among individuals at clinical high risk for psychosis. *Schizophrenia Research*, *108*, 176–181.

Tillman, R., & Geller, B. (2003). Definitions of rapid, ultrarapid, and ultradian cycling and of episode duration in pediatric and adult bipolar disorders: A proposal to distinguish episodes from cycles. *Journal of Child and Adolescent Psychopharmacology*, *13*(3), 267–271.

Trower, P., Birchwood, M., Meaden, A., Byrne, S., Nelson, A., & Ross, K. (2004). Cognitive therapy for command hallucinations: Randomized controlled trial. *British Journal of Psychiatry*, *184*(4), 312–320.

Trygstad, L., Buccheri, R., Dowling, G., Zind, R., White, K., Griffin, J. J., Henderson, S., Suciu, L., Hippie, S., Kaas, M. J., Covert, C., & Herbert, P. (2002). Behavioral management of persistent auditory hallucinations in schizophrenia: Outcomes from a 10-week course. *Journal of the American Psychiatric Nurses Association*, *8*(3), 84–91.

Tseng, W. S., Mathews, D., & Elwyn, T. S. (2004). *Cultural competence in forensic mental health: A guide for psychiatrists, psychologists, and attorneys.* Brunner-Routledge.

Ullrich, S., Keers, R., & Coid, J. W. (2013). Delusions, anger, and serious violence: New findings from the MacArthur violence risk assessment study. *Schizophrenia Bulletin* (electronic publication ahead of print, September 18, 2013).

Vaillant, G. E. (1962). The prediction of recovery in schizophrenia. *The Journal of Nervous and Mental Disease*, *135*(6), 534–543.

Vaillant, G. E. (1964a). A historical review of the remitting schizophrenias. *The Journal of Nervous and Mental Disease*, *138*(1), 48–56.

Vaillant, G. E. (1964b). Prospective prediction of schizophrenic remission. *Archives of General Psychiatry*, *11*(5), 509–518.

Valle, R. (2020). Schizophrenia in ICD-11: Comparison of ICD-10 and DSM-5. *Revista de Psiquiatría y Salud Mental* (English Edition), *13*(2), 95–104.

van der Gaag, M., Cuijpers, A., Hoffman, T., Remijsen, M., de Haan, L., van Meijel, B., van Harten, P. N., Valmaggia, L., de Hert, M., & Wiersma, D. (2006). The five-factor model of the positive and negative syndrome scale I: Confirmatory factor analysis fails to confirm 25 published five-factor solutions. *Schizophrenia Research*, *85*(1–3), 273–279.

van der Meer, L., Costafreda, S., Aleman, A., & David, A. S. (2010). Self-reflection and the brain: A theoretical review and meta-analysis of neuroimaging studies with implications for schizophrenia. *Neuroscience & Biobehavioral Reviews*, *34*(6), 935–946.

Van Lieshout, R. J., & Goldberg, J. O. (2007). Quantifying self-reports of auditory verbal hallucinations in persons with psychosis. *Canadian Journal of Behavioural Sciences*, *39*(1), 73–77.

van Nierop, M., Lataster, T., Smeets, F., Gunther, N., van Zelst, C., de Graaf, R., ten Have, M., van Dorsselaer, S., Bak, M., Myin-Germeys, I., Viechtbauer, W., van Os, J., & van Winkel, R. (2014). Psychopathological mechanisms linking childhood traumatic experiences to risk of psychotic symptoms: Analysis of a large, representative population-based sample. *Schizophrenia Bulletin, 40*(Suppl. 2), S123–S130.

van Os, J., Gilvarry, C., Bale, R., van Horn, E., Tattan, T., & White, I. (1999). A comparison of the utility of dimensional and categorical representations of psychosis. *Psychological Medicine, 29*(3), 595–606.

van Os, J., & Kapur, S. (2009). Schizophrenia. *Lancet, 374,* 635–645.

van Os, J., Linscott, R. J., Myin-Germeys, I., Delespaul, P., & Krabbendam, L. (2009). A systematic review and meta-analysis of the psychosis continuum: Evidence for a psychosis proneness-persistence-impairment model of psychotic disorder. *Psychological Medicine, 39,* 179–195.

Van Putten, T., Crumpton, E., & Yale, C. (1976). Drug refusal in schizophrenia and the wish to be crazy. *Archives of General Psychiatry, 33*(12), 1443–1446.

vas Os, J., & Reininghaus, U. (2016). Psychosis as a transdiagnostic and extended phenotype in the general population. *World Psychiatry, 15*(2), 118–124. https://doi.org/10.1002/wps.20310

Vaskinn, A., Sundet, K., Ueland, T., Agartz, I., Melle, I., & Andreassen, O. A. (2013). Social cognition and clinical insight in schizophrenia and bipolar disorder. *The Journal of Nervous and Mental Disease, 201*(6), 445–451.

Ventriglio, A., Gentile, A., Bonfitto, I., Stella, E., Mari, M., Steardo, L., & Bellomo, A. (2016). Suicide in the early stage of schizophrenia. *Frontiers in Psychiatry,* 7, 208770.

Ventura, J., Liberman, R. P., Green, M. F., Shaner, A., & Mintz, J. (1998). Training and quality assurance with the structured clinical interview for DSM-IV (SCID-I/P). *Psychiatry Research,* 79(2), 163–173.

Viglione, D. J., Fauroat, L., & Khorram, A. (1994). Child thought-scale. In W. Perry (Chair), *New diagnostic measures of psychopathology.* Symposium conducted at annual meeting of Society for Personality Assessment.

Viglione, D. J., & Senecal, S. (2014, March). *Research and development of a scale to measure unusual beliefs and experiences among children and adolescents.* Paper presented at the annual meeting of the Society for Personality Assessment.

Vollema, M. G., & Ormel, J. (2000). The reliability of the structured interview for Schizotypy – revised (SIS-R). *Schizophrenia Bulletin, 26*(5), 619–629.

Vollema, M. G., & van den Bosch, R. J. (1995). The multidimensionality of Schizotypy. *Schizophrenia Bulletin, 21*(1), 19–31.

Vygotsky, L. S. (1962). *Thought and language.* MIT Press. (Original work published 1934)

Waring, E. M., Neufield, R. W., & Schaefer, B. (2003). The thought disorder questionnaire. *Canadian Journal of Psychiatry, 48*(1), 45–51.

Warren, J. I., Murrie, D. C., Stejskal, W., Colwell, L. H., Morris, J., Chauhan, P., & Dietz, P. (2006). Opinion formation in evaluating the adjudicative competence and restorability of criminal defendants: A review of 8,000 evaluations. *Behavioral Sciences & the Law,* 24(2), 113–132.

Waters, F. (2015). Passivity symptoms experience of alien control. In F. Waters & M. Stephane (Eds.), *The assessment of psychosis* (pp. 245–254). Routledge.

Waters, F., & Stephane, M. (2015). *The assessment of psychosis.* Routledge.

Waters, F. A., Badcock, J. C., & Maybery, M. T. (2003). Revision of the factor structure of the Launay–Slade Hallucination Scale (LSHS-R). *Personality and Individual Differences*, *35*(6), 1351–1357.

Wechsler, D. (1955). *Manual for the Wechsler adult intelligence scale*. The Psychological Corporation.

Wechsler, D. (2008). *Wechsler adult intelligence scale–(WAIS-IV)* (4th ed.). Pearson.

Wechsler, D. (2014). *Wechsler intelligence scale for children–(WISC-V)* (5th ed.). NCS Pearson.

Wechsler, D., & Hsiao-pin, C. (2011). *WASI-II: Wechsler abbreviated scale of intelligence* (2nd ed.). Pearson.

Weigel, L., Wehr, S., Galderisi, S., Mucci, A., Davis, J., Giordano, G. M., & Leucht, S. (2023). The brief negative symptom scale (BNSS): A systematic review of measurement properties. *Schizophrenia*, *9*(1), 45.

Weiner, I. B. (1966). *Psychodiagnosis in schizophrenia*. John Wiley & Sons.

Weiner, I. B. (1977). Approaches to Rorschach validation. In M. A. Rickers-Ovsiankina (Ed.), *Rorschach psychology* (pp. 575–608). Krieger.

Weiner, I. B. (2021). Rorschach Comprehensive System (RCS) for assessing disordered thought and perception. In I. B. Weiner & J. H. Kleiger (Eds.), *Psychological assessment of disordered thinking and perception* (pp. 137–150). American Psychological Association.

Weiner, I. B., & Kleiger, J. H. (2021). *The psychological assessment of disordered thinking and perception*. American Psychological Association.

Weisman, A. (1958). Reality sense and reality testing. *Behavioral Science*, *5*, 228–261.

Werner, H. (1957). The concept of development from a comparative and organismic view. In D. B. Harris (Ed.), *The concept of development* (pp. 125–148). University of Minnesota Press.

Wessely, S., Buchanan, A., Reed, A., Cutting, J., Everitt, B., Garety, P., & Taylor, P. J. (1993). Acting on delusions: I. Prevalence. *British Journal of Psychiatry*, *163*, 69–76.

Westermeyer, J. F., Harrow, M., & Marengo, J. (1991). Risk for suicide in schizophrenia and other psychotic and nonpsychotic disorders. *Journal of Nervous and Mental Disease*, *5*, 259–265.

Wilk, C. M., Gold, J. M., McMahon, R. P., Humber, K., Iannone, V. N., & Buchanan, R. W. (2005). No, it is not possible to be schizophrenic yet neuropsychologically normal. *Neuropsychology*, *19*(6), 778.

Williams, T. F., Powers, A. R., Ellman, L. M., Corlett, P. R., Strauss, G. P., Schiffman, J., Walz, J. A., Silverstein, S. M., Woods, S. W., Walker, E. F., Gold, J. M., & Mittal, V. A. (2022). Three prominent self-report risk measures show unique and overlapping utility in characterizing those at clinical high-risk for psychosis. *Schizophrenia Research*, *244*, 58–65.

Wing, J. K. (1970). A standard form of psychiatric present-state examination and a method for standardizing the classification of symptoms. In E. H. Hare & J. K. Wing (Eds.), *Psychiatric epidemiology: An international symposium* (pp. 93–108). Oxford University Press.

Witt, K., van Dorn, R., & Fazel, S. (2013). Risk factors for violence in psychosis: Systematic review and meta-regression analysis of 110 studies. *PloS One, 8*, e55942.

Wood, J. M., Nezworski, M. T., Lilienfeld, S. O., & Garb, H. N. (2003). *What is wrong with the Rorschach? Science confronts the controversial inkblot test.* Wiley & Sons.

Woods, S. W., Addington, J., Cadenhead, K. S., Cannon, T. D., Cornblatt, B. A., Heinssen, R., Perkins, D. O., Seidman, L. J., Tsuang, M. T., Walker, E. F., & McGlashan, T. H. (2009). Validity of the prodromal risk syndrome for first psychosis: Findings from the North American prodrome longitudinal study. *Schizophrenia Bulletin, 35*(5), 894–908.

Woods, S. W., Parker, S., Kerr, M. J., Walsh, B. C., Wijtenburg, S. A., Prunier, N., ... & Wood, S. J. (2024). Development of the PSYCHS: Positive SYmptoms and Diagnostic Criteria for the CAARMS Harmonized with the SIPS. *Early Intervention in Psychiatry, 18*(4), 255–272.

Woods, S. W., Walsh, B. C., Saksa, J. R., & McGlashan, T. H. (2010). The case for including attenuated psychotic symptoms syndrome in DSM-5 as a psychosis risk syndrome. *Schizophrenia Research, 123*(2–3), 199–207.

World Drug Report. (2019). United Nations publication, Sales No. E.19.XI.8.

World Health Organization. (1973). *Report of the international pilot study of schizophrenia* (Vol. 1). WHO.

World Health Organization. (1994). *International statistical classification of diseases and related health problems* (10th ed.). WHO.

World Health Organization. (2019). *International statistical classification of diseases and related health problems* (11th ed.). WHO.

Yalof, J. (2021). Neuropsychological measures for assessing disordered thought and perception. In I. B. Weiner & J. H. Kleiger (Eds.), *The psychological assessment of disordered thinking and perception* (pp. 223–240). American Psychological Association.

Young, D. A., Davila, R., & Scher, H. (1993). Unawareness of illness and neuropsychological performance in chronic schizophrenia. *Schizophrenia Research, 10*(2), 117–124.

Young, R. C., Biggs, J. T., Ziegler, V. E., & Meyer, D. A. (1978). A rating scale for mania: Reliability, validity, and sensitivity. *British Journal of Psychiatry, 133*, 429–435.

Youngstrom, E. A. (2007). Pediatric bipolar disorder. In E. Mash & R. Barkley (Eds.), *Assessment of childhood disorders* (4th ed., pp. 253–304). Guilford Press.

Yung, A. R., & McGorry, P. D. (1996a). The initial prodrome in psychosis: Descriptive and qualitative aspects. *Australian and New Zealand Journal of Psychiatry, 30*, 587–599.

Yung, A. R., & McGorry, P. D. (1996b). The prodromal phase of first-episode psychosis: Past and current conceptualizations. *Schizophrenia Bulletin, 22*(2), 353–370.

Yung, A. R., McGorry, P. D., McFarlane, C. A., Jackson, H. J., Patton, G. C., & Rakkar, A. (1996). Monitoring and care of young people at incipient risk of psychosis. *Schizophrenia Bulletin, 22*(2), 283–303.

Yung, A. R., & Nelson, B. (2013). The ultra-high risk concept: A review. *Canadian Journal of Psychiatry*, *58*(1), 5–12.

Yung, A. R., Phillips, L. J., McGorry, P. D., McFarlane, C. A., Francey, S., Harrigan, S., Patton, G. C., & Jackson, H. J. (1998). Prediction of psychosis. A step towards indicated prevention of schizophrenia. *British Journal of Psychiatry*, *172*(Suppl. 33), 14–20.

Yung, A. R., Phillips, L. J., McGorry, P. D., Ward, J. L., & Thompson, K. (2000). *Comprehensive assessment of at-risk mental states (CAARMS)*. University of Melbourne.

Yung, A. R., Phillips, L. J., Yuen, H. P., Francey, S. M., McFarlane, C. A., Hallgren, M., & McGorry, P. D. (2003). Psychosis prediction: 12-month follow up of a high-risk ('prodromal') group. *Schizophrenia Research*, *60*, 21–32.

Yung, A. R., Phillips, L. J., Yuen, H. P., & McGorry, P. D. (2004). Risk factors for psychosis in an ultra high-risk group: Psychopathology and clinical features. *Schizophrenia Research*, *67*(2–3), 131–142.

Yung, A. R., Woods, S. W., Ruhrmann, S., Addington, J., Schultze-Lutter, F., Cornblatt, B. A., Amminger, G. P., Bechdolf, A., Birchwood, M., Borgwardt, S., Cannon, T. D., de Haan, L., French, P., Fusar-Poli, P., Keshavan, M., Klosterkötter, J., Kwon, J. S., McGorry, P. D., McGuire, P., . . . McGlashan, T. H. (2012). Whither the attenuated psychosis syndrome? *Schizophrenia Bulletin*, *38*(6), 1130–1134.

Yung, A. R., Yuen, H. P., McGorry, P. D., Phillips, L. J., Kelly, D., Dell'Olio, M., Francey, S. M., Cosgrave, E. M., Killackey, E., Godfrey, K., & Buckby, J. (2005). Mapping the onset of psychosis: The comprehensive assessment of at-risk mental states. *Australia and New Zealand Journal of Psychiatry*, *39*, 964–971.

Zalsman, G., & Cohen, D. J. (1998). Multiplex developmental disorder. *The Israel Journal of Psychiatry and Related Sciences*, *35*(4), 300–306.

Zanelli, J., Mollon, J., Sandin, S., Morgan, C., Dazzan, P., Pilecka, I., . . . Reichenberg, A. (2019). Cognitive change in schizophrenia and other psychoses in the decade following the first episode. *American Journal of Psychiatry*, *176*(10), 811–819.

Zapf, P. A., Roesch, R., & Pirelli, G. (2013). Competency to stand trial. In I. B. Weiner & R. K. Otto (Eds.), *The handbook of forensic psychology* (4th ed., pp. 281–314). John Wiley & Sons.

Zigler, E., & Glick, M. (1984). Paranoid schizophrenia: An unorthodox view. *American Journal of Orthopsychiatry*, *54*, 43–70.

Zimmerman, M. (2008). To screen or not to screen: Conceptual issues in screening for psychiatric disorders in psychiatric patients with a focus on the performance of the psychiatric diagnostic screening questionnaire. *International Journal of Mental Health and Addiction*, *6*, 53–63.

Zingela, Z., Stroud, L., Cronje, J., Fink, M., & van Wyk, S. (2021). Assessment of catatonia and inter-rater reliability of three instruments: A descriptive study. *International Journal of Mental Health Systems*, *15*, 1–8.

INDEX

Note: Page in **bold** indicate a table on the corresponding page.